Dietary Components and
Immune Function

Dietary Components and Immune Function

Editor

Ping Zhang

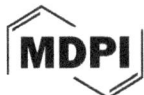

Basel • Beijing • Wuhan • Barcelona • Belgrade • Novi Sad • Cluj • Manchester

Editor
Ping Zhang
Center for Integrative Conservation
Xishuangbanna Tropical Botanical Garden
Chinese Academy of Sciences
Menglun
China

Editorial Office
MDPI AG
Grosspeteranlage 5
4052 Basel, Switzerland

This is a reprint of articles from the Special Issue published online in the open access journal *Nutrients* (ISSN 2072-6643) (available at: https://www.mdpi.com/journal/nutrients/special_issues/515Y5WR685).

For citation purposes, cite each article independently as indicated on the article page online and as indicated below:

Lastname, A.A.; Lastname, B.B. Article Title. *Journal Name* **Year**, *Volume Number*, Page Range.

ISBN 978-3-7258-1859-4 (Hbk)
ISBN 978-3-7258-1860-0 (PDF)
doi.org/10.3390/books978-3-7258-1860-0

© 2024 by the authors. Articles in this book are Open Access and distributed under the Creative Commons Attribution (CC BY) license. The book as a whole is distributed by MDPI under the terms and conditions of the Creative Commons Attribution-NonCommercial-NoDerivs (CC BY-NC-ND) license.

Contents

Preface vii

Nguyen Tien Dung, Takeshi Susukida, Sisca Ucche, Ka He, So-ichiro Sasaki, Ryuji Hayashi and Yoshihiro Hayakawa
Calorie Restriction Impairs Anti-Tumor Immune Responses in an Immunogenic Preclinical Cancer Model
Reprinted from: *Nutrients* **2023**, *15*, 3638, doi:10.3390/nu15163638 1

Dearbhla Finnegan, Restituto Tocmo and Christine Loscher
Targeted Application of Functional Foods as Immune Fitness Boosters in the Defense against Viral Infection
Reprinted from: *Nutrients* **2023**, *15*, 3371, doi:10.3390/nu15153371 10

Ping Zhang
The Role of Diet and Nutrition in Allergic Diseases
Reprinted from: *Nutrients* **2023**, *15*, 3683, doi:10.3390/nu15173683 49

Yuqian Wang, Lingeng Lu, Changquan Ling, Ping Zhang and Rui Han
Potential of Dietary HDAC2i in Breast Cancer Patients Receiving PD-1/PD-L1 Inhibitors
Reprinted from: *Nutrients* **2023**, *15*, 3984, doi:10.3390/nu15183984 74

Caterina Russo, Giovanni Enrico Lombardo, Giuseppe Bruschetta, Antonio Rapisarda, Alessandro Maugeri and Michele Navarra
Bergamot Byproducts: A Sustainable Source to Counteract Inflammation
Reprinted from: *Nutrients* **2024**, *16*, 259, doi:10.3390/nu16020259 95

Emilie Boucher, Caroline Plazy, Audrey Le Gouellec, Bertrand Toussaint and Dalil Hannani
Inulin Prebiotic Protects against Lethal *Pseudomonas aeruginosa* Acute Infection via γδ T Cell Activation
Reprinted from: *Nutrients* **2023**, *15*, 3037, doi:10.3390/nu15133037 115

Yasmine Y. Bouzid, Elizabeth L. Chin, Sarah S. Spearman, Zeynep Alkan, Charles B. Stephensen and Danielle G. Lemay
No Associations between Dairy Intake and Markers of Gastrointestinal Inflammation in Healthy Adult Cohort
Reprinted from: *Nutrients* **2023**, *15*, 3504, doi:10.3390/nu15163504 126

Xuefei Li, Zhengjie Lu, Yongjian Qi, Biao Chen and Bin Li
The Role of Polyunsaturated Fatty Acids in Osteoarthritis: Insights from a Mendelian Randomization Study
Reprinted from: *Nutrients* **2023**, *15*, 4787, doi:10.3390/nu15224787 138

Chen Wang, Dongfang Sun, Qi Deng, Lijun Sun, Lianhua Hu, Zhijia Fang, et al.
Elephantopus scaber L. Polysaccharides Alleviate Heat Stress-Induced Systemic Inflammation in Mice via Modulation of Characteristic Gut Microbiota and Metabolites
Reprinted from: *Nutrients* **2024**, *16*, 262, doi:10.3390/nu16020262 153

Ruonan Gao, Yilin Ren, Peng Xue, Yingyue Sheng, Qin Yang, Yuanyuan Dai, et al.
Protective Effect of the Polyphenol Ligustroside on Colitis Induced with Dextran Sulfate Sodium in Mice
Reprinted from: *Nutrients* **2024**, *16*, 522, doi:10.3390/nu16040522 175

Yuma Matsumoto, Mari Suto, Io Umebara, Hirofumi Masutomi and Katsuyuki Ishihara
Hydrophobic Components in Light-Yellow Pulp Sweet Potato (*Ipomoea batatas* (L.) Lam.) Tubers Suppress LPS-Induced Inflammatory Responses in RAW264.7 Cells via Activation of the Nrf2 Pathway
Reprinted from: *Nutrients* **2024**, *16*, 563, doi:10.3390/nu16040563 . . . . **188**

Dearbhla Finnegan, Monica A. Mechoud, Jamie A. FitzGerald, Tom Beresford, Harsh Mathur, Paul D. Cotter and Christine Loscher
Novel Fermentates Can Enhance Key Immune Responses Associated with Viral Immunity
Reprinted from: *Nutrients* **2024**, *16*, 1212, doi:10.3390/nu16081212 200

Preface

The link between nutrition and immune function has been known for a long time. For example, deficiencies in protein, zinc, and vitamin A lead to the impairment of immune cells and are correlated with increased risk of infection. In recent years, knowledge of the regulation of immune cells and immune mechanism-related diseases by dietary components has rapidly increased. The immune mechanism-mediated diseases that can be regulated by nutrients have expanded to cancer, autoimmune diseases, and allergies beyond infection. Newer cellular and molecular mechanisms are being elucidated. To reflect the newest developments in this field, this Special Issue collects 12 papers focused on the roles of nutrition and specific dietary components in systematic inflammation and local inflammatory responses in multiple tissues and immune cells. These papers highlight the roles played by dietary components such as dietary fiber, polyphenols, and polyunsaturated fatty acids in defense against viral infection, enhancing anti-tumor immune response in breast cancer and reducing inflammation in osteoarthritis, colitis, and allergic diseases through the modulation of immune function.

These findings will help physicians and researchers become aware of the critical roles played by dietary components in the prevention or treatment of a variety of inflammatory diseases. The potential of nutrition therapy to maintain proper immune function and health is great and worthy of further investigation.

Ping Zhang
Editor

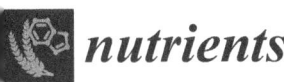

Brief Report

Calorie Restriction Impairs Anti-Tumor Immune Responses in an Immunogenic Preclinical Cancer Model

Nguyen Tien Dung [1,2], Takeshi Susukida [2], Sisca Ucche [2], Ka He [2], So-ichiro Sasaki [2], Ryuji Hayashi [1] and Yoshihiro Hayakawa [2,*]

[1] Department of Medical Oncology, Toyama University Hospital, University of Toyama, Toyama 930-0194, Japan; bs.dungnt@gmail.com (N.T.D.); hsayaka@med.u-toyama.ac.jp (R.H.)
[2] Section of Host Defences, Institute of Natural Medicine, University of Toyama, Toyama 930-0194, Japan; susukida@inm.u-toyama.ac.jp (T.S.); sisca.ucche@mail.ugm.ac.id (S.U.); d2168302@ems.u-toyama.ac.jp (K.H.); sasaki@inm.u-toyama.ac.jp (S.-i.S.)
* Correspondence: haya@inm.u-toyama.ac.jp; Tel.: +81-76-434-7620

Abstract: (1) Background: Although the important role of dietary energy intake in regulating both cancer progression and host immunity has been widely recognized, it remains unclear whether dietary calorie restriction (CR) has any impact on anti-tumor immune responses. (2) Methods: Using an immunogenic B16 melanoma cell expressing ovalbumin (B16-OVA), we examined the effect of the CR diet on B16-OVA tumor growth and host immune responses. To further test whether the CR diet affects the efficacy of cancer immunotherapy, we examined the effect of CR against anti-PD-1 monoclonal antibody (anti-PD-1 Ab) treatment. (3) Results: The CR diet significantly slowed down the tumor growth of B16-OVA without affecting both $CD4^+$ and $CD8^+$ T cell infiltration into the tumor. Although in vivo depletion of $CD8^+$ T cells facilitated B16-OVA tumor growth in the control diet group, there was no significant change in the tumor growth in the CR diet group with or without $CD8^+$ T cell-depletion. Anti-PD-1 Ab treatment lost its efficacy to suppress tumor growth along with the activation and metabolic shift of $CD8^+$ T cells under CR condition. (4) Conclusions: Our present results suggest that a physical condition restricted in energy intake in cancer patients may impair $CD8^+$ T cell immune surveillance and the efficacy of immunotherapy.

Keywords: calorie restriction; host immune response; $CD8^+$ T cell; immune checkpoint inhibitor

1. Introduction

The role of physical condition, including energy/food intake, diet, exercise, and weight, has been studied extensively in cancer progression. Diets high in calories, saturated fats, and refined sugars are associated with increased cancer risk and faster tumor growth, while diets high in fruits, vegetables, and whole grains are associated with reducing the risk of cancer and improving cancer outcomes [1–4]. Regular exercise has been shown to reduce inflammation, improve immune function and hormone regulation, and slow cancer growth [5,6]. In contrast, obesity is known to be associated with an increased risk of certain types of cancer and support aggressive tumor growth [7,8].

The correlation between physical condition and host immunity has also been studied recently. It has been reported that malnutrition and an unhealthy diet, characterized by a low intake of fruits, vegetables, and micronutrients, impair immune function and increase susceptibility to infections [9,10]. On the other hand, a diet rich in nutrients and phytochemicals, such as flavonoids, carotenes, and vitamins, is known to increase immune function and reduce inflammation [11,12]. Physical activity has also been shown to improve immune function by enhancing immune cell circulation and reducing inflammation [6,13]. Contrarily, obesity and a sedentary lifestyle were reported to impair immune function and increase the risk of infection [14,15]. Recent findings suggest the effect of dietary calorie intake has significant impact on cancer disease and therapy [16–19]. In general, calorie restriction (CR) is defined as the 20% to 40% reduction of the average daily caloric intake without incurring malnutrition or the deprivation of essential nutrients, and has been reported to affect cancer prevention and therapy [16–19].

In this study, we aim to investigate the effect of calorie restriction (CR) on anti-tumor immune responses in an immunogenic preclinical cancer model. We conducted a preclinical study using an immunogenic tumor model with B16 melanoma expressing ovalbumin (B16-OVA) and tested for the effect of CR on the host anti-tumor immune responses. B16-OVA model is one of the most well-established models used to monitor host $CD8^+$ T cell-dependent immune response. In addition, the effect of CR on immunotherapy with immune checkpoint blockade (ICB) was studied. Although the CR diet delayed tumor growth, the host anti-tumor immunity and the response to anti-PD-1 treatment were poor due to the alteration of $CD8^+$ T cells' number and function. These findings may contribute to understanding the response to ICB under energy restriction in cancer patients.

2. Materials and Methods

2.1. Cells

Murine melanoma cell line constitutively expressing ovalbumin, B16-OVA (MO4), was a kind gift from Dr. Shinichiro Fujii (Riken, Japan). Cells were cultured using Eagle's Minimum Essential Media (EMEM; Nissui, Tokyo, Japan) and supplemented with 2 mM L-glutamine, 10% fetal bovine serum, 100 U/mL penicillin, and 100 µg/mL streptomycin. Cells were all maintained at 37 °C in a humidified atmosphere of 95% air/5% CO_2.

2.2. Animals and Diet

All experiments were conducted using 7-week-old C57BL/6 mice which were purchased from CLEA Japan, Inc. (Tokyo, Japan). Mice were randomized into 2 groups using ad lib diet/CR diet, then each group was divided into 2 cages, with/without vehicles, and were group-housed and acclimatized to the animal facility environment for 7 days before experimentation, after which we measured daily food intake on average over the next 3 days. Animal rooms were maintained at 22.2 ± 1 °C and 30–70% humidity with a 12 h day/light cycles. On day 0, mice were subcutaneously inoculated with B16-OVA melanoma cells (10^5), then the CR group started fasting. Purified Rodent Diet with 10% fat (diet #D12450J, Research Diets, Inc., New Brunswick, NJ, USA) were fed for the entirety of the study, except a diet with 40% CR was customized and used for the CR group (diet # D16042001, Research Diets, Inc.). Tumors and body weight were measured 3 times weekly. Tumor growth was measured by a caliper square measuring along the longer axes (a) and the shorter axes (b) of the tumors. Tumor volumes (mm^3) were calculated by the formula: tumor volume (mm^3) = $ab2/2$. Tissues were collected between 8 a.m. and 12 p.m., ~14 h after the last meal. All experiments were approved (Animal Experiment Protocol: A209INM-4, A2022INM-5) and performed in accordance with the guidelines of Care and Use of Laboratory Animals of University of Toyama.

2.3. Antibody Treatment

For $CD8^+$ T cell depletion, B16-OVA-inoculated mice were pretreated with anti-CD8 antibody (clone 53.6.2, Bio X Cell, Lebanon, NH, USA) (0.25 mg/mouse i.p.) 2 times at 2 days prior day 0, and then again at days 7 and 14. For PD-1 blocking, B16-OVA-inoculated mice were treated with anti-PD-1 antibody (RMP1–14, BioXCell) (0.2 mg/mouse i.p.) at days 3, 6, and 9 from day 0.

2.4. Tumor-Infiltrating Lymphocyte (TIL) Isolation and Flow Cytometry

Tumor samples were cut into small pieces and digested in serum-free RPMI 1640 medium containing 2 mg/mL collagenase (Roche Diagnostics GmbH) and 0.1 mg/mL DNase I (Roche Diagnostics GmbH) for 1 h at 37 °C. The cells were then incubated with a saturating amount of fluorophore-conjugated antibodies against PE-Cy/7 CD45 (30-F11), FITC CD3ε (145-2C11), PerCP-Cy5.5 CD4 (GK1.5), APC CD8 (53-6.7), PE CD44 (IM7),

APC-Cy7 CD62L (MEL-14) were purchased from Biolegend (San Diego, CA, USA). FACS Canto II (BD Biosciences, Franklin Lakes, NJ, USA) was used for FACS analysis and data were analyzed using FlowJo software v.10 (BD Biosciences).

2.5. Real-Time CD8$^+$ T Cell Metabolic Analysis

After euthanizing the mice by cervical dislocation, cells were isolated by tumor-draining lymph node (tLN) from the mice fed with either a normal diet or CR diet. CD8$^+$ T cells were negatively selected using MojoSort™ mouse CD8 T cell Isolation Kit (BioLegend) according to the manufacturer's protocol. The isolated CD8+ T cell were seeded at the density of 5×10^5 cells/well in Poly-D-Lysine (Thermo Fisher Scientific, Waltham, MA, USA)-coated XFe24 plates in 500 μL Seahorse XF RPMI medium containing 1 mM pyruvate, 2 mM glutamine, and 10 mM glucose. ECAR and OCR were measured on an XFe24 Extracellular Flux analyzer (Agilent Technologies, Santa Clara, CA, USA) using the Seahorse XF Cell Mito Stress test kit (Agilent Technologies). The OCR and ECAR values were obtained at baseline and after the injections of oligomycin (final concentration 1 μM), FCCP (final concentration 1 μM), and antimycin/rotenone (final concentration 0.5 μM), respectively.

2.6. Statistical Analysis

Statistical analyses were performed using GraphPad Prism 8 Software (GraphPad Software, La Jolla, CA, USA). Significance was determined using either Bonferroni's test for multiple comparisons following one-way ANOVA or the unpaired two tailed t-test (Student's t-test). In all cases, p values of <0.05 were considered statistically significant. All data were obtained from the groups of 4–10 mice.

3. Results

3.1. Effect of CR on Host Anti-Tumor Immunity

We first examined the effect of CR on B16-OVA tumor growth. Mice were subcutaneously inoculated with B16-OVA cells, then subjected to a 40% CR condition from the day of tumor inoculation and monitored for tumor growth. The body weight change in CR-diet-fed mice is shown in Figure 1A by comparing control-diet-fed mice. There was a substantial decrease in the body weight in CR diet group, however, it was no more than 20% reduction and was reversible by regular feeding. As shown in Figure 1B, the growth of tumors was significantly impaired in mice fed with the CR diet compared to controls. To further determine the contribution of the host immune response, particularly CD8$^+$ T cells, for controlling tumor growth in mice fed with the control diet or the CR diet, mice were treated with anti-CD8 Ab to deplete CD8$^+$ T cells. In the control-diet-fed mice, anti-CD8 Ab treatment showed a trend to increase the growth of B16-OVA tumor (Figure 1C); however, it did not show any different tumor growth in the CR-diet-fed mice (Figure 1D). These results potentially implicate that the CR diet retards the growth of B16-OVA tumor. Although there were no statistically significant differences in both CD8+ T cell-depleted control diet and CR diet groups, the CR diet might also has a negative impact on the host anti-tumor immunity by CD8$^+$ T cells in controlling tumor growth.

3.2. Effect of CR on the Responsiveness to Immune Checkpoint Blockade

As CR-impaired host CD8$^+$ T cells display immunity against the B16-OVA tumor, we next tested whether CR affects the responsiveness to immune checkpoint blockade in tumor-bearing mice. B16-OVA tumor-bearing mice, either fed with the control diet or a 40% CR diet, were treated with anti-PD-1 Ab after the tumor inoculation. As shown in Figure 2A, anti-PD-1 Ab treatment significantly inhibited the growth of B16-OVA tumor in control-diet-fed mice. Contrarily, anti-PD-1 Ab treatment did not show any effect on the growth of the B16-OVA tumor in CR-fed-mice (Figure 2B), suggesting CR has a negative effect on the responsiveness to immune checkpoint blockade, presumably through a CD8$^+$ T cell-dependent anti-tumor immune response.

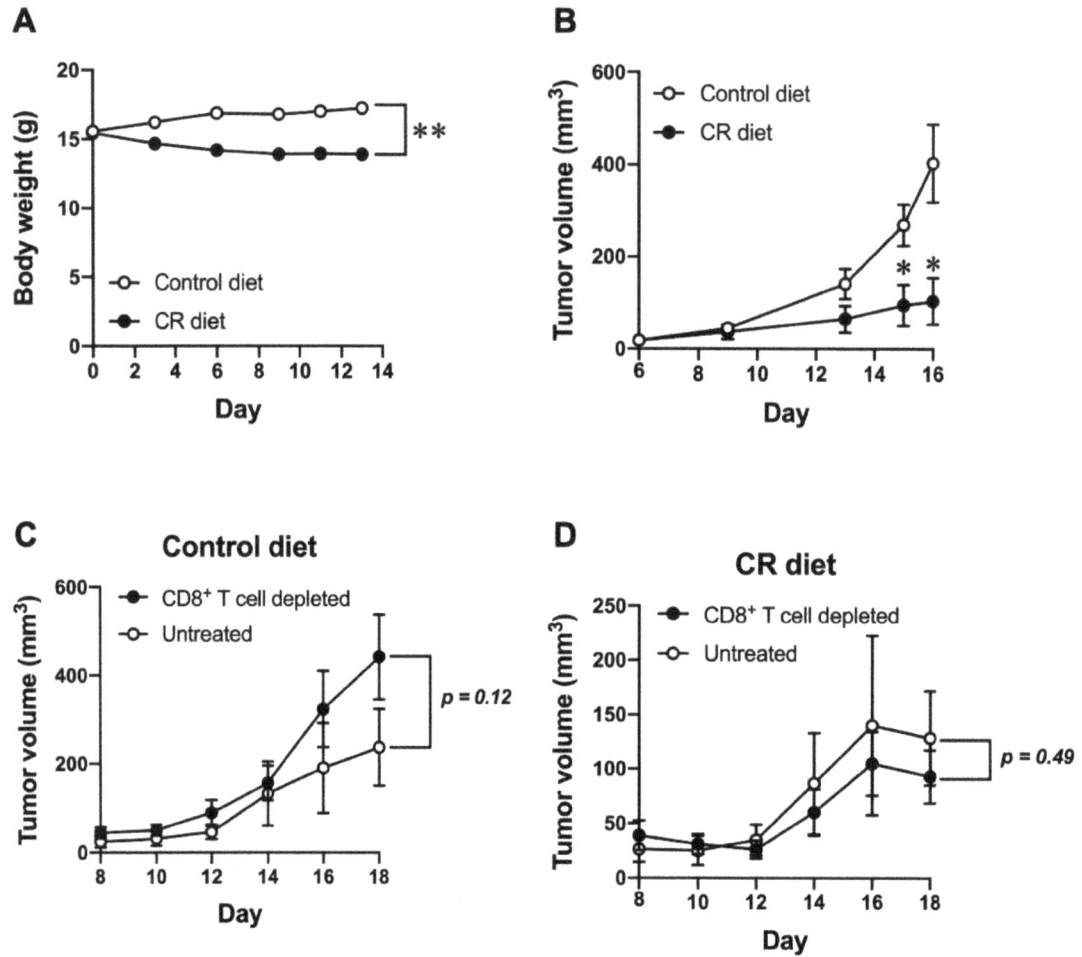

Figure 1. Effect of CR on tumor growth in the presence or absence of host CD8$^+$ T cell. (**A**) Body weight change in in control-diet-fed and CR-diet-fed C57BL/6J mice. (**B**) B16-OVA tumor size progression in control-diet-fed and CR-diet-fed C57BL/6J mice. (**C,D**) B16-OVA tumor size progression in control-diet-fed (**C**) and CR-diet-fed (**D**) mice with/without CD8$^+$ T cell depletion. Each plot represents the mean ± SEM (n = 4–21); * $p < 0.05$, ** $p < 0.01$, compared with control-diet-fed mice or antibody untreated group; indicated p values were obtained from a statistical comparison, the unpaired two tailed t-test (Student's t-test).

3.3. Effect of CR on the Population of Tumor-Infiltrating Lymphocytes (TILs)

In order to understand the effect of CR on CD8$^+$ T cell-dependent anti-tumor immune responses, we next examined the population of TILs in B16-OVA tumor-bearing mice fed with the control diet or the CR diet, and with or without anti-PD-1 Ab treatment. B16-OVA inoculated mice were fed with the control diet or the CR diet from day 0, and then treated with or without anti-PD-1 Ab (on days 3, 6, and 9). The tumor samples were collected on day 16 to isolate TILs, and subjected to flow cytometry analysis. There was no significant difference in the tumor infiltration of CD3$^+$ T cells (Figure 3A), the ratio of CD8$^+$/CD4$^+$ T cells (Figure 3B), or CD44high effector CD8$^+$ T cells (Figure 3C) between control-diet- and CR-diet-fed mice. In control-diet-fed mice, anti-PD-1 Ab treatment increased the population of those CD8$^+$ T cells in line with inhibiting the B16-OVA tumor growth (Figure 3). Although anti-PD-1 Ab treatment did not show an anti-tumor effect, it had a similar effect on the population of tumor-infiltrating CD8$^+$ T cells in CR-diet-fed mice (Figure 3). These results suggest that CR may not impair the anti-tumor effect of anti-PD-1 Ab treatment by affecting the presence of tumor-infiltrating effector CD8$^+$ T cells.

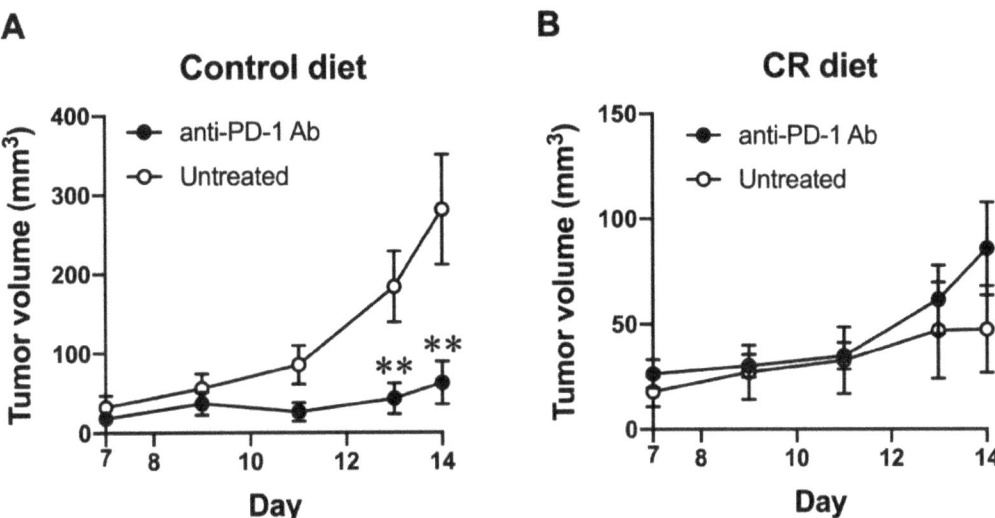

Figure 2. Effect of CR on the responsiveness to immune checkpoint blockade. (**A**,**B**) B16-OVA tumor size progression in control-diet-fed (**A**) and CR-diet-fed (**B**) C57BL/6J mice with/without anti-PD-1 antibody treatment (0.2 mg/mouse i.p.) at days 3, 6, and 9 from day 0. Each plot represents the mean ± SEM (n = 4–21); ** p < 0.01, compared with control-diet-fed mice or antibody-untreated group; indicated p values were obtained from a statistical comparison, the unpaired two tailed t-test (Student's t-test).

3.4. Effect of CR on the Metabolic Status of CD8$^+$ T Cell in B16-OVA Tumor-Bearing Mice

Considering that there was no significant effect of CR diet on the population of TILs, we sought to understand the metabolic status of CD8$^+$ T cells in B16-OVA tumor-bearing mice fed with the control or the CR diet, and also compared their response to anti-PD-1 Ab treatment using an extracellular flux analyzer. In CR-diet-fed mice, CD8$^+$ T cells in the B16-OVA tumor-draining lymph node (tLN) showed lower oxygen consumption rates (OCR, Figure 4A) and extracellular acidification rates (ECAR, Figure 4B) compared to control diet fed mice, suggesting the CR diet generally reduces the metabolic activity of CD8$^+$ T cells compared to the control diet. Upon anti-PD-1 Ab treatment, CD8$^+$ T cells in tLN of control-diet-fed mice showed lower OCR and higher ECAR compared to the untreated group, whereas those of CR-diet-fed mice did not show any difference (Figure 4). These results indicate that anti-PD-1 treatment activated and induced a metabolic shift of CD8$^+$ T cells to the glycolytic pathway under control-fed conditions; however, it cannot be recapitulated in CR-diet-fed mice.

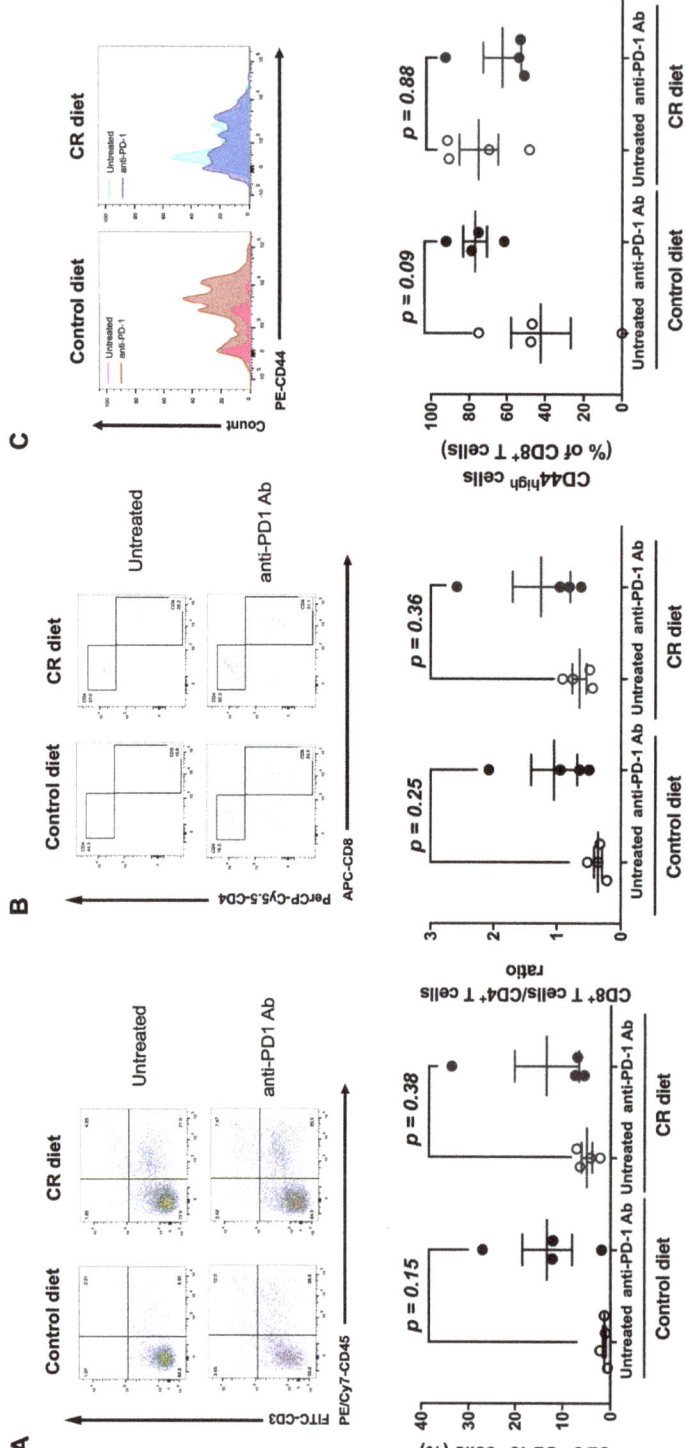

Figure 3. Effect of CR on the population of tumor-infiltrating lymphocytes (TILs). (**A**) Representative dot plots depicting (upper panel) or percentages (lower panel) of TILs expressing CD3 and CD45. B16-OVA-inoculated mice were treated with/without anti-PD-1 antibody (0.2 mg/mouse i.p.) at days 3, 6, and 9 from day 0. (**B**) Representative dot plots depicting (upper panels) or percentages (lower panel) of cells expressing CD4 and CD8 in the gated CD3$^+$CD45$^+$ TILs. (**C**) Representative histograms representing surface expression (upper panels) or median fluorescence intensity (MFI) values (lower panel) of CD44 on CD3$^+$CD8$^+$CD45$^+$ TILs derived from B16-OVA-inoculated mice. Each plot represents the mean ± SEM ($n = 4$); indicated p values were obtained from a statistical comparison; one-way ANOVA with Bonferroni's multiple comparisons correction.

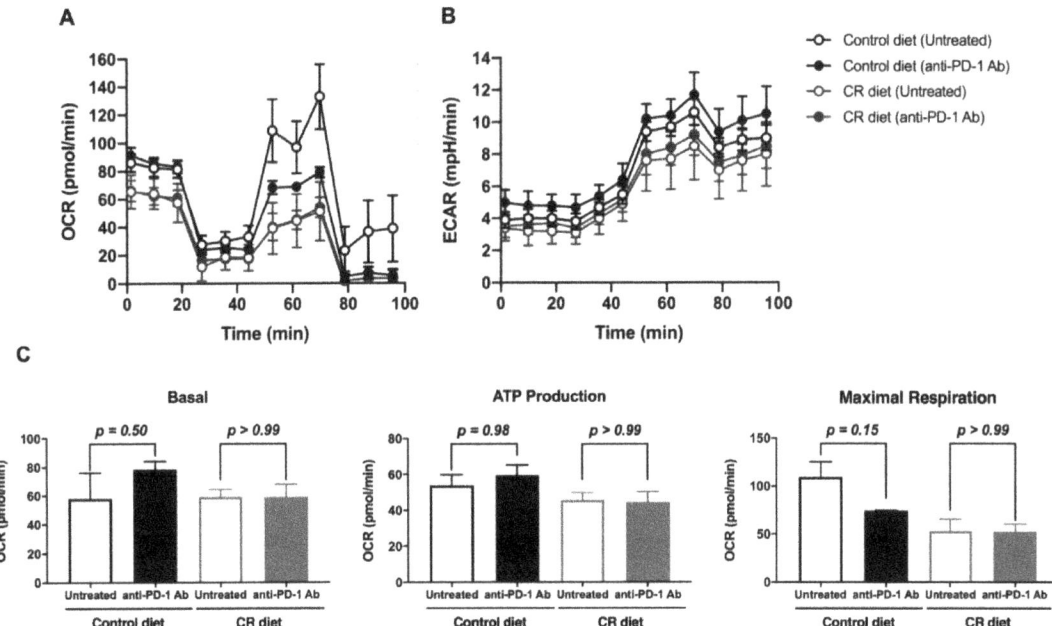

Figure 4. Effect of CR on the metabolic status of CD8$^+$ T cell in B16-OVA tumor-bearing mice. (**A**,**B**) The oxygen consumption rate (OCR) (**A**), the extracellular acidification rate (ECAR) (**B**), and the summary of respiration status and ATP production (**C**) of the isolated CD8$^+$ T cells from lymph nodes of each group was measured using a Seahorse XFe24 analyzer. Each plot represents the mean ± SEM (n = 3–4).

4. Discussion

To understand the importance of physical condition, particularly energy intake, in cancer progression, we studied the effect of CR on anti-tumor immune responses in the immunogenic B16-OVA melanoma model. CR significantly slowed down the tumor growth of B16-OVA without affecting both CD4$^+$ and CD8$^+$ T cell infiltration into the tumor. While the in vivo depletion of CD8$^+$ cells accelerated B16-OVA tumor growth in the normal diet group, there was no significant change in the tumor growth of the CR group with or without CD8$^+$ cells. Considering anti-PD-1 Ab lost its efficacy to suppress tumor growth under the CR condition along with the alteration of CD8$^+$ T cells' mitochondrial activity, the energy restricted physical condition in cancer patients may impair CD8$^+$ T cell immune surveillance and the efficacy of immunotherapy.

It has been known that CR reduces cancer risk and improves outcomes in preclinical and clinical studies. Calorie restriction activates molecular pathways that enhance cellular defenses, promote DNA repair, and reduce oxidative damage, which may contribute to its anticancer effects [20,21]. Additionally, CR has been shown to enhance the effectiveness of cancer treatments such as chemotherapy and radiation [22,23]. Indeed, some studies have demonstrated that calorie restriction can improve immune function and reduce inflammation, potentially contributing to increased health [21,24,25]. Several studies have also provided evidence indicating that calorie restriction can enhance immune function and alleviate inflammation, leading to potentially improved overall health [26,27]. CR has been shown to prevent mitochondrial dysfunction and enhance mitochondrial efficiency by reducing oxidative stress and inflammation, promoting mitochondrial biogenesis, and improving mitochondrial quality control mechanisms. Therefore, CR may improve cellular metabolism and energy production, reduce cellular damage, and contribute to improved health and longevity [28,29].

Contrary to the role of CR in cancer suppression, patients with sarcopenia or cachexia resulting from chronic caloric deficits may have a poorer response to immunotherapy, lower progression-free survival, and lower overall survival rates, according to some studies [30,31]. In line with our findings, those patients also showed a reduction in immune cell infiltration into the tumor microenvironment and impaired T cell activation [30,31]. In general, $CD8^+$ T cells use glycolysis during their differentiation to effector cells, and PD-1 ligation increases fatty acid oxidation (FAO) [32]. The mitochondrial activation of CD8+ T cells has been reported to enhance the efficacy of PD-1 blockade [33,34]. Therefore, it must be critical to balance between calorie restriction and maintaining an adequate calorie intake to avoid negative impacts on immune function and the subsequent response to cancer therapy.

5. Conclusions

In this study, we aim to investigate the effect of calorie restriction (CR) on anti-tumor immune responses in an immunogenic preclinical cancer model. Although the CR diet delayed tumor growth, the effect of anti-PD-1 treatment was poorer in CR mice. Although our presented study is still exploratory with a relatively low sample size and large data variations, our present results suggest that the energy restricted physical condition of cancer patients may impair $CD8^+$ T cell immune surveillance and the efficacy of immunotherapy.

Author Contributions: N.T.D. and T.S. planned and performed the experiments, analyzed the data and wrote the manuscript. S.U., K.H. and S.-i.S. coordinated the experiments. R.H. and Y.H. coordinated the experiments, and acquired the funding, Y.H. designed and supervised the experiments and wrote and edited the manuscript. All authors have read and agreed to the published version of the manuscript.

Funding: This study was partly supported by Yasuda Memorial Medical Foundation, and the Cooperative Research Project from the Institute of Natural Medicine, University of Toyama.

Institutional Review Board Statement: All experiments were approved (Animal Experiment Protocol: A209INM-4 (15 April 2019), A2022INM-5 (6 April 2022)) and performed in accordance with the guidelines of Care and Use of Laboratory Animals of University of Toyama.

Informed Consent Statement: Not applicable.

Data Availability Statement: The data presented in this study are available on request from the corresponding author.

Acknowledgments: We are grateful to all members of Hayakawa Laboratory for their support.

Conflicts of Interest: The authors declare no conflict of interest.

References

1. Mihaylova, M.M.; Chaix, A.; Delibegovic, M.; Ramsey, J.J.; Bass, J.; Melkani, G.; Singh, R.; Chen, Z.; William, W.J.; Shirasu-Hiza, M. When a calorie is not just a calorie: Diet quality and timing as mediators of metabolism and healthy aging. *Cell Metab.* **2023**, *35*, 1114–1131. [CrossRef] [PubMed]
2. Berger, N.A. Obesity and Cancer Pathogenesis. *Ann. N. Y. Acad. Sci.* **2014**, *1311*, 57–76. [CrossRef] [PubMed]
3. Schwingshackl, L.; Hoffmann, G. Adherence to Mediterranean Diet and Risk of Cancer: A Systematic Review and Meta-Analysis of Observational Studies. *Int. J. Cancer* **2014**, *135*, 1884–1897. [CrossRef] [PubMed]
4. Gonzalez, C.A.; Riboli, E. Diet and Cancer Prevention: Contributions from the European Prospective Investigation into Cancer and Nutrition (EPIC) Study. *Eur. J. Cancer* **2010**, *46*, 2555–2562. [CrossRef] [PubMed]
5. McTiernan, A. Mechanisms Linking Physical Activity with Cancer. *Nat. Rev. Cancer* **2008**, *8*, 205–211. [CrossRef] [PubMed]
6. Campbell, J.P.; Turner, J.E. Debunking the Myth of Exercise-Induced Immune Suppression: Redefining the Impact of Exercise on Immunological Health Across the Lifespan. *Front. Immunol.* **2018**, *9*, 648. [CrossRef] [PubMed]
7. Lauby-Secretan, B.; Scoccianti, C.; Loomis, D.; Grosse, Y.; Bianchini, F.; Straif, K. Body Fatness and Cancer—Viewpoint of the IARC Working Group. *N. Engl. J. Med.* **2016**, *375*, 794–798. [CrossRef]
8. Calle, E.E.; Rodriguez, C.; Walker-Thurmond, K.; Thun, M.J. Overweight, Obesity, and Mortality from Cancer in a Prospectively Studied Cohort of U.S. Adults. *N. Engl. J. Med.* **2003**, *348*, 1625–1638. [CrossRef]

9. Calder, P.C.; Carr, A.C.; Gombart, A.F.; Eggersdorfer, M. Optimal Nutritional Status for a Well-Functioning Immune System Is an Important Factor to Protect against Viral Infections. *Nutrients* **2020**, *12*, 1181. [CrossRef]
10. Bhaskaram, P. Immunobiology of Mild Micronutrient Deficiencies. *Br. J. Nutr.* **2001**, *85* (Suppl. 2), S75–S80. [CrossRef]
11. Gleeson, M.; Nieman, D.C.; Pedersen, B.K. Exercise, Nutrition and Immune Function. *J. Sports Sci.* **2004**, *22*, 115–125. [CrossRef] [PubMed]
12. Carr, A.C.; Maggini, S. Vitamin C and Immune Function. *Nutrients* **2017**, *9*, 1211. [CrossRef] [PubMed]
13. Simpson, R.J.; Kunz, H.; Agha, N.; Graff, R. Exercise and the Regulation of Immune Functions. *Prog. Mol. Biol. Transl. Sci.* **2015**, *135*, 355–380. [CrossRef] [PubMed]
14. Milner, J.J.; Beck, M.A. The Impact of Obesity on the Immune Response to Infection. *Proc. Nutr. Soc.* **2012**, *71*, 298–306. [CrossRef]
15. De Heredia, F.P.; Gómez-Martínez, S.; Marcos, A. Obesity, Inflammation and the Immune System. *Proc. Nutr. Soc.* **2012**, *71*, 332–338. [CrossRef] [PubMed]
16. Vidoni, C.; Ferraresi, A.; Esposito, A.; Maheshwari, C.; Dhanasekaran, D.N.; Mollace, V.; Isidoro, C. Calorie Restriction for Cancer Prevention and Therapy: Mechanisms, Expectations, and Efficacy. *J. Cancer Prev.* **2021**, *26*, 224–236. [CrossRef] [PubMed]
17. Brandhorst, S.; Longo, V.D. Fasting and Caloric Restriction in Cancer Prevention and Treatment. *Metab. Cancer* **2016**, *207*, 241–266. [CrossRef]
18. Pistollato, F.; Forbes-Hernandez, T.Y.; Iglesias, R.C.; Ruiz, R.; Zabaleta, M.E.; Dominguez, I.; Cianciosi, D.; Quiles, J.L.; Giampieri, F.; Battino, M. Effects of caloric restriction on immunosurveillance, microbiota and cancer cell phenotype: Possible implications for cancer treatment. *Semin. Cancer Biol.* **2021**, *73*, 45–57. [CrossRef]
19. Ibrahim, E.M.; Al-Foheidi, M.H.; Al-Mansour, M.M. Energy and caloric restriction, and fasting and cancer: A narrative review. *Support. Care Cancer* **2021**, *29*, 2299–2304. [CrossRef]
20. Longo, V.D.; Mattson, M.P. Fasting: Molecular Mechanisms and Clinical Applications. *Cell Metab.* **2014**, *19*, 181–192. [CrossRef]
21. Lee, C.; Longo, V.D. Fasting vs Dietary Restriction in Cellular Protection and Cancer Treatment: From Model Organisms to Patients. *Oncogene* **2011**, *30*, 3305–3316. [CrossRef] [PubMed]
22. Lee, C.; Raffaghello, L.; Brandhorst, S.; Safdie, F.M.; Bianchi, G.; Martin-Montalvo, A.; Pistoia, V.; Wei, M.; Hwang, S.; Merlino, A.; et al. Fasting Cycles Retard Growth of Tumors and Sensitize a Range of Cancer Cell Types to Chemotherapy. *Sci. Transl. Med.* **2012**, *4*, 124ra27. [CrossRef] [PubMed]
23. Safdie, F.; Brandhorst, S.; Wei, M.; Wang, W.; Lee, C.; Hwang, S.; Conti, P.S.; Chen, T.C.; Longo, V.D. Fasting Enhances the Response of Glioma to Chemo- and Radiotherapy. *PLoS ONE* **2012**, *7*, e44603. [CrossRef] [PubMed]
24. Johnson, J.B.; Summer, W.; Cutler, R.G.; Martin, B.; Hyun, D.-H.; Dixit, V.D.; Pearson, M.; Nassar, M.; Telljohann, R.; Maudsley, S.; et al. Alternate Day Calorie Restriction Improves Clinical Findings and Reduces Markers of Oxidative Stress and Inflammation in Overweight Adults with Moderate Asthma. *Free Radic. Biol. Med.* **2007**, *42*, 665–674. [CrossRef] [PubMed]
25. Martin, B.; Mattson, M.P.; Maudsley, S. Caloric Restriction and Intermittent Fasting: Two Potential Diets for Successful Brain Aging. *Ageing Res. Rev.* **2006**, *5*, 332–353. [CrossRef] [PubMed]
26. Topalian, S.L.; Taube, J.M.; Anders, R.A.; Pardoll, D.M. Mechanism-Driven Biomarkers to Guide Immune Checkpoint Blockade in Cancer Therapy. *Nat. Rev. Cancer* **2016**, *16*, 275–287. [CrossRef] [PubMed]
27. Raskov, H.; Orhan, A.; Christensen, J.P.; Gögenur, I. Cytotoxic CD8+ T Cells in Cancer and Cancer Immunotherapy. *Br. J. Cancer* **2021**, *124*, 359–367. [CrossRef] [PubMed]
28. López-Lluch, G.; Irusta, P.M.; Navas, P.; de Cabo, R. Mitochondrial biogenesis and healthy aging. *Exp. Gerontol.* **2008**, *43*, 813–819. [CrossRef]
29. Civitarese, A.E.; Smith, S.R.; Ravussin, E. Diet, Energy Metabolism and Mitochondrial Biogenesis. *Curr. Opin. Clin. Nutr. Metab. Care* **2007**, *10*, 679–687. [CrossRef]
30. Nishioka, N.; Uchino, J.; Hirai, S.; Katayama, Y.; Yoshimura, A.; Okura, N.; Tanimura, K.; Harita, S.; Imabayashi, T.; Chihara, Y.; et al. Association of Sarcopenia with and Efficacy of Anti-PD-1/PD-L1 Therapy in Non-Small-Cell Lung Cancer. *J. Clin. Med.* **2019**, *8*, 450. [CrossRef]
31. Li, S.; Wang, T.; Tong, G.; Li, X.; You, D.; Cong, M. Prognostic Impact of Sarcopenia on Clinical Outcomes in Malignancies Treated with Immune Checkpoint Inhibitors: A Systematic Review and Meta-Analysis. *Front. Oncol.* **2021**, *11*, 726257. [CrossRef]
32. Cao, J.; Liao, S.; Zeng, F.; Liao, Q.; Luo, G.; Zhou, Y. Effects of altered glycolysis levels on CD8+ T cell activation and function. *Cell Death Dis.* **2023**, *14*, 407. [CrossRef] [PubMed]
33. Chamoto, K.; Chowdhury, P.S.; Kumar, A.; Sonomura, K.; Matsuda, F.; Fagarasan, S.; Honjo, T. Mitochondrial activation chemicals synergize with surface receptor PD-1 blockade for T cell-dependent antitumor activity. *Proc. Natl. Acad. Sci. USA* **2017**, *114*, E761–E770. [CrossRef] [PubMed]
34. Chowdhury, P.S.; Chamoto, K.; Kumar, A.; Honjo, T. PPAR-Induced Fatty Acid Oxidation in T Cells Increases the Number of Tumor-Reactive CD8+ T Cells and Facilitates Anti–PD-1 Therapy. *Cancer Immunol. Res.* **2018**, *6*, 1375–1387. [CrossRef] [PubMed]

Disclaimer/Publisher's Note: The statements, opinions and data contained in all publications are solely those of the individual author(s) and contributor(s) and not of MDPI and/or the editor(s). MDPI and/or the editor(s) disclaim responsibility for any injury to people or property resulting from any ideas, methods, instructions or products referred to in the content.

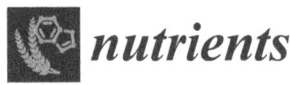

Review

Targeted Application of Functional Foods as Immune Fitness Boosters in the Defense against Viral Infection

Dearbhla Finnegan, Restituto Tocmo and Christine Loscher *

School of Biotechnology, Dublin City University, D09 DX63 Dublin, Ireland; dearbhla.finnegan7@mail.dcu.ie (D.F.); restituto.tocmo@dcu.ie (R.T.)
* Correspondence: christine.loscher@dcu.ie; Tel.: +353-(01)7008515

Abstract: In recent times, the emergence of viral infections, including the SARS-CoV-2 virus, the monkeypox virus, and, most recently, the Langya virus, has highlighted the devastating effects of viral infection on human life. There has been significant progress in the development of efficacious vaccines for the prevention and control of viruses; however, the high rates of viral mutation and transmission necessitate the need for novel methods of control, management, and prevention. In recent years, there has been a shift in public awareness on health and wellbeing, with consumers making significant dietary changes to improve their immunity and overall health. This rising health awareness is driving a global increase in the consumption of functional foods. This review delves into the benefits of functional foods as potential natural means to modulate the host immune system to enhance defense against viral infections. We provide an overview of the functional food market in Europe and discuss the benefits of enhancing immune fitness in high-risk groups, including the elderly, those with obesity, and people with underlying chronic conditions. We also discuss the immunomodulatory mechanisms of key functional foods, including dairy proteins and hydrolysates, plant-based functional foods, fermentates, and foods enriched with vitamin D, zinc, and selenium. Our findings reveal four key immunity boosting mechanisms by functional foods, including inhibition of viral proliferation and binding to host cells, modulation of the innate immune response in macrophages and dendritic cells, enhancement of specific immune responses in T cells and B cells, and promotion of the intestinal barrier function. Overall, this review demonstrates that diet-derived nutrients and functional foods show immense potential to boost viral immunity in high-risk individuals and can be an important approach to improving overall immune health.

Keywords: functional food; viral immunity; COVID-19; immune fitness; health benefits; elderly; obese; chronic disease; boosting immune system; fermentates; milk hydrolysates

1. Introduction

In recent years, as a result of the increase in awareness of the impact of diet on health, there has been a significant shift in the interest of consumers towards food that improves immune health. Food is a critical influencer of a healthy, disease-free, high-quality life. Given that global dietary risk factors are estimated to cause 11 million deaths and 255 million disability-adjusted life years annually [1], food has become fundamental to longevity more than ever. It is a long-known fact that what we eat influences our body, and vital nutrients are essential for growth, cellular function, tissue development, energy, and immune defense [2]. There is growing evidence that food can act as an immunomodulator, and certain nutrients and foods have been highlighted to improve immune defense and to increase resistance to infection while maintaining immune tolerance [3]. Furthermore, deficiency in certain nutrients leads to malnutrition and results in the development of diseases. Often, these diseases result from nutritional inadequacies, which impair immune function.

A poor diet can compromise the immune system, leaving the host more susceptible to pathogenic infection, including viral infections. With the recent viral outbreaks, including the SARS-CoV-2 virus, the monkeypox virus, and, most recently, the Langya virus, boosting the immune system is increasingly important. As seen with the COVID-19 pandemic, viruses have the capability of spreading rapidly from person to person, causing devastating damage to humanity due to their potential for high transmissibility. Therefore, there is an urgent need to explore new ways of enhancing viral immunity. Food has long been known to provide antiviral protection and, therefore, can be used as a first-line strategy to boost the immune system in the form of functional foods to enhance protection against new, emerging viral infections as well as well-established viruses, including the influenza virus [4–11].

Used in conjunction with hygiene practices and an active lifestyle, functional foods may provide additional, naturally sourced antiviral protection. In this review, we discuss the current trends in health and wellbeing in relation to the growing interest in functional foods, especially in Europe. We present the concept of boosting immune fitness with a focus on individuals at high risk of viral infections. Moreover, we discuss the mechanisms by which diet-derived nutrients and functional foods can boost immunity in high-risk individuals, and how diet-based strategies can be an important approach to improving overall immune health. Finally, we present future perspectives on how functional foods, especially fermented foods, can be further developed for boosting immune fitness.

2. Trends in Health and Wellbeing: A Focus on Functional Foods

The increased popularity and global explosion within the Health and Wellbeing industry are evidenced by the booming economic figures in data from 2015 to 2017, showing a growth rate of 6.4% [12]. This growth was expected to continue at this pace, and the global wellness industry had a net worth of an estimated USD 4.75 trillion in 2019 [12]. The total Healthy Eating, Nutrition, and Weight Loss sector comes to an estimated USD 702 billion, making it the second largest sector of the industry [12].

These trends in the Health and Wellbeing industry reflect trends seen in the food industry, with an increasing demand for healthy foods, in turn driving the revolution that is the development of food products that can impart additional health benefits to their consumers, i.e., the functional food industry. The functional food industry is growing at a phenomenal rate, with a worldwide growth rate of 10.34% from 2016 to 2021 based on data gathered from Euromonitor [13]. Furthermore, this growth rate is expected to increase further, nearly doubling that of 2016–2021, with an expected worldwide growth rate of 19.17% from 2021 to 2026 [13]. The retail sales value of the functional food industry in Europe in 2021 was dominated by the UK, which held the largest value, followed by France and Germany (Figure 1) [14]. The popularity of functional foods worldwide is on the rise, with the USA, Europe, and Japan being the regions holding the greatest retail sales values [14]. An annual increase in market size for Ireland, Eastern and Western Europe, the USA, and worldwide has been observed (Table 1) with future predictions in market size for 2022–2026. Figure 2 shows the percentage hold Ireland, Eastern and Western Europe, and the USA have in the worldwide functional food market, with Europe and the USA making up over a third of the worldwide functional food market at a combined 33.67% of the total market size.

This annual growth rate was expected to continue for the foreseeable future; however, in late 2019 and early 2020, the catastrophic news of a global COVID-19 pandemic further ignited global interest in the Health and Wellness industry. The rapid growth and boom within the functional food industry are clear evidence that, globally, we are now looking to food as a source of immune support when food is so well known to aid in anti-viral immunity and overall immune support [4–11]. Seeking functional food sources with immunomodulatory capabilities could potentially be a game changer to naturally aid our management of viral infection.

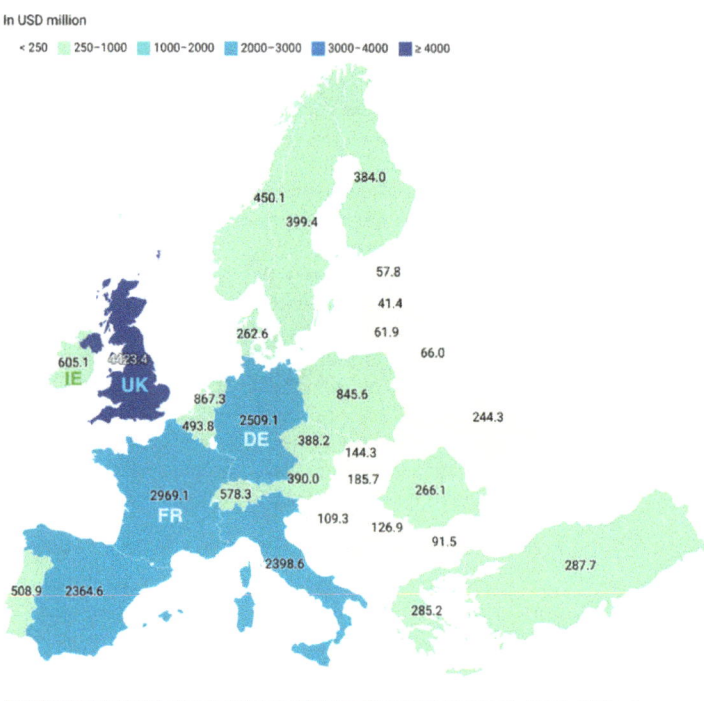

Figure 1. Retail sales value of functional foods in Europe in 2021 [13]. Two-letter country abbreviations included for markets of interest. Adapted from [14].

Table 1. Functional food market size in Ireland, Eastern Europe, Western Europe, and the world.

Year	2016	2017	2018	2019	2020	2021	2022	2023	2024	2025	2026
Ireland	494.97	510.65	519.51	531.83	554.24	584.79	585.71	591.82	617.89	646.61	679
Eastern Europe	4142	4727.30	4967.70	4999	4921	5211.80	5530.50	5745.60	5977.00	6234.30	6498.10
Western Europe	20,689.50	20,695.50	21,568.80	20,661.60	21,537.40	23,032.30	23,526.50	23,906.90	24,444.30	25,130.70	25,803.50
USA	31,902.50	31,708.50	31,007.50	30,956.90	32,053.90	31,512.30	32,940.60	34,148.30	35,239.50	36,210.90	37,164.30
World	159,040.10	164,365.30	168,157.20	168,477.90	168,919.00	177,395.00	184,464.70	192,846.20	201,417.00	201,355.60	219,467.80

Market values from 2016 to 2021 in USD million. Predicted market values for 2022–2026 in USD million. Data obtained from Euromonitor International, a market research provider (2022).

Due to the current economic climate and a recent global pandemic, the immune support and health supplements market is expected to grow even further, at a compound annual growth rate of over 9% from 2019 to 2025 [15]. With an estimated six-month immunity provided by the vaccines as antiviral therapy for the prevention of COVID-19 infection, alternative methods to augment protection against viral invasion are highly desirable [16,17].

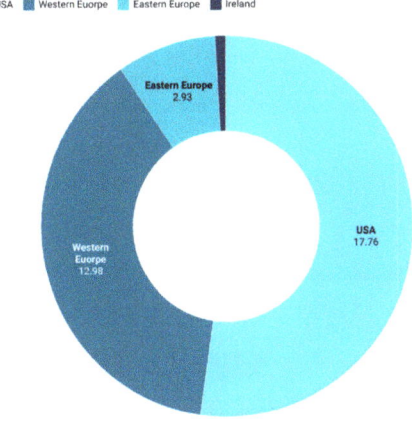

Figure 2. Percentage hold of various regions of the worldwide functional food market size for 2021. Data obtained from Euromonitor International, a market research provider (2022) [13]. Created with Datawrapper.

3. Boosting Immune Fitness in High-Risk Individuals

In this section, we highlight the importance of boosting the immunity of high-risk individuals. We first present the concept of immune fitness, followed by an overview of the key features of the innate and adaptive immune system of three highly vulnerable cohorts with a focus on gut immunity. Understanding the changes in the immune responses of these cohorts is critical to furthering the development of functional foods targeted at boosting viral immunity.

3.1. Immune Fitness

Immune fitness describes the capacity of the body to respond to health challenges, such as infection, via activation of the appropriate immune response in order to prompt disease resolution, prevent pathogen infection, and promote health, thereby ensuring quality of life [18]. Immune fitness refers to a resilient immune system with the "built-in" capacity to adapt to challenges by establishing, maintaining, and regulating an appropriate immune response [19]. This means that the individual's immune system is robust enough to eliminate harmful pathogens, such as viruses and bacteria, while simultaneously being able to tolerate harmless ones, such as food antigens. In doing so, this prevents the body from entering into a hyporesponsive state of weakened immunity, leading to increased infection, and from entering into a hyperresponsive state, leading to allergy and autoimmune disease (Figure 3) [19]. Immune fitness can be viewed as the establishment of core lifestyle habits that can improve your immune capacity, including good eating habits, good social relationships, abstinence from smoking, limiting alcohol consumption, and controlling stress levels, all of which can slow down the process of aging on the immune system [20].

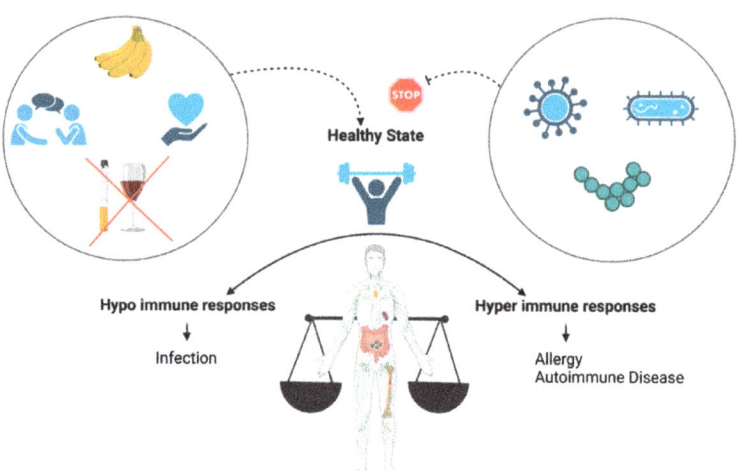

Figure 3. Maintaining immune fitness. Good diet, social relationships, stress control, and not smoking or drinking all aid in maintaining a healthy immune system to enable the immune system to fight off pathogens and recognise harmless food antigens. The ability and resilience of the immune system to fight off and manage such challenges are encapsulated by the immune fitness of the individual. Hypo immune responses lead to the development of infections. Hyper immune responses lead to the development of allergy and autoimmune disease. Created with BioRender.com.

As we age, the immune system changes, and chronic low-grade inflammation develops, termed "inflammageing", which, in turn, contributes to the pathogenesis of age-related disease [21]. The immune system responds more slowly and less effectively; thus, there is increased risk of infection due to less effective immune defenses. This gradual deterioration in the immune system caused by advanced aging is termed immunosenescence [20]. Nutrition is closely linked to proper functioning of the immune system, meaning what we eat has a huge influence over our immune response, making us more or less likely to suffer from infections or inflammatory disease [22]. It is long understood that the plant-based Mediterranean diet, consisting largely of cereals, legumes, vegetables, fruits, olive oil, and nuts, provides fibre with prebiotic activity, polyunsaturated fatty acids with anti-inflammatory properties, bioactive compounds with antioxidative properties, and vitamins and minerals, all aiding in the modulation of the microbiota, the activation of the host immunity, and, ultimately, promoting health and disease prevention [23]. On the other hand, the Western diet is associated with high animal protein, digestible sugars, and fat, while also being low in fibre [24]. Observational studies have linked the Western diet to the risk and development of inflammatory bowel diseases (IBDs), including Crohn's Disease (CD) and ulcerative colitis (UC), as well as other immune diseases, including asthma and allergy, while also coinciding with an increase in autoimmune diseases [25–28]. Furthermore, the Western diet is a key contributor to the global obesity epidemic, which causes low-grade activation of the immune system [28]. Therefore, the differing effects of the Mediterranean and Western diets demonstrate that differing dietary patterns have differential effects on the immune system and overall immune fitness. Individuals who are considered immunocompromised are those with weakened immune systems [29]. These people have a reduced ability to fight infections and other diseases. Certain conditions, like cancer, diabetes, AIDS, some genetic conditions, and even simply malnutrition, result in an individual becoming immunocompromised [30]. Not only this; often, the treatments for various diseases like cancer, including radiation therapy or stem cell therapy, result in immunosuppression [29]. The immunocompromised are a highly vulnerable group with reduced immune system response and thus require boosting of their immune fitness in order to help tackle any immune challenges they may face.

In this review, we examine the effect of functional foods on the immune fitness of three core vulnerable populations within our society: the elderly, the obese, and the immunocompromised. Challenges arise in the fight against viruses, such as COVID-19, in the elderly population, obese individuals, and for those who suffer from chronic underlying conditions, as these individuals have an already weakened immune system. Individuals that are older and have underlying conditions are at an increased risk of severe infection due to their already weakened immune systems [31]. It is the low-grade inflammation within the immune systems of the elderly and the obese that makes them vulnerable to infection [32,33]. The aging process is inevitable; however, there are other factors one can consider to keep the body as fit and healthy as possible to manage weight and to support the immune system in order to protect against viral invasion. Immune fitness encapsulates how one's immune system is built in terms of its resilience, fragility, and chronic immune disorder morbidity [34]. Immune fitness can be influenced by a variety of factors, including biological factors, such as the epigenome and microbiome, lifestyle factors, such as sleep, diet, and exercise, and other psychosocial factors, like stress response and the social environment [34]. Therefore, it is critical that we look for natural ways of boosting the immune fitness of the elderly, the obese, and the immunocompromised to ensure the immune system is in a prime state for fighting against viral infection by virtue of maintaining a healthy lifestyle.

3.1.1. Immune Response in the Elderly

The elderly are classed in the extremely vulnerable group of individuals at risk of contracting viral infections, including COVID-19 infection, while people less than 65 years old have been shown to have a smaller risk of COVID-19 deaths, even in pandemic epicentres [35]. Not only are the elderly at increased risk of susceptibility to infectious disease, but they are also seen to have reduced vaccine efficacy [36]. As we age, there is an increased dysregulation of the immune system, both innate and adaptive, due to the accumulation of damage over the years at a molecular, cellular, and organ-based level, which results in the increased risk of disease and higher rates of morbidity and mortality [37]. The degree to which the immune system is affected by the aging process is referred to as immunosenescence [38]. The degree of immunosenescence can be slowed down by optimising the immune fitness of the individual [39].

As we age, the innate immune system is highly affected. The mucosal immune system of the gastrointestinal tract, which provides the first line of defense against ingested pathogens by deciphering between harmless antigens and generating tolerance towards them or being able to mount a rapid protective immune response against dangerous pathogens, becomes significantly compromised in the elderly [40]. The intestinal mucosa provides innate immunity by virtue of the gut-associated lymphoid tissue (GALT), constituted by Peyer's patches, lymphoid follicles, and mesenteric lymph nodes [41]. In aged GALT, reductions in mucus secretion and defensins are reported, indicative of impaired gut function [42]. Aging brings about an increase in the innate cells of the intestine with an elevation of pro-inflammatory mediators, i.e., pro-inflammatory cytokines (IL-6, TNF-α, IFN-γ, and IL-1β) and C-reactive protein, contributing to the low-grade inflammation associated with aging, as well as a link to poorer cognitive performance [43]. Aged dendritic cells show significant decreases in IL-12p70 and IL-15 production and decreased expression of co-stimulatory factors CD80/CD86 [44,45], affecting their ability to present antigens that activate cells of the adaptive immune system. Furthermore, a link to reduced expression of IL-22 and IL-17 cytokines results in increased intestinal barrier permeability in the elderly [46]. Furthermore, an increase in IL-6 and TNF-α is associated with the increase in paracellular permeability of the microbiome as well as metabolic endotoxemia, which contributes to the low-grade chronic inflammatory state seen in aging [47]. Changes in the gut microbiome are often associated with aging, where a decrease in microbiota diversity is observed, and an increase in pro-inflammatory commensals is seen at the expense of beneficial microbes [48]. Such dysbiosis leads to alterations in microbiota-associated metabolite levels, impaired function and integrity of the gastrointestinal tract, and increased leaky gut [48]. In addition, reductions in chewing ability, dentition, taste, digestion, and intestinal transit time affect dietary choices and food digestion as we age, contributing directly or indirectly to microbiota alterations [49]. Therefore, as we age, the integrity and functioning of the gut are compromised, leading to increased permeability of the gut by virtue of its decreased integrity, meaning the elderly are at increased risk of viral infection due to this weakened first line of physical defense.

The adaptive arm of the immune system is highly affected by aging, with some key changes seen, such as decreased T cell function, the central defect of immunosenescence, as well as decreased production of T cell populations. Aging is associated with declined IL-2 production and expression of T cell receptors, resulting in decreased T cell proliferation, as well as altered signaling pathways associated with T cell activation, i.e., the NF-κB pathway [37,50]. T cell function is therefore already impaired in an older individual; thus, contracting COVID-19 and the associated T cell exhaustion (Tex) puts these individuals at a much greater risk of a poor outcome. Similarly, B cell function is affected by the aging process, making the elderly defective in their ability to produce optimal antibody responses [51]. These defects include reduced somatic hypermutation of the antibody variable region, reduced binding, reduced class switch recombination responsible for the generation of a secondary response of class switched antibodies, reduced neutralization capacity and binding specificity of secreted antibodies, increased frequencies of inflammatory B cell subsets and shorter telomers, and increased epigenetic modifications that are associated with lower antibody responses [51]. Furthermore, there is an obvious effect seen on B cell function in an aged immune system. The number of competent B cells significantly decreases with age, while the percentage of terminally differentiated and senescent memory $CD27^-$ B cells increases [52]. Thus, the elderly have an impaired antibody function, which only further serves as a potential risk factor for contracting viral pathogens.

The gut undergoes several changes in the adaptive immune response as a result of aging. On a cellular level, the ability of dendritic cells to initiate T cell responses is impaired due to defective priming by dendritic cells of the mucosal tissue, while antigen-specific T cell responses in the gut are reduced [44]. The expression of co-inhibitory molecules CTLA-4 and PD-1 in lamina propria $CD4^+$ T cells, which control homeostasis and antigen-specific responses, is significantly lower in the elderly [53–55]. Furthermore, older Th1 and Th17 cells proliferate to a lesser degree compared to their younger T subset counterparts, while higher levels of spontaneous death among older $CD4^+$ T cells are observed [54].

Immunoglobulin A (IgA) is the dominant class of antibody secreted by the intestinal mucosa, and it plays a key role in the regulation of the gut microbiota [56]. IgA is a major class of antibody secreted by the gut mucosa and is key to the maintenance of intestinal homeostasis [57], gut immunity, regulating the mucosal immune response, maintaining the microbiome [58], and activating the gut microbiome to promote protection from inflammation [59]. T cells regulate the magnitude and nature of microbiota-specific IgA via IgA-committed B cell responses [40]. However, these become senescent as we age, and it is therefore suggested to be a contributing factor in the decreased antigen-specific IgA responses associated with aging [56]. This reduction in IgA response is, in turn, thought to contribute to the decline in gut and intestinal immunity as we age. Specifically, this reduction in IgA is linked to the decreased small intestinal CCL25 and the increase in colonic CCL28 associated with advanced aging and the deterioration of gut immunity [58].

Overall, the elderly have a unique pro-inflammatory predisposition. They experience a constant low-grade inflammation (LGI) that leads to the chronic systemic inflammation that is strongly associated with the elderly population and is the causative factor of many age-related illnesses, such as cardiovascular disease and stroke, and autoimmune disorders, such rheumatoid arthritis [60]. Thus, in the context of viral infection, such as COVID-19, an elderly individual will already have a heightened inflammatory response and is at a significantly higher risk of having a more severe outcome from viral infection.

3.1.2. Immune Response in Obese Individuals

Obesity is an excessive accumulation of adipose tissue, clinically defined as constituting a body mass index (BMI) > 30 kg/m^2 [61]. Obesity is linked to a reduced oxygen saturation of the blood by compromised ventilation in the base of the lungs [62]. It is characterised by chronic low-grade systemic inflammation, with an increased pro-inflammatory cytokine profile in adipose tissue and infiltration of leukocytes, such as macrophages, into the adipose tissue [63]. Such chronic inflammation results in impaired insulin signaling in adipocytes, causing insulin resistance and further contributing to the development of metabolic disorders, such as cardiovascular disease, type 2 diabetes, and hypertension [64].

Obesity has long been known to be linked to an increase in susceptibility to viral infections, including influenza A virus and swine flu [65]. Comorbidities linked to obesity can result in an increased risk of worse prognosis for COVID-19 and may even require mechanical breathing [66]. Obese individuals are more likely to suffer from other independent risk factors for severe COVID-19 than normal-weight-bearing individuals, including heart disease, lung disease, and diabetes [67] due to their added weight, poorer diet, and reduced exercise compromising their metabolic health. Even when vaccinated, obese adults tend to contract viral infections more easily than healthy weight individuals. For example, obese individuals are twice as likely to develop influenza or influenza-like illness compared with healthy weight adults post influenza vaccination [68]. Therefore, the risk of contracting COVID-19 and other viral infections in obese individuals is higher because they already have decreased lung capacity and difficulty breathing, as well as chronic low-grade inflammation. This risk of contracting a viral infection puts them at a greater risk of increased susceptibility, poorer prognosis, increased severity of disease, and increased mortality rates.

Innate immunity is highly affected in the gut of obese individuals, making them more vulnerable to viral diseases. Macrophages are key players in innate immunity. They are major mediators of inflammation within adipose tissues and are the most abundant immune cells that contribute to obesity via the infiltration of adipose tissue and subsequent secretion of inflammatory cytokines in response to obesity [69,70]. A lean profile is associated with the "alternatively activated" M2 macrophage phenotype, while an obese profile is associated with the "classically activated" M1 macrophage phenotype [69]. It is the breach of the intestinal barrier that induces microbe-associated molecular patterns to stimulate intestinal epithelial cells (IECs) and macrophage, and dendritic cells to produce proinflammatory cytokines, such as IL-1, IL-6, IL-12, IL-18, and IL-23, which result in the intestinal cytokine profile associated with diet-induced obesity and often resulting in insulin resistance [71,72]. Intestinal permeability is increased as a result of obesity by virtue of a high-fat diet that sparks an imbalance in the gut microbiota diversity and alters the microbial composition [71,73]. This imbalance initiates an innate immune response triggered when pathogens cross the intestinal barrier with greater ease [71,73]. This increased intestinal permeability is due to the reduced expression of epithelial tight junction proteins, such as zonula occludens 1 (ZO-1) and claudins [74]. IFN-γ-secreting immune cells, i.e., M1 macrophages [69], are in part responsible for barrier permeability, as IFN-γ reduces ZO-1 expression in intestinal epithelial cells [75]. Similarly, IL-1β has been linked to the increase in intestinal epithelial tight junction permeability [76]. Macrophages are recruited due to the secretion of chemokines and the activation of pattern-recognition receptors (PRRs), such as toll-like receptors (TLRs), that recognise unique danger signals for the differentiation of pathogens for the neutralization of pathogens or clearing of stressed cells induced by obesity [69].

Obese adipose tissues have been noted to have increased macrophage accumulation and higher TNF-α and IL-6 cytokine levels; thus, obesity is associated with an accumulation of immune cells that, overall, contribute to a state of LGI, dysregulated metabolism, and insulin resistance as a result of this pro-inflammatory state [77]. Furthermore, the bone marrow, which is the site where immune cells develop, is affected by obesity in that ectopic fat accumulates here, thus affecting immune cell development [78]. Circulating PBMCs have been shown to secrete higher levels of TNF-α and lower levels of the anti-inflammatory cytokine IL-10 in obese individuals, which further establishes this permanent state of chronic inflammation [79]. In addition, TLR activation of PBMCs becomes impaired in obese people, with a decreased ability to produce antiviral type I IFNs, IFN-α, and IFN-β [80]. The chemoattractant monocyte chemoattractant protein-1 (MCP-1) is secreted by adipose tissue and macrophages and is more abundant in obese individuals than in lean individuals [81]. MCP-1 is stimulated by the presence of IL-1β, TNF-α, IL-8, IL-4, and IL-6, and thus further aids in the macrophage recruitment to adipose tissue seen in obesity [81].

It has been proven that obesity-related disease progression and severity are highly correlated with pro-inflammatory T and B cell phenotypes within the gut [69]. Gut resident T cells include CD8$^+$ T cells and CD4$^+$ T cells consisting of Th1 cells, Th2 cells, Th17 cells, Tfh cells, and Treg cells [82]. It is the CD4$^+$ Th17 and Treg cells that are most abundant in mucosal tissue [83]. Normal lean homeostatic conditions within the intestinal immune environment lead to immune cells, which are dominated by tolerogenic and mucosal-barrier-maintaining cells, such as IL-10-producing Treg cells, IL-22-producing lymphoid cells, and IL-17-protective Th17 cells, as well as IgA$^+$ antibody-secreting cells producing secretory IgA to interface within the lamina propria [84]. Diet-induced obesity in mice demonstrates a shift in the inflammatory response within the intestinal immune environment, which leads to increases in Th1 and CD8$^+$ T cells, a decrease in the aforementioned tolerogenic cell types Th17 and Treg [83], a decrease in intestinal homing CCR2$^+$ macrophage, a decrease in intestinal intra-epithelial CD8$\alpha\beta^+$ T cells, and an increase in IL-2, via small intestinal group 2 innate lymphoid cells. These all promote diet-induced obesity via intestinal dysfunction that enables dysregulated glucose homeostasis [84]. Obesity is associated with fewer intestinal IgA$^+$ immune cells and secreting less secretory IgA and IgA-promoting immune mediators, which results in dysfunctional glucose metabolism of the microbiome [85]. IgA is a critical B-cell-induced antibody that controls intestinal and adipose tissue inflammation, intestinal permeability, microbial encroachment, and the composition of the intestinal microbiome [85]. Limiting IgA secretion greatly impacts the gut immune system, further showing the detrimental effects associated with obesity on the gut. IgA is essential for gut homeostasis, and reduced levels demonstrated in obesity results in altered gut microbiota and further suggests a crucial supporting role for intestinal immunity as a key modulator of the systemic glucose metabolism microbiome [85].

The increased Th1 and Th17 subpopulations in obese individuals further contribute to the heightened proinflammatory state, which is detrimental to the body when under viral attack. Therefore, obese individuals are already in a state of LGI, cytokine dysregulation and T cell pro-inflammatory activation, putting them at higher risk of poorer prognosis in the event of contracting viral diseases, including COVID-19.

3.1.3. Immune Response in People with Underlying Chronic Conditions

People with underlying health conditions are at serious risk of contracting viral infections that may result in the need for hospitalisation, intensive care, ventilators, or mechanical machinery to help them survive, as they are at a higher risk of death due to the severity of the illness [86]. The weakened immune system puts these individuals at great risk for contracting viral infections as they have medical conditions and/or are undergoing treatments for medical conditions that suppress their immune system. Examples of immunocompromised cohorts include individuals suffering from CD or UC, HIV patients, cancer patients, and organ transplant recipients whose underlying conditions only serve to amplify the effects of COVID-19 [86]. In this section, we focus our discussion on the key features of the gut immunity in people living with HIV and those with IBD.

HIV is a virus that attacks the individual's immune system and weakens its ability to fight infection and disease, thus putting the HIV-positive individual at a higher risk of contracting other viral infections and suffering from poorer clinical outcomes. HIV damages the immune system by infecting CD4 cells that help fight off infection and protect the body from disease [87]. HIV affects approximately 37.7 million people worldwide, while 680,000 people died of HIV-related illness worldwide in 2020 [88,89], with no known cure [90].

HIV infection alters the components of the gut microbiome and changes the host immune responses to gut microbes, which means the gut plays a critical role in the immune systems of HIV-positive individuals [91]. HIV is associated with a chronic inflammatory state represented by increased soluble IL-6 and high-sensitivity CRP, D-dimer, and cystatin C levels even after antiretroviral therapy [92]. The gut epithelial barrier integrity, including intestinal fatty acid binding protein and zonulin-1 levels, as well as innate immune activation and inflammation through markers like soluble CD14 levels, kynurenine/tryptophan ratio, and TNF receptor 1 levels, are highly affected in HIV infection, with increased levels being strong independent predictors of mortality [93]. The gradual loss of CD4 T cells in HIV has a knock-on effect for the innate immunity provided by the gut, as the poor CD4 cell recovery within the lamina propria results in the disruption of the gut mucosal barrier integrity. Therefore, the first line of innate defense against invading pathogens becomes weakened, and there is a subsequent loss in cytokines secreted, which are needed for the support of normal barrier function [94].

The leaky gut barrier leads to systemic inflammation due to increased circulation of microbial components in the bloodstream as well as an increase in exposure of the resident gut mucosal T cell population to new antigens, meaning the gut barrier dysfunction seen with HIV infection may originate in the gut lamina propria and its resident CD4 T cells [91]. Lamina propria T cells are thought to be more susceptible to HIV infection due to the high levels of activation and expression of HIV receptors like CCR5 [95]. HIV infection is associated with the gradual loss of peripheral $CD4^+$ T cells, largely through the accelerated proliferation, expansion, and death of T cells, and this high T cell turnover results in the depletion and exhaustion of the regenerative capacity of the hyperactive immune system, leading to opportunistic infections, malignancies, and, ultimately, death [96]. It is this exhaustion of the immune system that leads to the subsequent development of acquired immunodeficiency syndrome (AIDS), whereby the immune system is unable to maintain the high rate of T cell production it requires for proper functioning [96]. This hyperactivation of the immune system on naïve T cells, whether antigen-specific, induced by cytokines, or by viral gene products, may lead to the increased consumption of both $CD4^+$ and $CD8^+$ naïve T cells through apoptosis of activated T cells or differentiation towards memory phenotypes [96–98]. Decreases in sigmoid IL-22-producing $CD4^+$ T cells, which are essential for the sigmoid mucosa integrity, are also observed in HIV infection, thereby worsening epithelial barrier dysfunction and increasing microbial translocation [91,94].

IBD is associated with gut discomfort as a result of immunological imbalances within the intestinal mucosa associated with cells of the adaptive immune system [99]. IBDs arise as a result of the immune system responding to self-antigens and triggering chronic inflammation in patients with diseases like UC and CD. The prevalence of IBDs is on the rise [100,101], with these chronic digestive diseases affecting over 10 million people worldwide; they have no known cause or cure [102].

With the modern diet consisting of greater meat and animal product consumption, observational studies have linked such dietary patterns to the risk and development of IBDs like that of CD and UC [27]. IBD is associated with the disruption of the integrity of the epithelial cells of the intestinal lumen bacteria, which are necessary to communicate with the immune system [103]. IECs are key players within the mucosal barrier, preventing the influx of antigens, the invasion of pathogens and commensal microorganisms, and maintaining tolerance to alimentary antigens and commensal microbiota, while also playing a crucial role in the activation of cellular innate and adaptive immune responses, producing cytokines and chemokines, and keeping the epithelial barrier intact [103,104]. Macrophages play a crucial role in the regulation of gut homeostasis within the intestinal mucosa, and when this macrophage function becomes disrupted, this leads to chronic intestinal inflammation [103]. Regulation of intestinal gut inflammation is largely due to the M2 macrophages that produce IL-10 [103]. Dysregulation in IL-10 function leads to a decrease in the secretion of this anti-inflammatory cytokine and is therefore linked to the pathogenesis of IBDs, particularly for UC [105]. Nucleotide-binding oligomerisation domain 2 (NOD2) is a protein encoded by the caspase recruitment domain-containing protein (CARD), which is an intracellular microbial sensor that acts as a potent activator and regulator of inflammation [99]. NOD2 mutation or deficient expression is often associated with IBDs, including CD, through increased expression of inflammatory factors [106]. TLR signaling helps protect the epithelial barrier and aids in tolerance to commensal bacteria; however, a malfunction in the TLR signaling associated with IBDs induces an intestinal inflammatory response through the activation of the NF-κB transcription factor, which regulates the expression of key inflammatory cytokines IL-1, IL-2, IL-6, IL-12, and TNF-α [104].

Inflammatory disorders, such as IBDs, are largely associated with issues with the adaptive immune system and consist of alterations in the autophagy of cells, antigen processing, regulation of cell signaling, and T cell homeostasis [99]. The imbalance of Th1 and Th2 cytokine release by the intestinal mucosa determines the development and persistence of inflammatory responses leading to chronic inflammatory disease [107]. Key Th1 cytokines linked to the development of IDBs are TNF-α [108], TGF-β [109], IFN-γ [110], IL-6 [103], IL-12, and IL-18 [111], as well as the response to self-antigens [99]. Similarly, Th17-related cytokines, such as IL-17 and IL-22, play a role in the development and establishment of IBDs [111,112]. Thus, T cells and their subsets may have excessive increases in the chemokines and cytokines that lead to the worsening or maintenance of mucosal inflammation [111]. Treg cells are associated with the pathogenesis of IBD [113]. $CD4^+$ and $CD25^+$ Treg cells play a role in immune regulation and IBD treatment in mice models, whereby these cells are recruited to the intestinal lymphatic tissues and lamina propria, playing a key role in maintaining intestinal homeostasis [111,114]. Reduction of Treg cells can result in the development of IBD [115]. In patients with IBDs, there is a dysregulation in the amount of antibodies produced and secreted from B cells [116]. UC is characterised by the infiltration of IgG-producing plasma cells via the CD184 receptor of inflamed mucosa, further exacerbating inflammation through the activation of intestinal $CD14^+$ macrophages [103,117]. CD is characterised by high levels of IgG1, IgG2, and IgG3 in both serum and intestinal mucosa [118]. Similarly, higher levels of IgM are associated with IBD pathogenesis [119].

Immunocompromised individuals with uncontrolled HIV and those who suffer from IBDs are in a state of chronic T cell exhaustion and chronic low-grade inflammation. These conditions show how highly affected the gut becomes when the body is in a weakened state of immunity and demonstrate the vulnerability of the host to further viral infection. Dietary interventions that enhance immune fitness may benefit people suffering from these conditions.

4. Functional Foods as Immune Fitness Boosters in the Context of Viral Infection

The concept of functional foods is thought to have first arisen in Japan less than 40 years ago, with the Japanese initiating the concept of functional food science based on the words of the ancient Chinese, in which they stated that "Medicine and food are isogenic" [120]. This area of food science research gained huge interest and popularity; however, the term "functional food" is still not recognised as a unique regulatory product category by the FDA and has no legal definition [121]. While the area of functional foods is rapidly emerging and has yet to be legally defined in EU or Irish food legislation, it is regulated through existing food legislation instead [122]. There are many global definitions of what a functional food is (Table 2). For the purpose of this review, we define a functional food to be a "Natural or processed foods that contains known or unknown biologically-active compounds; which, in defined, effective, non-toxic amounts, provide a clinically proven and documented health benefit for the prevention, management, or treatment of chronic disease" [123].

Table 2. Definitions of the term "functional food" and their originating regions.

Country	Definition	Reference
EU	A product which is shown in a satisfactory manner that, in addition to adequate nutritional effects, induces beneficial effects on one or more target functions of the organism, significantly improving the health status and welfare or reducing the risk of disease.	[124]
USA	Foods that, by virtue of the presence of physiologically active components, provide a health benefit beyond basic nutrition	[125]
Canada	Similar in appearance to conventional food, consumed as part of the usual diet, with demonstrated physiological benefits, and/or to reduce the risk of chronic disease beyond basic nutritional functions	[126]
Japan	Known as Foods for Specified Health Use, these are foods composed of functional ingredients that affect the structure and/or function of the body and are used to maintain or regulate specific health conditions, such as gastrointestinal health, blood pressure, and blood cholesterol levels	[127]

A recent review by Zhang et al. [128] noted the importance of vitamins A, B2, B3, B6, C, D, E, omega-3 polyunsaturated fatty acids, selenium, zinc, and iron in the fight against viral infections. These are key traditional functional food components that potentially have the ability to help in the protection against viral infections. In this review, we focus on milk proteins, fermentation products, other plant-derived products, Zinc, selenium, and vitamin D as functional foods with the potential to combat viral infections. In this section, we highlight their interactions with the immune system and the mechanisms underlying their immune-boosting activities.

4.1. Whole Milk Proteins and Hydrolysates

There are two groups of proteins in milk: casein and whey. Casein comprises 80% of total bovine milk protein, and the remaining 20% is whey protein. Whey is the major by-product generated from the cheese making industry [129] and is composed of β-lactoglobulin, α-lactalbumin, serum albumin, immunoglobulins, lactoferrin, and transferrin. Casein, on the other hand, is composed of various protein fractions, including αs1, αs2, β-, and κ caseins [130]. Milk-derived proteins can work in a variety of ways to act as antiviral molecules. These traditional antiviral mechanisms include binding to structural viral proteins to prevent host–cell interactions, interfering with viral entry through viral and/or cell surface interaction, as well as by interfering with certain viral enzymes required for viral replication [130]. Most of the antiviral properties attributed to milk are associated with whey proteins, largely lactoferrin; however, casein has also been shown to exert some antiviral activity towards viruses [131].

4.1.1. Whey

Most whey proteins have been shown to prevent viral infection [130]. Whey protein from human breastmilk was shown to effectively inhibit both SARS-CoV-2 and its related pangolin coronavirus via blocking viral attachment and viral replication at entry into the cytoplasm and post entry points, as well as by inhibiting infectious viral production [132]. Specifically, whey protein of human breastmilk significantly inhibited the RNA-dependent RNA polymerase (rdRp) activity of SARS-CoV-2 in a dose-dependent manner [132]. This is thought to be due to the rich lactoferrin content, well known for its antimicrobial effects, as well as other components found in breastmilk. Lactoferrin is a naturally occurring nontoxic glycoprotein that has been proven to help protect against viral infections, including SARS-CoV, which is closely related to SARS-CoV-2, which causes COVID-19 [133]. Lactoferrin has demonstrated the ability to inhibit many viruses, including hepatitis B and C viruses (HBV and HCV), herpes simplex viruses 1 and 2, HIV, human cytomegalovirus, human papilloma virus (HPV), enteroviruses, adenoviruses, influenza viruses, parainfluenza viruses, and rotaviruses [134]. For example, it inhibits the activity of reverse transcriptase, protease and integrase, and HIV-1 enzymes, which allow viral replication to occur; thus, lactoferrin can inhibit the viral replication of HIV [134,135].

Lactoferrin has immunomodulatory and anti-inflammatory properties that can be used to confer protection in host systems by modifying host responses to infections through its iron-binding capacity, its direct interaction with cell surfaces, its ability to promote immune cell activation, differentiation, and proliferation, as well as its ability to downregulate immune responses via anti-inflammatory cytokine activity [136]. For example, lactoferrin induces the expression of type I interferon IFN-α/β, known potent antiviral cytokines and immunomodulators, and inhibits viral replication [137]. It has also been shown to lower IL-6 and TNF-α, key players in the cytokine storm [44].

Another potential mechanism is through the inhibition of ACE2 and S glycoprotein. ACE2 is the receptor and main landing site for SARS-CoV-2 on host cells via the spike protein [138]. This spike protein, the S glycoprotein, plays an essential role in virus attachment, fusion, and entry into host cells [139]. Thus, through inhibition of the surface S glycoprotein, ACE2 receptor binding can be prevented, thereby inhibiting viral attachment and subsequent infection. A study by Fan et al. [132] revealed that whey can slightly block the affinity of ACE2 and the S glycoprotein.

In an observational study by Serrano et al. [140], they were able to elucidate a potential dose for the prevention and treatment of COVID-19 infection using liposomal lactoferrin, Lactyferrin™, as follows: a dose of 64–96 mg (20–30 mL) every 6 h daily (256–384 mg/d), which can be increased to 128 mg every 6 h (512 mg) if needed to cure COVID-19, while a dose of 64 mg two to three times daily can prevent COVID-19 (128–192 mg/d). This study allowed for complete and fast recovery of all 75 patients within the first 4–5 days, while smaller doses prevented individuals directly in contact with the patient from ever becoming infected. In another study, low COVID-19 incidence rates and lesser severity in children and infants were attributed to lactoferrin present in breastmilk and lactoferrin-containing infant formulas widely used in this population [141]. Table 3 summarises the immune boosting functions and mechanisms of action of whey and casein.

4.1.2. Casein

Bovine κ-Casein has been proven to have a direct inhibitory effect on the binding of viral particles via glycan residues against human rotavirus (HRV) [142]. This direct binding of viral particles results in 50–70% inhibition of viral activity against HRV, with the remaining 30–50% of uninhabitable activity hypothesised to be due to the fact there may be several key molecules involved in the cell entry process of viral attachment and replication [142]. In contrast, separate studies have shown that casein (the unmodified form) had no inhibitory effect on HIV-1 [143,144]. However, chemically modified casein inhibited HIV-1 via the direct binding of the HIV-1 gp 120 envelope glycoprotein and through direct binding of the CD4 cell receptor [145].

Table 3. Summary of immune mechanisms enhanced by milk-derived proteins.

Immune-Active Components	Immune-Boosting Functions	Mechanism	Reference
Whey/Lactoferrin	Antiviral	- Blocks viral attachment, replication, and production - Inhibits rdRp activity of SARS-CoV-2 - Inhibits reverse transcriptase, protease, integrase, and HIV-1 enzyme activity, inhibiting viral replication - ACE2 inhibitor	[132,134,135]
	Immunomodulator	- Promotes immune cell activation, differentiation, and proliferation - Induces type I interferon IFN-α/β - Promotes promoting CD4+ T cells into Th1 cells, stimulates neutrophil aggregation, activates phagocytosis, and increases activity of NK cells - Enhances antigen expression ability of B cells and regulates T cell function	[136,137,146,147]
	Anti-inflammatory	- Lowers IL-6 and TNF-α	[44]
Casein	Antiviral	- Inhibits viral binding in HRV via glycan residues - Some protease and integrase inhibitory activity - Potent inhibition of HIV-1 via direct binding of glycoprotein and CD4 cell receptor, inhibiting HIV-1 infection	[142,144,145]

4.2. Fermented Dairy Products

It is well documented that fermented foods can be used to support and boost immune responses in humans. For example, kefir, a fermented dairy product, has been noted for its antiviral and anti-inflammatory potential [148]. It can inhibit ACE levels and cholesterol metabolism, aid in wound healing, suppress tumour growth, alter the immune system to improve allergy symptoms, suppress viral activity via modulation of immune responses, and cause disruption of viral adhesion, as well as acting as an anti-inflammatory agent inhibiting proinflammatory cytokines like that of IL-1β, TNF-α, and IL-6 [148]. All of these are indicated in the low-grade inflammation seen within the elderly, obese, and immunocompromised populations, as well as being the key contributors to the cytokine storm of COVID-19 infection. Thus, kefir could be considered for its antiviral activity in the fight against COVID-19, largely through its ACE inhibitory abilities and its proinflammatory cytokine-reducing capabilities. Kefir is thought to exert this antiviral activity by direct probiotic–virus interaction and trapping, production of antiviral inhibitory metabolites, and/or via stimulation of the immune system for the development of bacteriocins, lactic acid, and hydrogen peroxide as antiviral agents [149]. Kefir modulates gut microbiota composition, regulates low-grade inflammation, controls intestinal permeability, and regulates gut homeostasis [150]; thus, it is a potentially powerful functional food for the elderly and IBD-immunocompromised and obese individuals whose gut immunity is compromised. Kefir improves serum zonulin levels, which are critical for the regulation of intestinal permeability and the modulation of tight junctions [151]. Furthermore, kefir could act against obesity by inhibiting enzymes related to the digestion of carbohydrates and lipids that result in less energy release [150].

Yogurt is a fermented milk product containing cultures of Lactobacillus bulgaricus and Streptococcus thermophilus [152]. Yogurt-derived peptides are known for their ACE inhibitory effects [153] and, therefore, may be effective in counteracting viral infection. Various in vitro and in vivo studies have shown that the bioactive peptides in yogurt have direct antiviral effects [153]. In addition to these antiviral effects, yogurt has been linked with improvements in gut health, reduced chronic inflammation by enhancing innate and adaptive immune responses, and improved intestinal barrier function [154]. Yogurt upregulates the expression of autophagy, tight junction proteins, and anti-microbial peptide-related genes, which all play a key role in maintaining a healthy gut barrier function through interaction with the intestinal epithelium [155]. Yogurt has inhibitory effects on colon cancer, restores gut homeostasis, and, therefore, prevents the development of and control of IBDs [156]. Decreases in TNF-α are associated with the consumption of LAB [157]. Therefore, yogurt is considered useful for the control of low-grade inflammation seen in the elderly, obese, and immunocompromised; for example, those suffering from type 2 diabetes [157]. Furthermore, yogurt also increases anti-inflammatory cytokine IL-10 while simultaneously reducing proinflammatory IL-17 and IL-12 [158], thus playing a key anti-inflammatory role crucial in the elderly, obese, and immunocompromised; in particular, those with IBDs.

Koumiss is a traditional fermented dairy product made from fermented mare's milk originating in Mongolia [159,160]. Koumiss has been shown to have immunomodulatory capabilities by virtue of its ability to reduce TNF-α [161], a key player in the low-grade inflammation seen among the elderly, obese, and immunocompromised, as well as being a key contributor to the cytokine storm seen in COVID-19 infection. Koumiss has been shown to increase IFN-γ [161], and these IFN-γ secreting cells play a critical role in maintaining the gut barrier function. Furthermore, Koumiss is capable of inducing gut mucosal responses by enhancing the production of sIgA and therefore has effects on both the innate and adaptive immune responses [161]. SIgA prevents infection by inhibiting the attachment of bacteria and viruses within the gastrointestinal system [162].

Overall, fermented dairy products could be considered functional foods with the potential to protect against viral infection. These fermented foods can be highly beneficial for the elderly and obese and immunocompromised individuals through the modulation of gut microbiota composition and their overall antiviral abilities by virtue of their ACE inhibitory role, their direct viral inhibitory mechanisms, their gastrointestinal system maintenance, and their contribution to enhanced epithelial gut barrier function. Table 4 summarises the immune boosting functions and mechanisms of action of fermented food products, kefir, yoghurt, and Koumiss.

Furthermore, one food component of interest of late are fermentates. A fermentate generally refers to "a powdered preparation, derived from a fermented [food] product and which can contain the fermenting microorganisms, components of these microorganisms, culture supernatants, fermented substrates, and a range of metabolites and bioactive components" [163]. For example, an oral fermentation product known as EpiCor, derived from *Saccharomyces cerevisiae* (*S. cerevisiae*), showed the potential of enhancing the immune system to protect and aid in defense against cold/flu-like symptoms [164,165]. In these two 12-week randomized, double-blind, placebo-controlled trials, it was proven that this oral over-the-counter fermentate has the ability to reduce the incidence of cold and flu-like symptoms in both individuals with and without a history of influenza vaccination [165]. These studies show the potential of fermentates for the protection and prevention of viral infections and thus warrant further investigation into their potential uses against COVID-19 as well as other viral infections.

Table 4. Summary of immune mechanisms enhanced by fermented dairy products.

Immune-Active Components	Immune-Boosting Functions	Mechanism	Reference
Kefir	Antiviral	- Inhibits ACE levels and suppresses viral activity - Directs probiotic–virus interaction and trapping, production of antiviral inhibitory metabolites, and development of lactic acid and hydrogen peroxide as antiviral agents	[148,149,153]
	Immunomodulator	- Antioxidant - Enhances cholesterol metabolism, aids in wound healing, suppresses tumour growth, and improves allergy - Modulates gut microbiota composition, controls intestinal permeability, and regulates gut homeostasis - Improves zonulin levels and regulates intestinal permeability and modulation of tight junctions	[148,150,151]
	Anti-inflammatory	- Inhibits IL-1β, TNF-α, and IL-6	[148]
Yogurt	Antiviral	- ACE inhibitor - Antithrombotic	[166]
	Immunomodulator	- Improves gut health and intestinal barrier function - Upregulates expression of autophagy, tight junction proteins, and anti-microbial peptide-related genes for gut barrier health	[153–155]
	Anti-inflammatory	- Decrease TNF-α - Decreases IL-17 and IL-12 and increases IL-10	[157,158]
Koumiss	Antiviral	- Enhanced SigA production, inhibiting the attachment of viruses in the gastrointestinal tract	[161,162]
	Immunomodulator	- Maintains healthy gastric intestinal systems, regulates cholesterol and sugar levels, controls blood pressure, and produces important vitamins - Increases IFN-γ secreting cells to maintain gut barrier function	[161,167]
	Anti-inflammatory	- Decreases TNF-α	[161]

4.3. Plant-Derived Functional Foods

Plant-based functional foods are becoming increasingly more popular with the growing interest in vegetarian and vegan diets. Plant-based functional foods are derived from natural or unprocessed plant foods or may be derived from plant foods modified via biotechnological means [168,169]. Plants have been long known to have medicinal properties reducing the risk of developing a range of illnesses, including diabetes, cancer, cardiovascular disease, hyperlipidaemia, and hyperuricemia, by virtue of their immunomodulatory capabilities [170].

Virgin coconut oil (VCO) comes from the coconuts of coconut palm trees (Cocos nucifera) and is rich in nutrients, vitamins, and minerals, including vitamin E, palmitic acid, lauric acid, monolaurin, plant sterols, and bioactive compounds, including polyphenols, sterols, and tocopherols [171–173]. VCO has been noted for its anti-inflammatory, analgesic, [174], gut microbiota modulator [175], anti-stress, antioxidant [176], and antimicrobial activities [177]. Therefore, VCO is a potent functional food that possesses many desirable qualities that could aid in the boosting of immune fitness among the elderly, obese, and immunocompromised and could aid in the protection against viral infection and the promotion of gut homeostasis.

Recently, VCO has been highlighted as a potential antiviral functional food with the ability to lower CRP levels among suspect and probable COVID-19-infected patients, aiding in faster recovery from viral infection [171]. VCO has the ability to increase the phagocytotic activity of the innate immune macrophage [178] and has been shown to suppress and inhibit key inflammatory cytokines TNF-α, IFN-γ, IL-6, IL-8, and IL-5 [179]. Thus, it could be useful for the control of low-grade inflammation seen within the elderly and obese and immunocompromised individuals, as well as for the control of the cytokine storm observed in COVID-19 infection. VCO has been observed to have a positive effect on the adaptive immune response via the increased $CD4^+$ T cell concentration, which is observed in HIV-positive individuals when supplementation with VCO is prescribed for 3×15 mL/day for 6 weeks [180], thus highlighting its importance as a functional food for the immunocompromised, including HIV-positive individuals. Similarly, VCO has been shown to increase $CD4^+$ and $CD8^+$ T cells in doxorubicin-induced immunosuppressed rats [181], showing its potential use for the elderly and immunocompromised and obese individuals, whose T cell levels are often compromised. Furthermore, more animal studies have shown the link between VCO consumption and increased adaptive immunity, where increased VCO consumption led to an increase in IgA in the spleen and Peyer's patch cells of the small intestine [182].

Extra virgin olive oil (EVOO) is the least processed variety of olive oil, extracted from olives of the olive tree (Olea europaea) [183]. EVOO is rich in vitamins and minerals, including vitamin E, vitamin K, polyunsaturated fatty acids, oleic acid, and phenolic compounds like that of oleuropein and hydroxytyrosol [184–186]. In the US, a patent has been created that uses a naturally occurring secoiridoid glucoside oleuropein compound from Oleaceae plants in the treatment of viral diseases, such as hepatitis, mononucleosis, shingles, herpes, influenza, the common cold, and viral types causing leukemia [187]. Similarly, daily consumption of 50 g of EVOO in elderly HIV-positive individuals, without antiretroviral treatment, has been shown to improve lipid profiles and alpha diversity of intestinal microbiota, largely through the increase in *Bifidobacteriaceae* and *Gardnerella* species, and to decrease proinflammatory genera, such as *Dethiosulfovibrionaceae* [188]. In another study, high-sensitivity C reactive protein (CRP) concentrations were lowered in HIV-positive individuals receiving antiretroviral therapy after daily consumption of 50 mL EVOO [189]. Positive effects are seen on gut microbiota when EVOO is consumed via the reduction in pathogenic bacteria, the stimulation of beneficial bacteria, and the increase in the production of microbially produced short-chain fatty acids (SCFAs) to exert a wide range of anti-inflammatory effects [190]. EVOO influences intestinal mucosa and supports gut homeostasis by encouraging intestinal IgA production [191]. Polyphenolic compounds from EVOO have been linked to reduced T cell activation and proliferation as well as reduced proinflammatory cytokine secretion [192]. Other molecules in EVOO, such as oleuropein, reach the large intestine as unmodified compounds that the human colonic microbiota then catabolize to hydroxytyrosol; thus, there is much higher content of bioactive polyphenols present in the gut [186]. Therefore, EVOO could play a critical role in the control of viral infection seen in immunocompromised individuals like that of HIV sufferers, as well as the elderly and obese, where their viral immunity is already weakened. Table 5 summarises the immune boosting functions and mechanisms of action of plant-derived VCO, and EVOO.

Table 5. Summary of immune mechanisms enhanced by plant-derived functional foods.

Immune-Active Components	Immune-Boosting Functions	Mechanism	Reference
Virgin Coconut Oil	Antiviral	- Faster recovery from COVID-19 - Disrupts the virus envelope, inhibits pathogen maturation, prevents assembly and budding of viral progeny, prevents pathogens from directly binding to the host cells, and inhibits production of viral particles	[171,173,193]
	Immunomodulator	- Antioxidant - Increases phagocytosis of innate macrophage - Anti-ulcerative, reduces gastric juice, reduces total acid output, reduces ulcer scoring, and increases gastric wall mucous secretion - Increases CD4+ T cell concentration in HIV patients - Increases CD4+ and CD8+ T cells - Increases IgA in spleen and Peyer's patch cells in small intestine	[178,180–182,193]
	Anti-inflammatory	- Lowers CRP levels - Inhibits TNF-α, IFN-γ, IL-6, IL-8, and IL-5	[171,179]
Extra Virgin Olive Oil	Antiviral	- Antioxidant	[194].
	Immunomodulator	- Improves lipid profiles and alpha diversity of intestinal microbiota - Reduces pathogenic gut microbiota and increases beneficial bacteria - Influences intestinal mucosa, supports gut homeostasis, and encourages intestinal IgA production - Reduces T cell activation and proliferation - Increases production of SCFA in gut	[188,190–192]
	Anti-inflammatory	- Lowers CRP concentrations in HIV patients - Reduces proinflammatory cytokine secretion - Reduces IL-6, TNF-α, metalloprotease secretion, COX-2, and α-smooth-actin levels - Inhibits IL-8, IL-6, NF-kB activation, and iNOS induction	[189,190,192,195,196]

4.4. Polyunsaturated Fatty Acids (PUFA)-Rich Foods

PUFAs act as substrates for proinflammatory and anti-inflammatory mediators, including prostaglandins, leukotrienes, thromboxanes, protectins, and resolvins [197], as well as for specialized pro-resolving lipid mediators (SPMs), which are critical chemical mediators needed for the stimulation of the resolution of inflammatory responses [198]. Omega-3 PUFA eicosapentaenoic acid (EPA) and docosahexaenoic acid (DHA) act as the substrate for SPM, while, in contrast, omega-6 PUFA arachidonic acid (AA) is the substrate for eicosanoids, including leukotrienes and prostaglandins, generated through the lipoxygenase and cyclooxygenase pathways [199]. Key sources of these omega-3 fatty acids are oily fish, such as salmon, mackerel, and trout, while omega-6 is found in meat, poultry, and eggs. A single lean fish meal, such as one serving of cod, could provide about 0.2 to 0.3 g of these omega-3 fatty acids, while a single oily fish meal, like one serving of salmon or mackerel, could provide 1.5 to 3.0 [200]. However, regardless of their wide availability, Western diets are often deficient in omega-3 PUFAs [129]. It is suggested that a dose of 60–90 mg of omega-3 PUFA could aid in the recovery of the gut microbiota and boost immunity [201].

Omega-3 PUFA has effects on both the innate and adaptive immune responses to aid in the tackling of invading viral particles. Omega-3 PUFAs upregulate the activation and improve the function of immune cells. For example, omega-3 PUFAs can induce cytokine and chemokine secretion and promote phagocytosis in macrophages [202]. Other effects of omega-3 PUFAs include increasing neutrophil function by enhancing migration, phagocytic capacity, and the production of reactive free radicals to kill microbes; promoting antigen presenting cells (APCs) that, in turn, activate T cells; inducing antibodies production in B cells; and boosting the first-line defense by activating dendritic cells, natural killer cells, mast cells, basophils, and eosinophils [197]. Long chain AA, EPA, and DHA have been shown to enhance epithelial barrier integrity as well as reduce IL-4-mediated permeability in gut [203]. A diet containing 18 g of fish oil/day for 12 weeks increased colonic concentrations of EPA and DHA while decreasing mucosal AA content in IBD [204]. Omega-3 PUFAs have the ability to modulate the gut microbiota [205] and have been shown to increase the abundance of several genera of gut microbes, including *Bifidobacterium* and *Roseburia* [206], of which a reduction in *Bifidobacterium* and *Lactobacillus* is implicated in many metabolic disorders and preserve a lean phenotype. Thus, omega-3 PUFAs are useful in the treatment and management of obesity [205,207]. *Bifidobacterium* and *Lactobacillus* have also been shown to improve clinical symptoms in IBDs [193]. These gut microbiota are critical for the continuous stimulation of resident macrophage within the intestine to release IL-10 for the promotion of Treg cells and the prevention of excessive Th17 cell activity [208]. Omega-3 PUFAs have been shown to increase triglyceride levels in patients with HIV, thus preventing lipid disorders, which could put the already at-risk individual at increased susceptibility to other diseases, including cardiovascular disease [209]. This increase in triglycerides through omega-3 supplementation could therefore be applied to the elderly population, too.

Omega-3-derived pro-resolving mediator protectin D1 has been associated with antiviral effects and inhibiting influenza viral replication in experimental models and thus warrants further investigation for its additive effect as a potential antiviral treatment for other lethal infections, such as COVID-19 [199]. Omega-3 PUFAs, including DHA-derived protectins and EPA-derived RvE1, have antiviral properties, with protectin D1 isomer (PDX) suppressing influenza virus replication through inhibition of the nuclear export of viral mRNA [210]. A link has been found between the supportive role of specialized pro-resolving mediators (SPM) in ARDS and acute lung injury [211]. Omega-3 supplementation has been shown to significantly improve ARDS patient status, including shorter duration of mechanical ventilation, shorter ICU stay, and significant decrease in ARDS mortality, and infectious complications remained unchanged [199]. These studies highlight the potential of omega-3 PUFAs as natural therapeutics for the treatment and prevention of viral infection, including influenza and COVID-19, and are thus of critical importance for the already at-risk elderly, obese, and immunocompromised individuals via their direct inhibition of viral replication.

It is hypothesised that by increasing omega-3 PUFAs and decreasing omega-6 PUFAs, one can skew the immune response in favour of the resolution of inflammation by favouring higher concentrations of resolvin/protectin rather than leukotriene/prostaglandin [199,212]. Omega-3 FAs are known to produce less pro-inflammatory cytokines; thus by increasing their intake as part of the diet, one could decrease viral entry, boost immune function, and even decrease the severity of disease in COVID-19 patients by virtue of altering the overdrive in immune response seen as the resultant cytokine storm [197]. Proinflammatory mediator gene activation is controlled by NF-kB, a transcription factor expressed in almost all cell types. Peroxisome proliferator-activated receptor (PPAR)-γ, an anti-inflammatory transcription factor, is activated by omega-3 PUFAs and leads to the inhibition of NF-kB activation; thus, the proinflammatory mediators cannot be transcribed [3,213]. NF-κB transcriptional activity and upstream cytoplasmic signaling events are downregulated by omega-3 FAs, EPA, and DHA [214]. Omega-3 FAs, EPA, and DHA downregulate the production of proinflammatory cytokines IL-1β, IL-6, and TNF-α associated with the aetiology of metabolic syndrome in THP-1-derived macrophages [214]. In particular, DHA has been linked to exerting an anti-inflammatory profile better than that observed from EPA [215]. Omega-3 PUFAs have been shown to reduce the ability of peripheral blood monocytes to produce TNF-α, IL-2, IL-1α, and IL-1β and to decrease mononuclear cell proliferation [216–218]. Thus, omega-3 PUFAs have the ability to decrease some of the key pro-inflammatory cytokines seen in the gut of the elderly, obese, and immunocompromised, which are exhibited as the chronic low-grade inflammation so detrimental to these at-risk individuals for increased susceptibility to viral infection. Omega-3 PUFAs are particularly potent in their ability to increase the IFN-γ /IL-4 ratio [219]. Stress-induced abnormalities in the intestine can be counteracted by DHA and EPA, reducing proinflammatory IFN-γ, TNF-α, IL-1β, and IL-6 while also increasing the expression of ZO-1, Z0-3 occluding, and E-cadherin [201,220]. Therefore, by increasing in particular DHA [221], one can inhibit the transcription of these proinflammatory genes by targeting their transcription factors and therefore aid in the modulation of the inflammatory process, thereby blocking the pathway and decreasing the cytokine storm seen in COVID-19 infection or decreasing the chronic low-grade inflammation seen in the elderly, obese, and immunocompromised. Mucous SIgA and serum IL-10 are increased at 60–90 mg doses of omega-3 PUFA [201], thus further exemplifying their potent anti-inflammatory effect. Further studies of the effect of omega-3 PUFA on dendritic cell function have demonstrated their role in increasing IL-10, suppressing IL-12, and enhancing the expression of CD40, CD80, CD86, and MHC II [215]. This suggests that omega-3 PUFAs could aid in the reduction of proinflammatory cytokines and the increase in anti-inflammatory IL-10 in the gut of the elderly, obese, and immunocompromised and potentially aid in the management of the chronic low-grade inflammation observed within these populations, as well as through inhibition of signaling pathways to control the hyperactivation of the inflammatory response.

It is thought that it is not only the COVID-19-induced cytokine storm that contributes to the overactive immune response that is so detrimental to the host individual, but also the so-called "eicosanoid storm", which is characterized by increased levels of proinflammatory lipid mediators that are key to the development of severe infection [222]. Eicosanoids contribute to inflammation in a variety of ways, including the recruitment of inflammatory cells, vasodilation, and broncho- and vasoconstriction, as well as increased vascular permeability [199]. Studies have suggested that along with the cytokine storm, the eicosanoid storm of proinflammatory lipid mediators also contributes to the hyperinflammation that is so prevalent and detrimental to the COVID-19 infection [223]. Therefore, targeting of proinflammatory eicosanoid lipoxygenase and cyclooxygenase signaling pathways could provide a means of potential protective intervention against COVID-19 infection. Table 6 summarises the immune boosting functions and mechanisms of action of Omega-3, and Omega-6 PUFA.

Table 6. Summary of immune mechanisms enhanced by polyunsaturated fatty acids (PUFA)-rich foods.

Immune-Active Components	Immune-Boosting Functions	Mechanism	Reference
Omega-3 PUFA e.g., EPA, DHA Omega-6 PUFA e.g., AA	Antiviral	- Pro-resolving mediator protectin D1 inhibits influenza virus replication - PDX suppresses influenza virus replication by inhibition of nuclear export of viral mRNA	[199,210]

Table 6. Cont.

Immune-Active Components	Immune-Boosting Functions	Mechanism	Reference
	Immunomodulator	- Upregulates the activation and improves the function of macrophage to promote cytokine and chemokine secretion and improve phagocytosis - Enhances neutrophil migration and production of free radicals, enhances T cell production through APCs, improves B cell function to produce more antibodies - Enhances CD40, CD80, CD86, and MHCII - Improves first-line cellular defense, producing more dendritic cells, NK cells, mast cells, basophils, and eosinophils - Enhances epithelial barrier integrity - Modulates the gut microbiota, increasing microbes including Bifidobacterium, Roseburia, and Lactobacillus - Increases triglyceride levels in patients with HIV - Improvements in ARDS patients through SPM - Increases mucous SIgA - Reduces IL-4-mediated permeability in the intestine	[197,199,201–203,205,206,209,211,215]
	Anti-inflammatory	- Activates PPAR-γ transcription factor, inhibits NF-kB activation - Reduces production of TNF-α, IL-2, IL-6, IL-1α, and IL-1β and decreases mononuclear cell proliferation - Suppresses IL-12, increases IL-10 - Increases IFN-γ/IL-4 ratio - Reduces IFN-γ and increases expression of ZO-1, Z0–3, and E-cadherin - Reduces omega-6 eicosanoids and aids in the resolution of eicosanoid storm	[3,199,201,203,214–220,224]

4.5. Vitamin-D-Enriched Foods

Vitamin D is a crucial vitamin that helps regulate the amount of calcium and phosphate in the body in order to keep the bones and teeth strong and healthy, prevent the harmful effects of excess vitamin A, and prevent diseases like rickets and osteoporosis [225,226]. Furthermore, vitamin D is needed for muscle movement, nerve functioning, and for the immune system in helping to fight off invading bacteria and viruses [226]. The main source of vitamin D is from sunlight on our skin; however, it is also found naturally in foods, such as oily fish like salmon and sardines, as well as being sourced from eggs [225]. The vitamin D receptor is expressed on immune cells, including B cells, T cells, and APCs, which can synthesize the active vitamin D metabolite and therefore can potentially modulate both the innate and adaptive immune response, as deficiency in vitamin D is associated with increased susceptibility to infection [227]. It has been reported that poor nutrition and/or lack of sun exposure observed through low vitamin D levels contributes to severe disease and the progression of ARDS in some patients infected with COVID-19, while, similarly, low vitamin D levels in the active form of 1,25-dihydroxyvitamin D (1,25OHD) allow for proinflammatory molecules to trigger the subsequent development of ARDS in patients with COVID-19-associated pneumonia [228]. McCartney suggests that Irish adults should have an intake of 20–25 micrograms (800–1000 iu) of vitamin D per day for the duration of the COVID-19 pandemic [229], taken with food in order to achieve the critical 50 nanomoles per litre blood of vitamin D where immunity against COVID-19 can be enhanced [230]. These studies suggest that vitamin D is of critical importance to the elderly, obese, and immunocompromised, whose innate and adaptive immune responses are already weakened.

Vitamin D is predominantly present in the skin and thus functions in its active form, 1,25-dihydroxyvitamin D, along with vitamin D receptor (1,25OHD or VDR) to aid the immune system by maintaining tight junctions, gap junctions, and adherens junctions in the innate immune system [231]. Vitamin D supports the integrity of the epithelial barrier via the increased expression of VDR-associated intracellular junction proteins that constitute tight junctions between epithelial cells and include occludin, claudin, vinculin, ZO-1, and ZO-2 [232]. VDR is expressed in various tissues, including the skin, parathyroid gland, adipocyte, small intestines, and colon [233], and thus is widely expressed within the body, including within the gut; this means it could act as a therapeutic target where gut immunity is weakened. Vitamin D and VDR deficiency are associated with the pathogenesis of IBDs and is linked to elevated claudin-2 junction protein in inflammatory responses and therefore plays a critical role in intestinal barrier function [234]. VDR influences individual bacterial taxa, including *Parabacteroides*, where a much lower abundance of *Parabacteroides* are seen in UC and CD patients [235]. The downregulation of VDR or the inability to produce the active form of vitamin D is associated with a decrease in *Lactobacillus* in the gut and an increase in Proteobacteria [233], suggesting the influence of vitamin D on gut microbiota. Taken together, reductions in the levels of VDR and vitamin D are associated with dysfunctional intestinal integrity, intestinal barrier function, and gut microbiota composition; therefore, increased vitamin D consumption as a functional food component could aid in viral immunity and gut health for at-risk populations like the elderly and obese and immunocompromised individuals.

Active vitamin D suppresses Th1-mediated immune responses, inhibiting the production of inflammatory cytokines including IL-2 and IFN-γ while simultaneously promoting a Th2 response by producing anti-inflammatory cytokines IL-4 and IL-10 for indirect inhibition of the Th1 cells [231,236]. Furthermore, it induces Treg cells for the inhibition of the inflammatory process for the overall inhibition of a viral attack [231]. Deficiency in vitamin D negatively impacts Treg differentiation and weakens its function, thus leading to the triggering of autoimmune diseases, including IBDs [237]. Correcting vitamin D deficiency has been associated with suppressed CD26 adhesion molecules used for COVID-19 cell adhesion and invasion, as well as being linked to the ability to attenuate IFN-γ and IL-6 inflammatory responses, both of which are highly correlated with critically ill, ventilated COVID-19 patients [229] and within the elderly, obese, and immunocompromised.

Taken together, these mechanisms of antiviral activity via the suppression of proinflammatory markers could potentially be applied to the chronic low-grade inflammation seen in the elderly, obese, and immunocompromised, or for the cytokine storm that occurs during COVID-19 infection. These mechanisms work via the targeting of cell surface adhesion molecules for the suppression and/or inhibition of the otherwise dangerously proinflammatory state leading to chronic disease persistence or viral infection. Table 7 summarises the immune boosting functions and mechanisms of action of vitamin-D enriched foods.

Table 7. Summary of immune mechanisms enhanced by vitamin-D-enriched foods.

Immune-Active Components	Immune-Boosting Functions	Mechanism	Reference
1,25-dihydroxyvitamin D and vitamin D receptor (1,25OHD or VDR)	Antiviral	- Suppresses CD26 adhesion molecules, inhibits COVID-19 cell adhesion and invasion	[229],
	Immunomodulator	- Maintains tight, gap, and adherens junctions - Supports integrity of epithelial barrier and increases expression of VDR-associated intracellular junction proteins, including occludin, claudin, vinculin, ZO-1, and ZO-2 - Improves gut barrier function - Influences gut microbiota - Induces B cell proliferation and the secretion of IgE and IgM, enables formation of memory B cells and B cell apoptosis promotion	[231–234,238]
	Anti-inflammatory	- Suppresses Th1-mediated immune responses (inhibits IL-2 and IFN-γ), promotes Th2 response (produces IL-4 and IL-10) - Induces Treg cells - Attenuates IL-6	[229,231,236]

4.6. Zinc-Enriched Foods

Zinc is a key micronutrient involved in the maintenance of a healthy immune system, directly affecting aspects of the innate and adaptive immune responses [239]. Zinc can be found in food sources including oyster, red meat, and poultry, as well as in smaller amounts in beans, nuts, and whole grains [240]. Zinc deficiency occurs frequently in the elderly and the obese, as well as those with chronic diseases, such IBDs [241–243]. Zinc supplementation has been shown to have protective effects against viruses like the common cold and to result in fewer infectious incidents, including pneumonia in the elderly [50]. Zinc deficiency is responsible for 16% of all deep respiratory infections worldwide [244], which suggests a link between deficiency in zinc and the risk of infection and severe prognosis of COVID-19. This suggests a possible role for supplementation as a treatment or preventative antiviral measure [245].

Zinc enhances mucociliary clearance of viruses like the coronaviruses, removing the viral particle and reducing the risk of secondary infections; it is also essential for preserving tissue barrier integrity and important in protecting against viral entry into a host [245]. Zinc deficiency has been associated with reduced first responder cellular chemotaxis and phagocytosis, while supplementation has proven to enhance this [239]. Zinc has the potential to increase the cytotoxic activity of natural killer cells (NK), which are capable of attacking the cells that have abnormal or unusual proteins in the plasma, by infecting the cells and causing the microorganisms within the cells to be released and destroyed through phagocytosis by neutrophils and macrophages [246]. Furthermore, zinc deficiency is linked to altered MHCI recognition by NK cells and thus influences NK lytic abilities [239]. MHCI recognition is needed to allow NK cells to function to their best ability in order to kill the invading virus. Macrophage function becomes reduced when an individual is zinc deficient and when oxidative burst becomes impaired, while, in addition, neutrophil granulocytes cause reduced chemotactic activity and decreased numbers [247]. Zinc deficiency is associated with the pathogenesis of CD due to poor zinc absorption in the gastrointestinal lumen of the small intestine [248]. Zinc deficiency is associated with decreases in transepithelial resistance and alterations in the tight and adherens junctions, including ZO-1, occluding, β-catenin, and E-cadherin, leading to the disruption of membrane barrier integrity and the subsequent infiltration of neutrophils [249]. Furthermore, zinc-dependent alterations in gene expression by pneumocytes also affect viral entry: whereby zinc binding the ACE2 active centre becomes essential for enzymatic activity, zinc homeostasis might affect ACE2 expression, which is regulated by Sirt-1 and which zinc decreases; thus, this might decrease ACE2 expression and subsequent viral entry into cells [245].

In addition to this, zinc directly inhibits viral replication for many viral infections, including influenza, HIV, *papillaviridae*, *picornaviridae*, *Herpesviridae*, *metapneumovirus*, and coronavirus (SARS-CoV); thus, due to their similarity, it is estimated that this is likely to also be true for SARS-CoV-2 [243,245]. The mechanism by which it is thought to do so is by preventing fusion with the host membrane, decreasing viral polymerase function, impairing protein translation and processing, blocking particle release, and destabilising the viral envelope [243]. Long-term zinc supplementation at nutritional levels delays immunological failure, decreases diarrhea, and decreases rates of opportunistic infection over time in HIV-positive patients [250]. It is thought that zinc can inhibit HIV reverse transcriptase presumably via the competitive displacement of one or more Mg^{2+} ions bound to the reverse transcriptase, with zinc promoting the formation of a highly stable, slowly progressing reverse transcriptase complex [251]. Low-dose supplementation of zinc in combination with zinc ionophores, such as pyrithione and hionkitol, can decrease RNA synthesis in influenza, poliovirus, picornavirus, equine arteritis virus, and SARS-CoV by directly inhibiting RNA-dependant RNA polymerase (rdRp) [245,252].

Zinc deficiency influences the adaptive immune system, causing T cell lymphopenia [253]. Too high or too low levels of zinc have been linked to the inhibition of nicotinamide adenine dinucleotide phosphate (NADPH) oxidases, which enable the destruction of invading pathogens [254]. Thus, it is important to strike a balance in the levels of zinc in the body to reach an optimal zinc homeostasis to avoid immunosuppression via supplying zinc in either excess or deficient quantities. Zinc deficiency is characterised by an increase in proinflammatory cytokines like IL-1β, IL-6, and TNF-α, all of which are elevated during COVID-19 infection [239], and chronic low-grade inflammation within the gut of the elderly, obese, and immunocompromised. Similarly, zinc deficiency results in increased IL-8 and thus plays a critical role in gut inflammation [249]. Zinc acts as an anti-inflammatory to maintain immune tolerance via the induction of Treg cell development and mitigates the development of proinflammatory Th17 and Th9 cells, thus limiting the inflammatory response and controlling low-grade inflammation seen in the elderly, obese, and immunocompromised [246]. Zinc, when supplemented with antiretroviral therapy in HIV patients, has been shown to increase $CD4^+$ T cell counts as opposed to antiretroviral treatment alone [243]. Managing proinflammatory cytokines is key to the prevention of the cytokine storm and chronic low-grade inflammation seen in the elderly, obese, and immunocompromised. Zinc possesses antiviral and anti-inflammatory activity through its ability to inhibit NF-κB signaling and the modulation of regulatory T-cell functions and thus can limit the cytokine storm in COVID-19 and chronic low-grade inflammation [255].

It has been observed that there is a clear link between zinc deficiency and viral infections, including HIV and COVID-19 [256,257]. Patients in the at-risk group for contracting COVID-19 and who are at risk of a poorer prognosis of COVID-19 have been highly interlinked to lower zinc levels [256,257]. Such groups include individuals with chronic obstructive pulmonary disorder (COPD), bronchial asthma cardiovascular diseases, autoimmune diseases like UC and CD, and kidney diseases, dialysis patients, as well as those with comorbidities, such as obesity, diabetes, cancer, atherosclerosis, liver cirrhosis, immunosuppression, and known liver damage [256,257]. Thus, it is important to consider the possible role that zinc homeostasis has in the prevention and protection from contracting COVID-19 and other viral infections, as it is clear that it plays a critical role in antiviral immunity, where its deficiency is already seen to be strongly correlated with poorer clinical outcomes and is therefore of critical importance to the already at-risk elderly, obese, and immunocompromised populations. Table 8 summarises the immune boosting functions and mechanisms of action of zinc enriched foods.

Table 8. Summary of immune mechanisms enhanced by zinc-enriched foods.

Immune-Active Components	Immune-Boosting Functions	Mechanism	Reference
Zn^{2+}	Antiviral	- Enhances mucociliary clearance of viruses, removes the viral particle, reduces risk of secondary infections, preserves tissue barrier integrity to prevent viral entry - Inhibits ACE2 - Inhibits viral fusion with host membrane, decreases viral polymerase function, impairs protein translation and processing, blocks particle release, and destabilises the viral envelope - Inhibits HIV reverse transcriptase - Decreases RNA synthesis of viruses by direct inhibition of rdRp	[243,245,251,252]
	Immunomodulator	- Increases first responder cellular chemotaxis and phagocytosis - Increases cytotoxic activity of NK cells - Influences NK lytic abilities via MHCI recognition by NK cells - Regulates transepithelial resistance and tight and adherens junctions, including ZO-1, occluding, β-catenin, and E-cadherin, thus influencing membrane barrier integrity - Modulates NADPH oxidases - Stimulates production of IgG - Increases premature and immature B cells and affects antibody production	[239,246,247,249,254,258]
	Anti-inflammatory	- Reduces IL-1β, IL-6, and TNF-α - Decreases IL-8 - Induces Treg cell development, mitigates Th17 and Th9 - Inhibits NF-κB signaling and modulates Treg cell function - Increases CD4+ T cell counts in HIV patients	[239,243,246,249,255]

4.7. Selenium-Enriched Foods

Selenium is a ubiquitous element to sulfur that is found in nature and can be sourced organically from food [259]. Selenium constitutes 25 selenoproteins that play critical roles in reproduction, thyroid hormone metabolism, DNA synthesis, protein folding, mitochondrial health, and, most importantly, protection from oxidative damage and defense against viral infection [260–262]. Selenium deficiency is a risk factor for several chronic diseases associated with oxidative stress and inflammation, including IBDs [263], as well as being associated with obesity [264]. Selenium functions by virtue of its selenocysteine-active centre [261]. Rich sources of selenium include eggs, fish, corns like wheat, maize, and rice, chicken liver, garlic, onions, broccoli, yeast bran, coconut fruits, Brazil nuts, and seafood, and it is an essential component of all living organisms [265]. Selenium deficiency is reported to affect 500 million to 1 billion people worldwide, mainly due to inadequate dietary intake [261].

Selenium regulates the intestinal microflora, with increased gut microbiota diversity observed with increased dietary selenium, which in turn affects the gut microflora, influencing selenium bioavailability and selenoprotein expression [266–268]. Increases in proinflammatory taxa, including *Turicibacter and Dorea*, are associated with IBD [269,270]. With moderate selenium consumption, microbiota including *Turicibacter and Dorea* can be regulated and intestinal damage can be improved [267,271]. Selenium deficiency affects the killing ability of NK cells [271].

Deficiency in selenium leads to increased viral pathogenesis via oxidative stress and redox signaling, which ultimately affects cell proliferation, apoptosis, and cytokine expression [272,273]. Oxidative stress is a result of viral infections causing a disruption to the equilibrium between reactive oxygen species (ROS) and their scavenging systems, thus causing an imbalance between ROS and the cellular antioxidant defense system [274].

Viral infections result in oxidative stress, enhancing the replication and accumulation of mutations in the viral RNA genome, which ultimately leads to increased virulence and damage to the host via this amplification loop [274]. Deficiency in selenium has been associated with mutations in the viral genome that result in highly virulent forms of the viral particle, as well as being linked with increased susceptibility and pathogenicity of viral infections [274]. Selenoproteins are essential for an effective immune response to infections [261], largely through the critical selenoproteins, glutathione peroxidase and thioredoxin reductases, that provide antiviral defense by virtue of their redox signaling and homeostatic activities [262]. Selenium's antiviral activity is largely controlled by antioxidant factors, including glutathione peroxidase (GPXs) regulation by selenocysteine [272]. Furthermore, selenium has been shown to demonstrate an inhibitory effect on HIV via the antioxidative effects of GPX and other selenoproteins, with low selenium levels being correlated to HIV-infected individuals and further disease progression [275]. Similarly, selenium deficiency is seen in patients with hepatitis B and C viruses, and increases in selenium would help see better treatment response [276]. Selenite acts as an oxidant, which has important implications for selenium's antiviral properties, in that selenite reacts readily with sulfhydryl groups in the active site of viral protein disulphide isomerase (PDI), converting them to inactive disulphide; thus, the viral hydrophobic spike loses its ability to undergo the exchange reaction with disulphide groups of the cell membrane proteins and therefore renders the virus unable to enter the healthy cell cytoplasm, preventing viral entry into the cell [277,278].

Selenium status has been found to positively correlate with the survival of patients with COVID-19 compared with non-survivors, while overall selenium levels are lower in patients with COVID-19 than their healthy control counterparts [261]. This suggests the importance of adequate selenium levels in the prevention of COVID-19 and could further suggest its relevance as an antiviral for other viral infections. These viral mechanisms contribute to the oxidative stress associated with many RNA viral infections, the increased viral replication and hence increased mutation rate, and the higher pathogenicity or even higher mortality seen in selenium-deficient patients with COVID-19; thus, there is a clear association being reported between cure rates for COVID-19 and selenium status, as observed through the examination of city-based population selenium statuses of different Chinese cities [279]. Similarly, these findings have been clinically confirmed in Germany, where serum selenium levels were shown to be highly correlated with COVID-19 outcomes in hospitalised patients; 65% of those who died had low selenium compared to only 39% of those who survived, and very low selenium levels were present in 44.4% of patients. Most importantly, the lowest selenium levels were strongly associated with mortality, thus highlighting the importance of selenium in the defense and protection against severe clinical outcomes in COVID-19 patients [280].

Furthermore, selenium is a well-known NF-kB inhibitor and thus plays a critical role in reducing viral-induced apoptosis; it could also influence the mitigation of the cytokine storm in COVID-19 infection [281,282] and chronic low-grade inflammation seen in the gut of the elderly, obese, and immunocompromised by virtue of the interruption of the signaling pathway responsible for the chronic proinflammatory state. NF-kB is the central mediator of immune and inflammatory responses critically responsible for the proinflammatory cytokine production involved in the life-threatening cytokine storm [282] and chronic low-grade inflammation within the gut. Supplementing at-risk groups, including the elderly, obese, and immunocompromised, with 200 mcg selenium supplementation daily for three weeks, followed by a maintenance dose of less than or equal to 200 mcg μg for the duration of the active circulation of COVID-19, as well as the documentation of serum selenium levels in COVID-19-hospitalised patients for the systemic addition of selenium upon hospitalisation at the earliest stage possible, could aid in the management of the cytokine storm [282].

Selenium deficiency is linked to increases in proinflammatory cytokines IL-6, IL-8, IFN-γ, and TNF-α, while decreases in anti-inflammatory cytokines IL-2, IL-10, IL-17, IL-

1β, IFN-α, and IFN-β have been observed in many tissues, including the gastrointestinal tract [283,284]. Selenium supplementation increases the polarization of macrophages from the M1 to M2 phenotype, favouring inflammatory resolution, playing a critical role in IBDs [285]. This suggests selenium's role as an anti-inflammatory capable of managing the chronic low-grade inflammation seen in the gut of the elderly, obese, and immunocompromised through regulation of the proinflammatory immune response via cytokine production and their signaling pathways.

Selenium plays a key role in the proliferation and differentiation of CD4+ Th cells [271]. Increases in selenium result in increased Treg cell differentiation from naïve CD4+ T cells through TCR stimulation [271]. Therefore, increased selenium may play a role in managing the chronic inflammation of IBDs and low-grade inflammation seen in the gut of the elderly, obese, and immunocompromised by virtue of its regulatory role in T cell differentiation. Table 9 summarises the immune boosting functions and mechanisms of action of selenium enriched foods.

Table 9. Summary of immune mechanisms enhanced by selenium-rich foods.

Immune-Active Components	Immune-Boosting Functions	Mechanism	Reference
Selenite Selenoproteins	Antiviral	- Resists viral genome mutations, prevents development of highly virulent forms of viral particles, decreases susceptibility and pathogenicity of viral infections - Antiviral defense through redox signaling and homeostatic activity - Antioxidant - Inhibits HIV and slows HIV disease progression - Improves treatment response in HBV and HBC patients - Prevents viral entry to cell via interaction of sulfhydryl in active site of viral PDI	[262,272,274–278]
	Immunomodulator	- Regulates intestinal microflora, increases gut microbiota diversity, influences selenium bioavailability and selenoproteins' expression - Modulates microbiota, including Turicibacter and Dorea, and improves intestinal damage - Improves NK killing ability - Inhibits NF-kB	[266–268,271]
	Anti-inflammatory	- Decreases IL-6, IL-8, IFN-γ, and TNF-α - Increases IL-2, IL-10, IL-17, IL-1β, IFN-α, and IFN-β - Increases polarisation of M1 to M2 phenotype - Enhances CD4+ Th proliferation and differentiation - Increases Treg cell differentiation	[271,281–285]

5. Conclusions and Outlook

In summary, the COVID-19 pandemic has led to a focus on potential treatment and prevention methods to control, limit, and halt the spread of the virus, which causes an array of symptoms and illnesses, including mild to severe symptoms, such as ARDS, multiple organ failure, and, ultimately, death. An examination of the added risk of other comorbidities and age is an important challenge in the fight against COVID-19. In this review, we examined the potential of functional foods as natural sources of immune-boosting reinforcements at a time when antiviral vaccines are under strain due to rapid mutation and high turnaround for boosters due to their low 6-month immunity. Various studies have started to reveal that milk proteins, dairy fermentation products, and food products containing PUFAs, vitamin D, selenium, and Zinc may be used in the development of functional foods with the potential to combat not only COVID-19 but also other viral infections via their immune-modulating capabilities (Figure 4). This review, therefore, stresses the importance of supporting immune fitness by means of healthy eating and increased functional food intake, particularly for at-risk individuals, including the elderly, the obese, and those who are already immunocompromised.

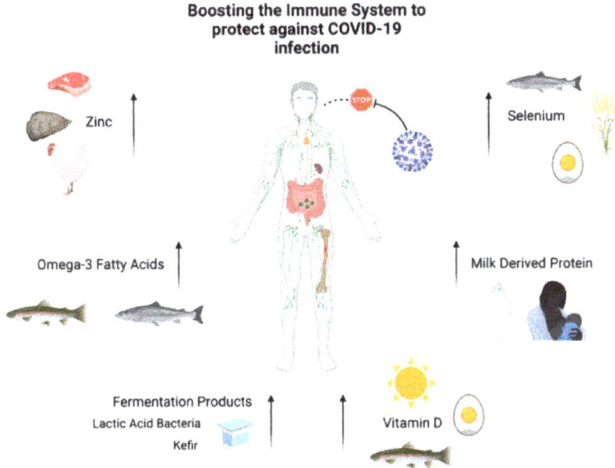

Figure 4. Summary of functional foods capable of boosting the immune system and inhibiting COVID-19 infection. Functional foods with properties capable of inhibiting viral infection and their key food sources. Arrows indicate increasing food component consumption to aid in preventing COVID-19 infection. Created using BioRender.com.

Author Contributions: Conceptualization, D.F. and C.L.; writing—original draft preparation, D.F. and R.T.; writing—review and editing, D.F., R.T. and C.L.; project administration, D.F. and C.L.; funding acquisition, C.L. All authors have read and agreed to the published version of the manuscript.

Funding: C.L. and D.F. are supported by Enterprise Ireland (Grant #: TC20180025). R.T is funded by the Marie Skłodowska-Curie/Enterprise Ireland Career-Fit Plus Program (Grant #: MF2021 0255).

Institutional Review Board Statement: Not applicable.

Informed Consent Statement: Not applicable.

Data Availability Statement: No new data were created or analysed in this study. Data sharing is not applicable to this article.

Conflicts of Interest: The authors declare no conflict of interest.

References

1. Fadnes, L.T.; Økland, J.-M.; Haaland, Ø.A.; Johansson, K.A. Estimating Impact of Food Choices on Life Expectancy: A Modeling Study. *PLoS Med.* **2022**, *19*, e1003889. [CrossRef]
2. Koithan, M.; Devika, J. New Approaches to Nutritional Therapy. *J. Nurse Pract.* **2010**, *6*, 805–806. [CrossRef]
3. Wu, D.; Lewis, E.D.; Pae, M.; Meydani, S.N. Nutritional Modulation of Immune Function: Analysis of Evidence, Mechanisms, and Clinical Relevance. *Front. Immunol.* **2018**, *9*, 3160. [CrossRef]
4. Atherton, J.G.; Kratzing, C.C.; Fisher, A. The Effect of Ascorbic Acid on Infection of Chick-Embryo Ciliated Tracheal Organ Cultures by Coronavirus. *Arch. Virol.* **1978**, *56*, 195–199. [CrossRef]
5. Chihara, G.O.R.O. Medical Aspects of Lentinan Isolated from Lentinus Edodes (Berk.) Sing. In *Mushroom Biology and Mushroom Products*; Chinese University Press: Hong Kong, 1993; pp. 261–266.
6. Tochikura, T.S.; Nakashima, H.; Hirose, K.; Yamamoto, N. A Biological Response Modifier, PSK, Inhibits Human Immunodeficiency Virus Infection in Vitro. *Biochem. Biophys. Res. Commun.* **1987**, *148*, 726–733. [CrossRef]

7. Takehara, M.; Kuida, K.; Mori, K. Antiviral Activity of Virus-like Particles FromLentinus Edodes (Shiitake). *Arch. Virol.* **1979**, *59*, 269–274. [CrossRef]
8. Hayashi, T.; Hayashi, K.; Maeda, M.; Kojima, I. Calcium Spirulan, an Inhibitor of Enveloped Virus Replication, from a Blue-Green Alga Spirulina Platensis. *J. Nat. Prod.* **1996**, *59*, 83–87. [CrossRef]
9. Khan, Z.; Bhadouria, P.; Bisen, P.S. Nutritional and Therapeutic Potential of Spirulina. *Curr. Pharm. Biotechnol.* **2005**, *6*, 373–379. [CrossRef]
10. Schandalik, R.; Gatti, G.; Perucca, E. Pharmacokinetics of Silybin in Bile Following Administration of Silipide and Silymarin in Cholecystectomy Patients. *Arzneimittelforschung* **1992**, *42*, 964–968.
11. Rahman, M.M.; Mosaddik, A.; Alam, A.K. Traditional Foods with Their Constituent's Antiviral and Immune System Modulating Properties. *Heliyon* **2021**, *7*, e05957. [CrossRef]
12. Wellness Creative Co Health & Wellness Industry Statistics 2022 [Latest Market Data & Trends]. Wellness Creative Co 2019. Available online: https://www.wellnesscreatives.com/wellness-industry-statistics/ (accessed on 1 July 2022).
13. Euromonitor International, a Market Research Provider Market Sizes. 2022. Available online: https://www-portal-euromonitor-com.dcu.idm.oclc.org/portal/statisticsevolution/index (accessed on 1 July 2022).
14. Sørensen, H.M.; Rochfort, K.D.; Maye, S.; MacLeod, G.; Brabazon, D.; Loscher, C.; Freeland, B. Exopolysaccharides of Lactic Acid Bacteria: Production, Purification and Health Benefits towards Functional Food. *Nutrients* **2022**, *14*, 2938. [CrossRef] [PubMed]
15. Research and Markets. *Immune Health Supplements Market—Global Outlook and Forecast 2020–2025*; Research and Markets: Dublin, Ireland, 2021.
16. Health Service Executive. *How Long Does Immunity Last after COVID-19 Vaccination? Does Immunity Wane Faster in Certain Sub-Populations? How Safe and Effective Are Booster Doses of COVID-19 Vaccine?* HLI (Health Library Ireland): Dublin, Ireland, 2021.
17. Thomas, S.J.; Moreira, E.D.; Kitchin, N.; Absalon, J.; Gurtman, A.; Lockhart, S.; Perez, J.L.; Pérez Marc, G.; Polack, F.P.; Zerbini, C.; et al. Safety and Efficacy of the BNT162b2 MRNA COVID-19 Vaccine through 6 Months. *N. Engl. J. Med.* **2021**, *385*, 1761–1773. [CrossRef]
18. van de Loo, A.J.A.E.; Kerssemakers, N.; Scholey, A.; Garssen, J.; Kraneveld, A.D.; Verster, J.C. Perceived Immune Fitness, Individual Strength and Hangover Severity. *Int. J. Environ. Res. Public Health* **2020**, *17*, 4039. [CrossRef]
19. Danone Nutricia Research. *Immune Fitness: Working towards a Resilient Immune System*; Danone Nutricia Research: Utrecht, The Netherlands, 2022.
20. Villar-Álvarez, F.; de la Rosa-Carrillo, D.; Fariñas-Guerrero, F.; Jiménez-Ruiz, C.A. Immunosenescence, Immune Fitness and Vaccination Schedule in the Adult Respiratory Patient. *Open Respir. Arch.* **2022**, *4*, 100181. [CrossRef] [PubMed]
21. Franceschi, C.; Garagnani, P.; Parini, P.; Giuliani, C.; Santoro, A. Inflammaging: A New Immune–Metabolic Viewpoint for Age-Related Diseases. *Nat. Rev. Endocrinol.* **2018**, *14*, 576–590. [CrossRef]
22. Christ, A.; Lauterbach, M.; Latz, E. Western Diet and the Immune System: An Inflammatory Connection. *Immunity* **2019**, *51*, 794–811. [CrossRef]
23. Pérez-Cano, F.J. Mediterranean Diet, Microbiota and Immunity. *Nutrients* **2022**, *14*, 273. [CrossRef]
24. Cordain, L.; Eaton, S.B.; Sebastian, A.; Mann, N.; Lindeberg, S.; Watkins, B.A.; O'Keefe, J.H.; Brand-Miller, J. Origins and Evolution of the Western Diet: Health Implications for the 21st Century. *Am. J. Clin. Nutr.* **2005**, *81*, 341–354. [CrossRef]
25. Bach, J.-F. The Effect of Infections on Susceptibility to Autoimmune and Allergic Diseases. *N. Engl. J. Med.* **2002**, *347*, 911–920. [CrossRef]
26. Eder, W.; Ege, M.J.; von Mutius, E. The Asthma Epidemic. *N. Engl. J. Med.* **2006**, *355*, 2226–2235. [CrossRef]
27. Lewis, J.D. The Role of Diet in Inflammatory Bowel Disease. *Gastroenterol. Hepatol.* **2016**, *12*, 51–53.
28. Wypych, T.P.; Marsland, B.J.; Ubags, N.D.J. The Impact of Diet on Immunity and Respiratory Diseases. *Ann. ATS* **2017**, *14*, S339–S347. [CrossRef]
29. NIH Definition of Immunocompromised—NCI Dictionary of Cancer Terms—NCI. Available online: https://www.cancer.gov/publications/dictionaries/cancer-terms/def/immunocompromised (accessed on 22 July 2022).
30. CDC CDC—Cryptosporidiosis—Fact Sheets—Infection—Immunocompromised Persons. Available online: https://www.cdc.gov/parasites/crypto/gen_info/infect_ic.html (accessed on 22 July 2022).
31. World Health Organization. *Clinical Management of Severe Acute Respiratory Infection (SARI) When COVID-19 Disease Is Suspected: Interim Guidance, 13 March 2020*; World Health Organization: Geneva, Switzerland, 2020.
32. Suardi, C.; Cazzaniga, E.; Graci, S.; Dongo, D.; Palestini, P. Link between Viral Infections, Immune System, Inflammation and Diet. *Int. J. Environ. Res. Public Health* **2021**, *18*, 2455. [CrossRef] [PubMed]
33. Mohammad, S.; Aziz, R.; Al Mahri, S.; Malik, S.S.; Haji, E.; Khan, A.H.; Khatlani, T.S.; Bouchama, A. Obesity and COVID-19: What Makes Obese Host so Vulnerable? *Immun. Ageing* **2021**, *18*, 1. [CrossRef] [PubMed]
34. Ashan, Maria., What is immune fitness, July 2022, News Medical Life Sciences. Available online: https://www.news-medical.net/health/What-is-Immune-Fitness.aspx (accessed on 26 July 2023).
35. Ioannidis, J.P.A.; Axfors, C.; Contopoulos-Ioannidis, D.G. Population-Level COVID-19 Mortality Risk for Non-Elderly Individuals Overall and for Non-Elderly Individuals without Underlying Diseases in Pandemic Epicenters. *Environ. Res.* **2020**, *188*, 109890. [CrossRef]
36. Oh, S.-J.; Lee, J.K.; Shin, O.S. Aging and the Immune System: The Impact of Immunosenescence on Viral Infection, Immunity and Vaccine Immunogenicity. *Immune Netw.* **2019**, *19*, e37. [CrossRef]

37. Pae, M.; Meydani, S.N.; Wu, D. The Role of Nutrition in Enhancing Immunity in Aging. *Aging Dis.* **2011**, *3*, 91–129.
38. Palmer, D.B. The Effect of Age on Thymic Function. *Front. Immunol.* **2013**, *4*, 316. [CrossRef]
39. Müller, L.; Pawelec, G. Aging and Immunity—Impact of Behavioral Intervention. *Brain Behav. Immun.* **2014**, *39*, 8–22. [CrossRef]
40. Mabbott, N.A.; Kobayashi, A.; Sehgal, A.; Bradford, B.M.; Pattison, M.; Donaldson, D.S. Aging and the Mucosal Immune System in the Intestine. *Biogerontology* **2015**, *16*, 133–145. [CrossRef]
41. Faria, A.M.C.; Mucida, D.; McCafferty, D.-M.; Tsuji, N.M.; Verhasselt, V. Tolerance and Inflammation at the Gut Mucosa. *Clin. Dev. Immunol.* **2012**, *2012*, 738475. [CrossRef]
42. Magrone, T.; Jirillo, E. The Interaction between Gut Microbiota and Age-Related Changes in Immune Function and Inflammation. *Immun. Ageing* **2013**, *10*, 31. [CrossRef] [PubMed]
43. Shemtov, S.J.; Emani, R.; Bielska, O.; Covarrubias, A.J.; Verdin, E.; Andersen, J.K.; Winer, D.A. The Intestinal Immune System and Gut Barrier Function in Obesity and Ageing. *FEBS J.* **2022**. [CrossRef] [PubMed]
44. Zimecki, M.; Właszczyk, A.; Zagulski, T.; Kübler, A. Lactoferrin Lowers Serum Interleukin 6 and Tumor Necrosis Factor Alpha Levels in Mice Subjected to Surgery. *Arch. Immunol. Ther. Exp.* **1998**, *46*, 97–104.
45. Wu, Y.; Xu, J.; Rong, X.; Wang, F.; Wang, H.; Zhao, C. Gut Microbiota Alterations and Health Status in Aging Adults: From Correlation to Causation. *Aging Med.* **2021**, *4*, 206–213. [CrossRef]
46. Walker, E.M.; Slisarenko, N.; Gerrets, G.L.; Kissinger, P.J.; Didier, E.S.; Kuroda, M.J.; Veazey, R.S.; Jazwinski, S.M.; Rout, N. Inflammaging Phenotype in Rhesus Macaques Is Associated with a Decline in Epithelial Barrier-Protective Functions and Increased pro-Inflammatory Function in CD161-Expressing Cells. *Geroscience* **2019**, *41*, 739–757. [CrossRef]
47. Thevaranjan, N.; Puchta, A.; Schulz, C.; Naidoo, A.; Szamosi, J.C.; Verschoor, C.P.; Loukov, D.; Schenck, L.P.; Jury, J.; Foley, K.P.; et al. Age-Associated Microbial Dysbiosis Promotes Intestinal Permeability, Systemic Inflammation, and Macrophage Dysfunction. *Cell Host Microbe* **2017**, *21*, 455–466.e4. [CrossRef]
48. Ragonnaud, E.; Biragyn, A. Gut Microbiota as the Key Controllers of "Healthy" Aging of Elderly People. *Immun. Ageing* **2021**, *18*, 2. [CrossRef]
49. Jeffery, I.B.; Lynch, D.B.; O'Toole, P.W. Composition and Temporal Stability of the Gut Microbiota in Older Persons. *ISME J.* **2016**, *10*, 170–182. [CrossRef]
50. Pae, M.; Wu, D. Nutritional Modulation of Age-Related Changes in the Immune System and Risk of Infection. *Nutr. Res.* **2017**, *41*, 14–35. [CrossRef]
51. Frasca, D.; Blomberg, B.B. Aging Induces B Cell Defects and Decreased Antibody Responses to Influenza Infection and Vaccination. *Immun. Ageing* **2020**, *17*, 37. [CrossRef]
52. Colonna-Romano, G.; Bulati, M.; Aquino, A.; Pellicanò, M.; Vitello, S.; Lio, D.; Candore, G.; Caruso, C. A Double-Negative (IgD−CD27−) B Cell Population Is Increased in the Peripheral Blood of Elderly People. *Mech. Ageing Dev.* **2009**, *130*, 681–690. [CrossRef] [PubMed]
53. Thangavelu, G.; Smolarchuk, C.; Anderson, C.C. Co-Inhibitory Molecules. *Self Nonself* **2010**, *1*, 77–88. [CrossRef] [PubMed]
54. Dillon, S.M.; Liu, J.; Purba, C.M.; Christians, A.J.; Kibbie, J.J.; Castleman, M.J.; McCarter, M.D.; Wilson, C.C. Age-Related Alterations in Human Gut CD4 T Cell Phenotype, T Helper Cell Frequencies, and Functional Responses to Enteric Bacteria. *J. Leukoc. Biol.* **2020**, *107*, 119–132. [CrossRef]
55. Dillon, S.M.; Thompson, T.A.; Christians, A.J.; McCarter, M.D.; Wilson, C.C. Reduced Immune-Regulatory Molecule Expression on Human Colonic Memory CD4 T Cells in Older Adults. *Immun. Ageing* **2021**, *18*, 6. [CrossRef] [PubMed]
56. Sugahara, H.; Okai, S.; Odamaki, T.; Wong, C.B.; Kato, K.; Mitsuyama, E.; Xiao, J.-Z.; Shinkura, R. Decreased Taxon-Specific IgA Response in Relation to the Changes of Gut Microbiota Composition in the Elderly. *Front. Microbiol.* **2017**, *8*, 1757. [CrossRef]
57. Peterson, D.A.; McNulty, N.P.; Guruge, J.L.; Gordon, J.I. IgA Response to Symbiotic Bacteria as a Mediator of Gut Homeostasis. *Cell Host Microbe* **2007**, *2*, 328–339. [CrossRef]
58. Nagafusa, H.; Sayama, K. Age-Related Chemokine Alterations Affect IgA Secretion and Gut Immunity in Female Mice. *Biogerontology* **2020**, *21*, 609–618. [CrossRef]
59. Nakajima, A.; Vogelzang, A.; Maruya, M.; Miyajima, M.; Murata, M.; Son, A.; Kuwahara, T.; Tsuruyama, T.; Yamada, S.; Matsuura, M.; et al. IgA Regulates the Composition and Metabolic Function of Gut Microbiota by Promoting Symbiosis between Bacteria. *J. Exp. Med.* **2018**, *215*, 2019–2034. [CrossRef]
60. Childs, C.E.; Calder, P.C.; Miles, E.A. Diet and Immune Function. *Nutrients* **2019**, *11*, 1933. [CrossRef]
61. González-Muniesa, P.; Mártinez-González, M.-A.; Hu, F.B.; Després, J.-P.; Matsuzawa, Y.; Loos, R.J.F.; Moreno, L.A.; Bray, G.A.; Martinez, J.A. Obesity. *Nat. Rev. Dis. Primers* **2017**, *3*, 17034. [CrossRef] [PubMed]
62. Ejaz, H.; Alsrhani, A.; Zafar, A.; Javed, H.; Junaid, K.; Abdalla, A.E.; Abosalif, K.O.A.; Ahmed, Z.; Younas, S. COVID-19 and Comorbidities: Deleterious Impact on Infected Patients. *J. Infect. Public Health* **2020**, *13*, 1833–1839. [CrossRef] [PubMed]
63. Kim, J.; Nam, J.-H. Insight into the Relationship between Obesity-Induced Low-Level Chronic Inflammation and COVID-19 Infection. *Int. J. Obes.* **2020**, *44*, 1541–1542. [CrossRef] [PubMed]
64. Kim, J.; Na, H.; Kim, J.-A.; Nam, J.-H. What We Know and What We Need to Know about Adenovirus 36-Induced Obesity. *Int. J. Obes.* **2020**, *44*, 1197–1209. [CrossRef]
65. Hulme, K.D.; Noye, E.C.; Short, K.R.; Labzin, L.I. Dysregulated Inflammation During Obesity: Driving Disease Severity in Influenza Virus and SARS-CoV-2 Infections. *Front. Immunol.* **2021**, *12*, 4356. [CrossRef]

66. Antunes, A.E.C.; Vinderola, G.; Xavier-Santos, D.; Sivieri, K. Potential Contribution of Beneficial Microbes to Face the COVID-19 Pandemic. *Food Res. Int.* **2020**, *136*, 109577. [CrossRef]
67. Wadman, M. Why COVID-19 Is More Deadly in People with Obesity—Even If They're Young. Available online: https://www.science.org/content/article/why-covid-19-more-deadly-people-obesity-even-if-theyre-young (accessed on 4 July 2022).
68. Neidich, S.D.; Green, W.D.; Rebeles, J.; Karlsson, E.A.; Schultz-Cherry, S.; Noah, T.L.; Chakladar, S.; Hudgens, M.G.; Weir, S.S.; Beck, M.A. Increased Risk of Influenza among Vaccinated Adults Who Are Obese. *Int. J. Obes.* **2017**, *41*, 1324–1330. [CrossRef]
69. McLaughlin, T.; Ackerman, S.E.; Shen, L.; Engleman, E. Role of Innate and Adaptive Immunity in Obesity-Associated Metabolic Disease. *J. Clin. Investig.* **2017**, *127*, 5–13. [CrossRef]
70. Weisberg, S.P.; McCann, D.; Desai, M.; Rosenbaum, M.; Leibel, R.L.; Ferrante, A.W. Obesity Is Associated with Macrophage Accumulation in Adipose Tissue. *J. Clin. Investig.* **2003**, *112*, 1796–1808. [CrossRef]
71. Winer, D.A.; Luck, H.; Tsai, S.; Winer, S. The Intestinal Immune System in Obesity and Insulin Resistance. *Cell Metab.* **2016**, *23*, 413–426. [CrossRef]
72. Maynard, C.L.; Elson, C.O.; Hatton, R.D.; Weaver, C.T. Reciprocal Interactions of the Intestinal Microbiota and Immune System. *Nature* **2012**, *489*, 231–241. [CrossRef]
73. Cani, P.D.; Amar, J.; Iglesias, M.A.; Poggi, M.; Knauf, C.; Bastelica, D.; Neyrinck, A.M.; Fava, F.; Tuohy, K.M.; Chabo, C.; et al. Metabolic Endotoxemia Initiates Obesity and Insulin Resistance. *Diabetes* **2007**, *56*, 1761–1772. [CrossRef] [PubMed]
74. Cani, P.D.; Bibiloni, R.; Knauf, C.; Waget, A.; Neyrinck, A.M.; Delzenne, N.M.; Burcelin, R. Changes in Gut Microbiota Control Metabolic Endotoxemia-Induced Inflammation in High-Fat Diet–Induced Obesity and Diabetes in Mice. *Diabetes* **2008**, *57*, 1470–1481. [CrossRef] [PubMed]
75. Luck, H.; Tsai, S.; Chung, J.; Clemente-Casares, X.; Ghazarian, M.; Revelo, X.S.; Lei, H.; Luk, C.T.; Shi, S.Y.; Surendra, A.; et al. Regulation of Obesity-Related Insulin Resistance with Gut Anti-Inflammatory Agents. *Cell Metab.* **2015**, *21*, 527–542. [CrossRef] [PubMed]
76. Al-Sadi, R.; Ye, D.; Dokladny, K.; Ma, T.Y. Mechanism of IL-1β-Induced Increase in Intestinal Epithelial Tight Junction Permeability. *J. Immunol.* **2008**, *180*, 5653–5661. [CrossRef]
77. Russo, L.; Lumeng, C.N. Properties and Functions of Adipose Tissue Macrophages in Obesity. *Immunology* **2018**, *155*, 407–417. [CrossRef]
78. Bredella, M.A.; Gill, C.M.; Gerweck, A.V.; Landa, M.G.; Kumar, V.; Daley, S.M.; Torriani, M.; Miller, K.K. Ectopic and Serum Lipid Levels Are Positively Associated with Bone Marrow Fat in Obesity. *Radiology* **2013**, *269*, 534–541. [CrossRef]
79. Dicker, D.; Salook, M.A.; Marcoviciu, D.; Djaldetti, M.; Bessler, H. Role of Peripheral Blood Mononuclear Cells in the Predisposition of Obese Individuals to Inflammation and Infection. *Obes. Facts* **2013**, *6*, 146–151. [CrossRef]
80. Teran-Cabanillas, E.; Montalvo-Corral, M.; Caire-Juvera, G.; Moya-Camarena, S.Y.; Hernández, J. Decreased Interferon-α and Interferon-β Production in Obesity and Expression of Suppressor of Cytokine Signaling. *Nutrition* **2013**, *29*, 207–212. [CrossRef]
81. Bruun, J.M.; Lihn, A.S.; Pedersen, S.B.; Richelsen, B. Monocyte Chemoattractant Protein-1 Release Is Higher in Visceral than Subcutaneous Human Adipose Tissue (AT): Implication of Macrophages Resident in the AT. *J. Clin. Endocrinol. Metab.* **2005**, *90*, 2282–2289. [CrossRef]
82. Field, C.S.; Baixauli, F.; Kyle, R.L.; Puleston, D.J.; Cameron, A.M.; Sanin, D.E.; Hippen, K.L.; Loschi, M.; Thangavelu, G.; Corrado, M.; et al. Mitochondrial Integrity Regulated by Lipid Metabolism Is a Cell-Intrinsic Checkpoint for Treg Suppressive Function. *Cell Metab.* **2020**, *31*, 422–437.e5. [CrossRef] [PubMed]
83. Zhou, H.; Wang, L.; Liu, F. Immunological Impact of Intestinal T Cells on Metabolic Diseases. *Front. Immunol.* **2021**, *12*, 639902. [CrossRef]
84. Khan, S.; Luck, H.; Winer, S.; Winer, D.A. Emerging Concepts in Intestinal Immune Control of Obesity-Related Metabolic Disease. *Nat. Commun.* **2021**, *12*, 2598. [CrossRef]
85. Luck, H.; Khan, S.; Kim, J.H.; Copeland, J.K.; Revelo, X.S.; Tsai, S.; Chakraborty, M.; Cheng, K.; Tao Chan, Y.; Nøhr, M.K.; et al. Gut-Associated IgA+ Immune Cells Regulate Obesity-Related Insulin Resistance. *Nat. Commun.* **2019**, *10*, 3650. [CrossRef]
86. CDC People with Certain Medical Conditions. Available online: https://www.cdc.gov/coronavirus/2019-ncov/need-extra-precautions/people-with-medical-conditions.html (accessed on 27 July 2022).
87. NIAID. The Effects of Highly Active Antiretroviral Therapy (HAART) on the Recovery of Immune Function in HIV-Infected Children and Young Adults. 2013. Available online: clinicaltrials.gov (accessed on 12 July 2023).
88. HIV.Gov Global Statistics. Available online: https://www.hiv.gov/hiv-basics/overview/data-and-trends/global-statistics (accessed on 27 July 2022).
89. WHO HIV/AIDS. Available online: https://www.who.int/data/gho/data/themes/hiv-aids (accessed on 27 July 2022).
90. *HIV Ireland Treatment*; HIV Ireland: Dublin, Ireland, 2022.
91. Liu, J.; Williams, B.; Frank, D.; Dillon, S.M.; Wilson, C.C.; Landay, A.L. Inside Out: HIV, the Gut Microbiome, and the Mucosal Immune System. *J. Immunol.* **2017**, *198*, 605–614. [CrossRef] [PubMed]
92. Neuhaus, J.; Jacobs, D.R., Jr.; Baker, J.V.; Calmy, A.; Duprez, D.; La Rosa, A.; Kuller, L.H.; Pett, S.L.; Ristola, M.; Ross, M.J.; et al. Markers of Inflammation, Coagulation, and Renal Function Are Elevated in Adults with HIV Infection. *J. Infect. Dis.* **2010**, *201*, 1788–1795. [CrossRef] [PubMed]

93. Hunt, P.W.; Sinclair, E.; Rodriguez, B.; Shive, C.; Clagett, B.; Funderburg, N.; Robinson, J.; Huang, Y.; Epling, L.; Martin, J.N.; et al. Gut Epithelial Barrier Dysfunction and Innate Immune Activation Predict Mortality in Treated HIV Infection. *J. Infect. Dis.* **2014**, *210*, 1228–1238. [CrossRef] [PubMed]
94. Fernandes, S.M.; Pires, A.R.; Ferreira, C.; Foxall, R.B.; Rino, J.; Santos, C.; Correia, L.; Poças, J.; Veiga-Fernandes, H.; Sousa, A.E. Enteric Mucosa Integrity in the Presence of a Preserved Innate Interleukin 22 Compartment in HIV Type 1–Treated Individuals. *J. Infect. Dis.* **2014**, *210*, 630–640. [CrossRef]
95. Lapenta, C.; Boirivant, M.; Marini, M.; Santini, S.M.; Logozzi, M.; Viora, M.; Belardelli, F.; Fais, S. Human Intestinal Lamina Propria Lymphocytes Are Naturally Permissive to HIV-1 Infection. *Eur. J. Immunol.* **1999**, *29*, 1202–1208. [CrossRef]
96. Hazenberg, M.D.; Hamann, D.; Schuitemaker, H.; Miedema, F. T Cell Depletion in HIV-1 Infection: How CD4+ T Cells Go out of Stock. *Nat. Immunol.* **2000**, *1*, 285–289. [CrossRef]
97. Unutmaz, D.; Pileri, P.; Abrignani, S. Antigen-Independent Activation of Naive and Memory Resting T Cells by a Cytokine Combination. *J. Exp. Med.* **1994**, *180*, 1159–1164. [CrossRef] [PubMed]
98. Swingler, S.; Mann, A.; Jacqué, J.-M.; Brichacek, B.; Sasseville, V.G.; Williams, K.; Lackner, A.A.; Janoff, E.N.; Wang, R.; Fisher, D.; et al. HIV-1 Nef Mediates Lymphocyte Chemotaxis and Activation by Infected Macrophages. *Nat. Med.* **1999**, *5*, 997–1003. [CrossRef] [PubMed]
99. de Mattos, B.R.R.; Garcia, M.P.G.; Nogueira, J.B.; Paiatto, L.N.; Albuquerque, C.G.; Souza, C.L.; Fernandes, L.G.R.; Tamashiro, W.M.d.S.C.; Simioni, P.U. Inflammatory Bowel Disease: An Overview of Immune Mechanisms and Biological Treatments. *Mediat. Inflamm.* **2015**, *2015*, 493012. [CrossRef] [PubMed]
100. CDC Prevalence of IBD | CDC. Available online: https://www.cdc.gov/ibd/data-and-statistics/prevalence.html (accessed on 19 July 2022).
101. Alatab, S.; Sepanlou, S.G.; Ikuta, K.; Vahedi, H.; Bisignano, C.; Safiri, S.; Sadeghi, A.; Nixon, M.R.; Abdoli, A.; Abolhassani, H.; et al. The Global, Regional, and National Burden of Inflammatory Bowel Disease in 195 Countries and Territories, 1990–2017: A Systematic Analysis for the Global Burden of Disease Study 2017. *Lancet Gastroenterol. Hepatol.* **2020**, *5*, 17–30. [CrossRef]
102. EFCCA About IBD (Inflammatory Bowel Diseases) Organisations | World IBD Day. Available online: https://worldibdday.org/about-us (accessed on 19 July 2022).
103. Hisamatsu, T.; Kanai, T.; Mikami, Y.; Yoneno, K.; Matsuoka, K.; Hibi, T. Immune Aspects of the Pathogenesis of Inflammatory Bowel Disease. *Pharmacol. Ther.* **2013**, *137*, 283–297. [CrossRef]
104. Silva, F.A.R.; Rodrigues, B.L.; Ayrizono, M.d.L.S.; Leal, R.F. The Immunological Basis of Inflammatory Bowel Disease. *Gastroenterol. Res. Pract.* **2016**, *2016*, e2097274. [CrossRef]
105. Franke, A.; Balschun, T.; Karlsen, T.H.; Sventoraityte, J.; Nikolaus, S.; Mayr, G.; Domingues, F.S.; Albrecht, M.; Nothnagel, M.; Ellinghaus, D.; et al. Sequence Variants in IL10, ARPC2 and Multiple Other Loci Contribute to Ulcerative Colitis Susceptibility. *Nat. Genet.* **2008**, *40*, 1319–1323. [CrossRef]
106. Negroni, A.; Pierdomenico, M.; Cucchiara, S.; Stronati, L. NOD2 and Inflammation: Current Insights. *J. Inflamm. Res.* **2018**, *11*, 49–60. [CrossRef]
107. Neurath, M.F.; Fuss, I.; Kelsall, B.L.; Presky, D.H.; Waegell, W.; Strober, W. Experimental Granulomatous Colitis in Mice Is Abrogated by Induction of TGF-Beta-Mediated Oral Tolerance. *J. Exp. Med.* **1996**, *183*, 2605–2616. [CrossRef]
108. Kam, L.Y.; Targan, S.R. TNF-Alpha Antagonists for the Treatment of Crohn's Disease. *Expert Opin. Pharmacother.* **2000**, *1*, 615–622. [CrossRef]
109. Monteleone, G.; Boirivant, M.; Pallone, F.; MacDonald, T.T. TGF-Beta1 and Smad7 in the Regulation of IBD. *Mucosal Immunol.* **2008**, *1* (Suppl. S1), S50–S53. [CrossRef]
110. Ghosh, S.; Chaudhary, R.; Carpani, M.; Playford, R. Interfering with Interferons in Inflammatory Bowel Disease. *Gut* **2006**, *55*, 1071–1073. [CrossRef] [PubMed]
111. Huang, Y.; Chen, Z. Inflammatory Bowel Disease Related Innate Immunity and Adaptive Immunity. *Am. J. Transl. Res.* **2016**, *8*, 2490–2497. [PubMed]
112. Monteleone, I.; Sarra, M.; Pallone, F.; Monteleone, G. Th17-Related Cytokines in Inflammatory Bowel Diseases: Friends or Foes? *Curr. Mol. Med.* **2012**, *12*, 592–597. [CrossRef] [PubMed]
113. Yamada, A.; Arakaki, R.; Saito, M.; Tsunematsu, T.; Kudo, Y.; Ishimaru, N. Role of Regulatory T Cell in the Pathogenesis of Inflammatory Bowel Disease. *World J. Gastroenterol.* **2016**, *22*, 2195–2205. [CrossRef]
114. Izcue, A.; Coombes, J.L.; Powrie, F. Regulatory T Cells Suppress Systemic and Mucosal Immune Activation to Control Intestinal Inflammation. *Immunol. Rev.* **2006**, *212*, 256–271. [CrossRef]
115. Boden, E.K.; Snapper, S.B. Regulatory T Cells in Inflammatory Bowel Disease. *Curr. Opin. Gastroenterol.* **2008**, *24*, 733–741. [CrossRef]
116. MacDermott, R.P.; Nash, G.S.; Bertovich, M.J.; Seiden, M.V.; Bragdon, M.J.; Beale, M.G. Alterations of IgM, IgG, and IgA Synthesis and Secretion by Peripheral Blood and Intestinal Mononuclear Cells from Patients with Ulcerative Colitis and Crohn's Disease. *Gastroenterology* **1981**, *81*, 844–852. [CrossRef]
117. Uo, M.; Hisamatsu, T.; Miyoshi, J.; Kaito, D.; Yoneno, K.; Kitazume, M.T.; Mori, M.; Sugita, A.; Koganei, K.; Matsuoka, K.; et al. Mucosal CXCR4+ IgG Plasma Cells Contribute to the Pathogenesis of Human Ulcerative Colitis through FcγR-Mediated CD14 Macrophage Activation. *Gut* **2013**, *62*, 1734–1744. [CrossRef]

118. Tsianos, E.V.; Katsanos, K. Do We Really Understand What the Immunological Disturbances in Inflammatory Bowel Disease Mean? *World J. Gastroenterol.* **2009**, *15*, 521–525. [CrossRef]
119. Hodgson, H.J.F.; Jewell, D.P. The Humoral Immune System in Inflammatory Bowel Disease. *Dig. Dis. Sci.* **1978**, *23*, 123–128. [CrossRef] [PubMed]
120. Arai, S.; Osawa, T.; Ohigashi, H.; Yoshikawa, M.; Kaminogawa, S.; Watanabe, M.; Ogawa, T.; Okubo, K.; Watanabe, S.; Nishino, H.; et al. A Mainstay of Functional Food Science in Japan—History, Present Status, and Future Outlook. *Biosci. Biotechnol. Biochem.* **2001**, *65*, 1–13. [CrossRef] [PubMed]
121. Taylor, C.L. Regulatory Frameworks for Functional Foods and Dietary Supplements. *Nutr. Rev.* **2004**, *62*, 55–59. [CrossRef]
122. FSAI. *Functional Food*; Food Safety Authority of Ireland: Dublin, Ireland, 2007.
123. Martirosyan, D.M.; Singh, J. A New Definition of Functional Food by FFC: What Makes a New Definition Unique? *Funct. Foods Health Dis.* **2015**, *5*, 209. [CrossRef]
124. FUFOSE. Scientific Concepts of Functional Foods in Europe Consensus Document. *Br. J. Nutr.* **1999**, *81*, S1–S27. [CrossRef]
125. ISI North America Technical Committee. Safety Assessment and Potential Health Benefits of Food Components Based on Selected Scientific Criteria. *Crit. Rev. Food Sci. Nutr.* **1999**, *39*, 203–206. [CrossRef] [PubMed]
126. Canada Health ARCHIVED. Policy Paper—Nutraceuticals/Functional Foods and Health Claims on Foods. Available online: https://www.canada.ca/en/health-canada/services/food-nutrition/food-labelling/health-claims/nutraceuticals-functional-foods-health-claims-foods-policy-paper.html (accessed on 12 August 2022).
127. Arai, S.; Morinaga, Y.; Yoshikawa, T.; Ichiishi, E.; KISO, Y.; Yamazaki, M.; Morotomi, M.; Shimizu, M.; Kuwata, T.; Kaminogawa, S. Recent Trends in Functional Food Science and the Industry in Japan. *Biosci. Biotechnol. Biochem.* **2002**, *66*, 2017–2029. [CrossRef] [PubMed]
128. Zhang, L.; Liu, Y. Potential Interventions for Novel Coronavirus in China: A Systematic Review. *J. Med. Virol.* **2020**, *92*, 479–490. [CrossRef] [PubMed]
129. Akintola, C.; Finnegan, D.; Hunt, N.; Lalor, R.; O'Neill, S.; Loscher, C. Nutrition Nutraceuticals: A Proactive Approach for Healthcare. In *Advances in Nutraceuticals and Functional Foods*; Apple Academic Press: Ontario, CA, USA, 2022; pp. 123–172. ISBN 978-1-00-327708-8.
130. Sun, H.; Jenssen, H.; Sun, H.; Jenssen, H. Milk Derived Peptides with Immune Stimulating Antiviral Properties. In *Milk Protein*; IntechOpen: London, UK, 2012.
131. Gallo, V.; Giansanti, F.; Arienzo, A.; Antonini, G. Antiviral Properties of Whey Proteins and Their Activity against SARS-CoV-2 Infection. *J. Funct. Foods* **2022**, *89*, 104932. [CrossRef]
132. Fan, H.; Hong, B.; Luo, Y.; Peng, Q.; Wang, L.; Jin, X.; Chen, Y.; Hu, Y.; Shi, Y.; Li, T.; et al. The Effect of Whey Protein on Viral Infection and Replication of SARS-CoV-2 and Pangolin Coronavirus in Vitro. *Signal Transduct. Target. Ther.* **2020**, *5*, 275. [CrossRef]
133. Chen, Y.; Liu, Q.; Guo, D. Emerging Coronaviruses: Genome Structure, Replication, and Pathogenesis. *J. Med. Virol.* **2020**, *92*, 418–423. [CrossRef] [PubMed]
134. Wajs, J.; Król, K.; Brodziak, A. *Milk and Dairy Products as a Source of Antiviral Compounds*; E-Wydawnictwo. Prawnicza i Ekonomiczna Biblioteka Cyfrowa. Wydział Prawa, Administracji i Ekonomii Uniwersytetu Wrocławskiego: Wroclaw, Poland, 2021. [CrossRef]
135. Senapathi, J.; Bommakanti, A.; Mallepalli, S.; Mukhopadhyay, S.; Kondapi, A.K. Sulfonate Modified Lactoferrin Nanoparticles as Drug Carriers with Dual Activity against HIV-1. *Colloids Surf. B Biointerfaces* **2020**, *191*, 110979. [CrossRef] [PubMed]
136. Legrand, D.; Elass, E.; Carpentier, M.; Mazurier, J. Interactions of Lactoferrin with Cells Involved in Immune FunctionThis Paper Is One of a Selection of Papers Published in This Special Issue, Entitled 7th International Conference on Lactoferrin: Structure, Function, and Applications, and Has Undergone the Journal's Usual Peer Review Process. *Biochem. Cell Biol.* **2006**, *84*, 282–290. [CrossRef] [PubMed]
137. Puddu, P.; Carollo, M.G.; Belardelli, F.; Valenti, P.; Gessani, S. Role of Endogenous Interferon and LPS in the Immunomodulatory Effects of Bovine Lactoferrin in Murine Peritoneal Macrophages. *J. Leukoc. Biol.* **2007**, *82*, 347–353. [CrossRef]
138. Bakhshandeh, B.; Sorboni, S.G.; Javanmard, A.-R.; Mottaghi, S.S.; Mehrabi, M.; Sorouri, F.; Abbasi, A.; Jahanafrooz, Z. Variants in ACE2; Potential Influences on Virus Infection and COVID-19 Severity. *Infect. Genet. Evol.* **2021**, *90*, 104773. [CrossRef]
139. Duan, L.; Zheng, Q.; Zhang, H.; Niu, Y.; Lou, Y.; Wang, H. The SARS-CoV-2 Spike Glycoprotein Biosynthesis, Structure, Function, and Antigenicity: Implications for the Design of Spike-Based Vaccine Immunogens. *Front. Immunol.* **2020**, *11*, 576622. [CrossRef]
140. Serrano, G.; Kochergina, I.; Albors, A.; Diaz, E.; Oroval, M.; Hueso, G.; Serrano, J.M. Liposomal Lactoferrin as Potential Preventative and Cure for COVID-19. *Int. J. Res. Health Sci.* **2020**, *8*, 8–15. [CrossRef]
141. Chang, R.; Ng, T.B.; Sun, W.-Z. Lactoferrin as Potential Preventative and Adjunct Treatment for COVID-19. *Int. J. Antimicrob. Agents* **2020**, *56*, 106118. [CrossRef]
142. Inagaki, M.; Muranishi, H.; Yamada, K.; Kakehi, K.; Uchida, K.; Suzuki, T.; Yabe, T.; Nakagomi, T.; Nakagomi, O.; Kanamaru, Y. Bovine κ-Casein Inhibits Human Rotavirus (HRV) Infection via Direct Binding of Glycans to HRV. *J. Dairy Sci.* **2014**, *97*, 2653–2661. [CrossRef]
143. Wang, H.; Ye, X.; Ng, T.B. First Demonstration of an Inhibitory Activity of Milk Proteins against Human Immunodeficiency Virus-1 Reverse Transcriptase and the Effect of Succinylation. *Life Sci.* **2000**, *67*, 2745–2752. [CrossRef]
144. Ng, T.B.; Ye, X.Y. A Polymeric Immunoglobulin Receptor-like Milk Protein with Inhibitory Activity on Human Immunodeficiency Virus Type 1 Reverse Transcriptase. *Int. J. Biochem. Cell Biol.* **2004**, *36*, 2242–2249. [CrossRef] [PubMed]

45. Ng, T.B.; Cheung, R.C.F.; Wong, J.H.; Wang, Y.; Ip, D.T.M.; Wan, D.C.C.; Xia, J. Antiviral Activities of Whey Proteins. *Appl. Microbiol. Biotechnol.* **2015**, *99*, 6997–7008. [CrossRef] [PubMed]
46. Wang, Y.; Wang, P.; Wang, H.; Luo, Y.; Wan, L.; Jiang, M.; Chu, Y. Lactoferrin for the Treatment of COVID-19 (Review). *Exp. Ther. Med.* **2020**, *20*, 272. [CrossRef]
47. Siqueiros-Cendón, T.; Arévalo-Gallegos, S.; Iglesias-Figueroa, B.F.; García-Montoya, I.A.; Salazar-Martínez, J.; Rascón-Cruz, Q. Immunomodulatory Effects of Lactoferrin. *Acta Pharmacol. Sin.* **2014**, *35*, 557–566. [CrossRef]
48. Hamida, R.S.; Shami, A.; Ali, M.A.; Almohawes, Z.N.; Mohammed, A.E.; Bin-Meferij, M.M. Kefir: A Protective Dietary Supplementation against Viral Infection. *Biomed. Pharmacother.* **2021**, *133*, 110974. [CrossRef] [PubMed]
49. Al Kassaa, I.; Hober, D.; Hamze, M.; Chihib, N.E.; Drider, D. Antiviral Potential of Lactic Acid Bacteria and Their Bacteriocins. *Probiotics Antimicrob. Proteins* **2014**, *6*, 177–185. [CrossRef]
50. Peluzio, M.d.C.G.; Dias, M.d.M.e.; Martinez, J.A.; Milagro, F.I. Kefir and Intestinal Microbiota Modulation: Implications in Human Health. *Front. Nutr.* **2021**, *8*, 638740. [CrossRef]
51. Pražnikar, Z.J.; Kenig, S.; Vardjan, T.; Bizjak, M.Č.; Petelin, A. Effects of Kefir or Milk Supplementation on Zonulin in Overweight Subjects. *J. Dairy Sci.* **2020**, *103*, 3961–3970. [CrossRef]
52. Freitas, M. Chapter 24—The Benefits of Yogurt, Cultures, and Fermentation. In *The Microbiota in Gastrointestinal Pathophysiology*; Floch, M.H., Ringel, Y., Allan Walker, W., Eds.; Academic Press: Boston, MA, USA, 2017; pp. 209–223. ISBN 978-0-12-804024-9.
53. Gouda, A.S.; Adbelruhman, F.G.; Sabbah Alenezi, H.; Mégarbane, B. Theoretical Benefits of Yogurt-Derived Bioactive Peptides and Probiotics in COVID-19 Patients—A Narrative Review and Hypotheses. *Saudi J. Biol. Sci.* **2021**, *28*, 5897–5905. [CrossRef]
54. Pei, R.; Martin, D.A.; DiMarco, D.M.; Bolling, B.W. Evidence for the Effects of Yogurt on Gut Health and Obesity. *Crit. Rev. Food Sci. Nutr.* **2017**, *57*, 1569–1583. [CrossRef]
55. Popovic, N.; Brdarić, E.; Djokic, J.; Dinic, M.; Veljovic, K.; Golić, N.; Terzic-Vidojevic, A. Yogurt Produced by Novel Natural Starter Cultures Improves Gut Epithelial Barrier In Vitro. *Microorganisms* **2020**, *8*, 1586. [CrossRef] [PubMed]
56. Wilkins, T.; Sequoia, J. Probiotics for Gastrointestinal Conditions: A Summary of the Evidence. *Am. Fam. Physician* **2017**, *96*, 170–178. [PubMed]
57. Mohamadshahi, M.; Veissi, M.; Haidari, F.; Shahbazian, H.; Kaydani, G.-A.; Mohammadi, F. Effects of Probiotic Yogurt Consumption on Inflammatory Biomarkers in Patients with Type 2 Diabetes. *Bioimpacts* **2014**, *4*, 83–88. [CrossRef] [PubMed]
58. De Moreno De Leblanc, A.; Chaves, S.; Perdigón, G. Effect of Yoghurt on the Cytokine Profile Using a Murine Model of Intestinal Inflammation. *Eur. J. Inflamm.* **2009**, *7*, 97–109. [CrossRef]
59. Yao, G.; Yu, J.; Hou, Q.; Hui, W.; Liu, W.; Kwok, L.-Y.; Menghe, B.; Sun, T.; Zhang, H.; Zhang, W. A Perspective Study of Koumiss Microbiome by Metagenomics Analysis Based on Single-Cell Amplification Technique. *Front. Microbiol.* **2017**, *8*, 165. [CrossRef] [PubMed]
60. Tang, H.; Ma, H.; Hou, Q.; Li, W.; Xu, H.; Liu, W.; Sun, Z.; Haobisi, H.; Menghe, B. Profiling of Koumiss Microbiota and Organic Acids and Their Effects on Koumiss Taste. *BMC Microbiol.* **2020**, *20*, 85. [CrossRef]
61. Ya, T.; Zhang, Q.; Chu, F.; Merritt, J.; Bilige, M.; Sun, T.; Du, R.; Zhang, H. Immunological Evaluation of Lactobacillus Casei Zhang: A Newly Isolated Strain from Koumiss in Inner Mongolia, China. *BMC Immunol.* **2008**, *9*, 68. [CrossRef]
62. Fukushima, Y.; Kawata, Y.; Hara, H.; Terada, A.; Mitsuoka, T. Effect of a Probiotic Formula on Intestinal Immunoglobulin A Production in Healthy Children. *Int. J. Food Microbiol.* **1998**, *42*, 39–44. [CrossRef]
63. Mathur, H.; Beresford, T.P.; Cotter, P.D. Health Benefits of Lactic Acid Bacteria (LAB) Fermentates. *Nutrients* **2020**, *12*, 1679. [CrossRef]
64. Moyad, M.A.; Robinson, L.E.; Zawada, E.T.; Kittelsrud, J.M.; Chen, D.-G.; Reeves, S.G.; Weaver, S.E. Effects of a Modified Yeast Supplement on Cold/Flu Symptoms. *Urol. Nurs.* **2008**, *28*, 50–55.
65. Moyad, M.A.; Robinson, L.E.; Zawada, E.T.; Kittelsrud, J.; Chen, D.-G.; Reeves, S.G.; Weaver, S. Immunogenic Yeast-Based Fermentate for Cold/Flu-like Symptoms in Nonvaccinated Individuals. *J. Altern. Complement. Med.* **2010**, *16*, 213–218. [CrossRef] [PubMed]
66. Nielsen, M.S.; Martinussen, T.; Flambard, B.; Sørensen, K.I.; Otte, J. Peptide Profiles and Angiotensin-I-Converting Enzyme Inhibitory Activity of Fermented Milk Products: Effect of Bacterial Strain, Fermentation PH, and Storage Time. *Int. Dairy J.* **2009**, *19*, 155–165. [CrossRef]
67. Kırdar, S.S. Therapeutics Effects and Health Benefits of the Caucasus Koumiss: A Review. *Annu. Res. Rev. Biol.* **2021**, *36*, 47–56. [CrossRef]
68. Jiang, L.-L.; Gong, X.; Ji, M.-Y.; Wang, C.-C.; Wang, J.-H.; Li, M.-H. Bioactive Compounds from Plant-Based Functional Foods: A Promising Choice for the Prevention and Management of Hyperuricemia. *Foods* **2020**, *9*, 973. [CrossRef] [PubMed]
69. Ferreira, I.C.F.R.; Morales, P.; Barros, L. *Wild Plants, Mushrooms and Nuts: Functional Food Properties and Applications*; John Wiley & Sons: Hoboken, NJ, USA, 2017; ISBN 978-1-118-94462-2.
70. Jiang, L.; Zhang, G.; Li, Y.; Shi, G.; Li, M. Potential Application of Plant-Based Functional Foods in the Development of Immune Boosters. *Front. Pharmacol.* **2021**, *12*, 637782. [CrossRef]
71. Angeles-Agdeppa, I.; Nacis, J.S.; Capanzana, M.V.; Dayrit, F.M.; Tanda, K.V. Virgin Coconut Oil Is Effective in Lowering C-Reactive Protein Levels among Suspect and Probable Cases of COVID-19. *J. Funct. Foods* **2021**, *83*, 104557. [CrossRef]
72. WebMD Coconut Oil: Is It Good for You? Available online: https://www.webmd.com/diet/coconut-oil-good-for-you (accessed on 3 August 2022).

173. Joshi, S.; Kaushik, V.; Gode, V.; Mhaskar, S. Coconut Oil and Immunity: What Do We Really Know about It so Far? *J. Assoc. Phys. India* **2020**, *68*, 67–72.
174. Intahphuak, S.; Khonsung, P.; Panthong, A. Anti-Inflammatory, Analgesic, and Antipyretic Activities of Virgin Coconut Oil. *Pharm. Biol.* **2010**, *48*, 151–157. [CrossRef]
175. Djurasevic, S.; Bojic, S.; Nikolić, B.; Dimkić, I.; Todorovic, Z.; Djordjevic, J.; Mitić-Ćulafić, D. Beneficial Effect of Virgin Coconut Oil on Alloxan-Induced Diabetes and Microbiota Composition in Rats. *Plant Foods Hum. Nutr.* **2018**, *73*, 295–301. [CrossRef]
176. Yeap, S.K.; Beh, B.K.; Ali, N.M.; Yusof, H.M.; Ho, W.Y.; Koh, S.P.; Alitheen, N.B.; Long, K. Antistress and Antioxidant Effects of Virgin Coconut Oil in Vivo. *Exp. Ther. Med.* **2015**, *9*, 39–42. [CrossRef]
177. Dumancas, G.; Viswanath, L.; Leon, A.; Ramasahayam, S.; Maples, R.; Hikkaduwa Koralege, R.; Don, U.; Perera, U.D.N.; Langford, J.; Shakir, A.; et al. Health Benefits of Virgin Coconut Oil. In *Vegetable Oil: Properties, Uses and Benefits*; Lybrate: Delhi, India, 2016.
178. Widianingrum, D.C.; Noviandi, C.T.; Salasia, S.I.O. Antibacterial and Immunomodulator Activities of Virgin Coconut Oil (VCO) against Staphylococcus Aureus. *Heliyon* **2019**, *5*, e02612. [CrossRef]
179. Varma, S.R.; Sivaprakasam, T.O.; Arumugam, I.; Dilip, N.; Raghuraman, M.; Pavan, K.B.; Rafiq, M.; Paramesh, R. In Vitro Anti-Inflammatory and Skin Protective Properties of Virgin Coconut Oil. *J. Tradit. Complement. Med.* **2018**, *9*, 5–14. [CrossRef]
180. Widhiarta, D.K.D. Virgin Coconut Oil for HIV—Positive People. *CORD* **2016**, *32*, 8. [CrossRef]
181. Silalahi, J.; Rosidah, R.; Yuandani, Y.; Satria, D. Virgin Coconut Oil Modulates Tcd4+ and Tcd8+ Cell Profile of Doxorubicin-Induced Immune-Suppressed Rats. *Asian J. Pharm. Clin. Res.* **2018**, *11*, 37. [CrossRef]
182. Komatsuzaki, N.; Arai, S.; Fujihara, S.; Wijesekara, R. Effect of Intake of Virgin Coconut Oil (*Cocos nucifera* L.) on the Spleen and Small Intestinal Immune Cells and Liver Lipid of Mice. *Ceylon J. Sci.* **2021**, *50*, 103. [CrossRef]
183. Link, R. Why Extra Virgin Olive Oil Is the Healthiest Fat on Earth. Available online: https://www.healthline.com/nutrition/extra-virgin-olive-oil (accessed on 3 August 2022).
184. Omar, S.H. Oleuropein in Olive and Its Pharmacological Effects. *Sci. Pharm.* **2010**, *78*, 133–154. [CrossRef] [PubMed]
185. Jimenez-Lopez, C.; Carpena, M.; Lourenço-Lopes, C.; Gallardo-Gomez, M.; Lorenzo, J.M.; Barba, F.J.; Prieto, M.A.; Simal-Gandara, J. Bioactive Compounds and Quality of Extra Virgin Olive Oil. *Foods* **2020**, *9*, 1014. [CrossRef]
186. Vrdoljak, J.; Kumric, M.; Vilovic, M.; Martinovic, D.; Tomic, I.J.; Krnic, M.; Ticinovic Kurir, T.; Bozic, J. Effects of Olive Oil and Its Components on Intestinal Inflammation and Inflammatory Bowel Disease. *Nutrients* **2022**, *14*, 757. [CrossRef]
187. Fredrickson, W.R. *Method and Composition for Antiviral Therapy*; World Intellectual Property Organization: Geneva, Switzerland, 2000.
188. Olalla, J.; García de Lomas, J.M.; Chueca, N.; Pérez-Stachowski, X.; De Salazar, A.; Del Arco, A.; Plaza-Díaz, J.; De la Torre, J.; Prada, J.L.; García-Alegría, J.; et al. Effect of Daily Consumption of Extra Virgin Olive Oil on the Lipid Profile and Microbiota of HIV-Infected Patients over 50 Years of Age. *Medicine* **2019**, *98*, e17528. [CrossRef]
189. Kozić Dokmanović, S.; Kolovrat, K.; Laškaj, R.; Jukić, V.; Vrkić, N.; Begovac, J. Effect of Extra Virgin Olive Oil on Biomarkers of Inflammation in HIV-Infected Patients: A Randomized, Crossover, Controlled Clinical Trial. *Med. Sci. Monit. Int. Med. J. Exp. Clin. Res.* **2015**, *21*, 2406. [CrossRef]
190. Millman, J.F.; Okamoto, S.; Teruya, T.; Uema, T.; Ikematsu, S.; Shimabukuro, M.; Masuzaki, H. Extra-Virgin Olive Oil and the Gut-Brain Axis: Influence on Gut Microbiota, Mucosal Immunity, and Cardiometabolic and Cognitive Health. *Nutr. Rev.* **2021**, *79*, 1362–1374. [CrossRef] [PubMed]
191. Martín-Peláez, S.; Castañer, O.; Solà, R.; Motilva, M.J.; Castell, M.; Pérez-Cano, F.J.; Fitó, M. Influence of Phenol-Enriched Olive Oils on Human Intestinal Immune Function. *Nutrients* **2016**, *8*, 213. [CrossRef]
192. Alvarez-Laderas, I.; Ramos, T.L.; Medrano, M.; Caracuel-García, R.; Barbado, M.V.; Sánchez-Hidalgo, M.; Zamora, R.; Alarcón-de-la-Lastra, C.; Hidalgo, F.J.; Piruat, J.I.; et al. Polyphenolic Extract (PE) from Olive Oil Exerts a Potent Immunomodulatory Effect and Prevents Graft-versus-Host Disease in a Mouse Model. *Biol. Blood Marrow Transplant.* **2020**, *26*, 615–624. [CrossRef] [PubMed]
193. Selverajah, M.; Zakaria, Z.A.; Long, K.; Ahmad, Z.; Yaacob, A.; Somchit, M.N. Anti-Ulcerogenic Activity of Virgin Coconut Oil Contribute to the Stomach Health of Humankind. *CELLMED* **2016**, *6*, 11.1–11.7. [CrossRef]
194. Tangney, C.C.; Rasmussen, H.E. Polyphenols, Inflammation, and Cardiovascular Disease. *Curr. Atheroscler. Rep.* **2013**, *15*, 324. [CrossRef] [PubMed]
195. Menicacci, B.; Cipriani, C.; Margheri, F.; Mocali, A.; Giovannelli, L. Modulation of the Senescence-Associated Inflammatory Phenotype in Human Fibroblasts by Olive Phenols. *Int. J. Mol. Sci.* **2017**, *18*, 2275. [CrossRef]
196. Serra, G.; Incani, A.; Serreli, G.; Porru, L.; Melis, M.P.; Tuberoso, C.I.G.; Rossin, D.; Biasi, F.; Deiana, M. Olive Oil Polyphenols Reduce Oxysterols -Induced Redox Imbalance and pro-Inflammatory Response in Intestinal Cells. *Redox Biol.* **2018**, *17*, 348–354. [CrossRef]
197. Hathaway, D.; Pandav, K.; Patel, M.; Riva-Moscoso, A.; Singh, B.M.; Patel, A.; Min, Z.C.; Singh-Makkar, S.; Sana, M.K.; Sanchez-Dopazo, R.; et al. Omega 3 Fatty Acids and COVID-19: A Comprehensive Review. *Infect. Chemother.* **2020**, *52*, 478–495. [CrossRef]
198. Chiang, N.; Serhan, C.N. Specialized Pro-Resolving Mediator Network: An Update on Production and Actions. *Essays Biochem.* **2020**, *64*, 443–462. [CrossRef]
199. Arnardottir, H.; Pawelzik, S.-C.; Öhlund Wistbacka, U.; Artiach, G.; Hofmann, R.; Reinholdsson, I.; Braunschweig, F.; Tornvall, P.; Religa, D.; Bäck, M. Stimulating the Resolution of Inflammation Through Omega-3 Polyunsaturated Fatty Acids in COVID-19: Rationale for the COVID-Omega-F Trial. *Front. Physiol.* **2021**, *11*, 1748. [CrossRef]

200. Calder, P.C. Marine Omega-3 Fatty Acids and Inflammatory Processes: Effects, Mechanisms and Clinical Relevance. *Biochim. Biophys. Acta* **2015**, *1851*, 469–484. [CrossRef] [PubMed]
201. Zhu, X.; Bi, Z.; Yang, C.; Guo, Y.; Yuan, J.; Li, L.; Guo, Y. Effects of Different Doses of Omega-3 Polyunsaturated Fatty Acids on Gut Microbiota and Immunity. *Food Nutr. Res.* **2021**, *65*. [CrossRef] [PubMed]
202. Eslamloo, K.; Xue, X.; Hall, J.R.; Smith, N.C.; Caballero-Solares, A.; Parrish, C.C.; Taylor, R.G.; Rise, M.L. Transcriptome Profiling of Antiviral Immune and Dietary Fatty Acid Dependent Responses of Atlantic Salmon Macrophage-like Cells. *BMC Genom.* **2017**, *18*, 706. [CrossRef] [PubMed]
203. Willemsen, L.E.M.; Koetsier, M.A.; Balvers, M.; Beermann, C.; Stahl, B.; van Tol, E.A.F. Polyunsaturated Fatty Acids Support Epithelial Barrier Integrity and Reduce IL-4 Mediated Permeability in Vitro. *Eur. J. Nutr.* **2008**, *47*, 183–191. [CrossRef]
204. Hillier, K.; Jewell, R.; Dorrell, L.; Smith, C.L. Incorporation of Fatty Acids from Fish Oil and Olive Oil into Colonic Mucosal Lipids and Effects upon Eicosanoid Synthesis in Inflammatory Bowel Disease. *Gut* **1991**, *32*, 1151–1155. [CrossRef]
205. Bellenger, J.; Bellenger, S.; Bourragat, A.; Escoula, Q.; Weill, P.; Narce, M. Intestinal Microbiota Mediates the Beneficial Effects of N-3 Polyunsaturated Fatty Acids during Dietary Obesity. *OCL* **2021**, *28*, 21. [CrossRef]
206. Watson, H.; Mitra, S.; Croden, F.C.; Taylor, M.; Wood, H.M.; Perry, S.L.; Spencer, J.A.; Quirke, P.; Toogood, G.J.; Lawton, C.L.; et al. A Randomised Trial of the Effect of Omega-3 Polyunsaturated Fatty Acid Supplements on the Human Intestinal Microbiota. *Gut* **2018**, *67*, 1974–1983. [CrossRef]
207. Costantini, L.; Molinari, R.; Farinon, B.; Merendino, N. Impact of Omega-3 Fatty Acids on the Gut Microbiota. *Int. J. Mol. Sci.* **2017**, *18*, 2645. [CrossRef]
208. Rivollier, A.; He, J.; Kole, A.; Valatas, V.; Kelsall, B.L. Inflammation Switches the Differentiation Program of Ly6Chi Monocytes from Antiinflammatory Macrophages to Inflammatory Dendritic Cells in the Colon. *J. Exp. Med.* **2012**, *209*, 139–155. [CrossRef]
209. Jackiewicz, A.; Czarnecki, M.; Knysz, B. Effect of Diet on Lipid Profile in HIV-Infected Patients. *HIV AIDS Rev.* **2018**, *17*, 159–163. [CrossRef]
210. Imai, Y. Role of Omega-3 PUFA-Derived Mediators, the Protectins, in Influenza Virus Infection. *Biochim. Biophys. Acta (BBA)—Mol. Cell Biol. Lipids* **2015**, *1851*, 496–502. [CrossRef] [PubMed]
211. Darwesh, A.M.; Bassiouni, W.; Sosnowski, D.K.; Seubert, J.M. Can N-3 Polyunsaturated Fatty Acids Be Considered a Potential Adjuvant Therapy for COVID-19-Associated Cardiovascular Complications? *Pharmacol. Ther.* **2021**, *219*, 107703. [CrossRef]
212. Thul, S.; Labat, C.; Temmar, M.; Benetos, A.; Bäck, M. Low Salivary Resolvin D1 to Leukotriene B4 Ratio Predicts Carotid Intima Media Thickness: A Novel Biomarker of Non-Resolving Vascular Inflammation. *Eur. J. Prev. Cardiol.* **2017**, *24*, 903–906. [CrossRef] [PubMed]
213. Calder, P.C.; Bosco, N.; Bourdet-Sicard, R.; Capuron, L.; Delzenne, N.; Doré, J.; Franceschi, C.; Lehtinen, M.J.; Recker, T.; Salvioli, S.; et al. Health Relevance of the Modification of Low Grade Inflammation in Ageing (Inflammageing) and the Role of Nutrition. *Ageing Res. Rev.* **2017**, *40*, 95–119. [CrossRef] [PubMed]
214. Mullen, A.; Loscher, C.E.; Roche, H.M. Anti-Inflammatory Effects of EPA and DHA Are Dependent upon Time and Dose-Response Elements Associated with LPS Stimulation in THP-1-Derived Macrophages. *J. Nutr. Biochem.* **2010**, *21*, 444–450. [CrossRef]
215. Draper, E.; Reynolds, C.M.; Canavan, M.; Mills, K.H.; Loscher, C.E.; Roche, H.M. Omega-3 Fatty Acids Attenuate Dendritic Cell Function via NF-KB Independent of PPARγ. *J. Nutr. Biochem.* **2011**, *22*, 784–790. [CrossRef]
216. Endres, S.; Meydani, S.N.; Ghorbani, R.; Schindler, R.; Dinarello, C.A. Dietary Supplementation with N-3 Fatty Acids Suppresses Interleukin-2 Production and Mononuclear Cell Proliferation. *J. Leukoc. Biol.* **1993**, *54*, 599–603. [CrossRef]
217. Meydani, S.N.; Endres, S.; Woods, M.M.; Goldin, B.R.; Soo, C.; Morrill-Labrode, A.; Dinarello, C.A.; Gorbach, S.L. Oral (n-3) Fatty Acid Supplementation Suppresses Cytokine Production and Lymphocyte Proliferation: Comparison between Young and Older Women. *J. Nutr.* **1991**, *121*, 547–555. [CrossRef]
218. Kim, W.; Khan, N.A.; McMurray, D.N.; Prior, I.A.; Wang, N.; Chapkin, R.S. Regulatory Activity of Polyunsaturated Fatty Acids in T-Cell Signaling. *Prog. Lipid Res.* **2010**, *49*, 250–261. [CrossRef]
219. Mizota, T.; Fujita-Kambara, C.; Matsuya, N.; Hamasaki, S.; Fukudome, T.; Goto, H.; Nakane, S.; Kondo, T.; Matsuo, H. Effect of Dietary Fatty Acid Composition on Th1/Th2 Polarization in Lymphocytes. *JPEN J. Parenter. Enter. Nutr.* **2009**, *33*, 390–396. [CrossRef]
220. Cao, W.; Wang, C.; Chin, Y.; Chen, X.; Gao, Y.; Yuan, S.; Xue, C.; Wang, Y.; Tang, Q. DHA-Phospholipids (DHA-PL) and EPA-Phospholipids (EPA-PL) Prevent Intestinal Dysfunction Induced by Chronic Stress. *Food Funct.* **2019**, *10*, 277–288. [CrossRef] [PubMed]
221. Weldon, S.M.; Mullen, A.C.; Loscher, C.E.; Hurley, L.A.; Roche, H.M. Docosahexaenoic Acid Induces an Anti-Inflammatory Profile in Lipopolysaccharide-Stimulated Human THP-1 Macrophages More Effectively than Eicosapentaenoic Acid. *J. Nutr. Biochem.* **2007**, *18*, 250–258. [CrossRef] [PubMed]
222. Dennis, E.A.; Norris, P.C. Eicosanoid Storm in Infection and Inflammation. *Nat. Rev. Immunol.* **2015**, *15*, 511–523. [CrossRef]
223. Hammock, B.D.; Wang, W.; Gilligan, M.M.; Panigrahy, D. Eicosanoids: The Overlooked Storm in Coronavirus Disease 2019 (COVID-19)? *Am. J. Pathol.* **2020**, *190*, 1782–1788. [CrossRef]
224. Calder, P.C. Omega-3 Fatty Acids and Inflammatory Processes: From Molecules to Man. *Biochem. Soc. Trans.* **2017**, *45*, 1105–1115. [CrossRef]
225. Health Service Executive. Vitamins and Minerals—Vitamin D. Available online: https://www2.hse.ie/conditions/vitamins-and-minerals/vitamin-d/ (accessed on 4 July 2022).

226. National Institute of Health Office of Dietary Supplements. Vitamin D. Available online: https://ods.od.nih.gov/factsheets/VitaminD-Consumer/ (accessed on 4 July 2022).
227. Aranow, C. Vitamin D and the Immune System. *J. Investig. Med.* **2011**, *59*, 881–886. [CrossRef]
228. Faul, J.L.; Kerley, C.P.; Love, B.; O'Neill, E.; Cody, C.; Tormey, W.; Hutchinson, K.; Cormican, L.J.; Burke, C.M. Vitamin D Deficiency and ARDS after SARS-CoV-2 Infection. *Ir. Med. J.* **2021**, *113*, 84.
229. McCartney, D.M.; Byrne, D.G. Optimisation of Vitamin D Status for Enhanced Immuno-Protection against COVID-19. *Ir. Med. J.* **2020**, *113*, 58. [PubMed]
230. Walsh, L. Please Take Vitamin D to Protect against COVID-19, Say Irish Experts. Available online: https://www.breakingnews.ie/ireland/please-take-vitamin-d-to-protect-against-covid-19-say-irish-experts-1069537.html (accessed on 4 July 2022).
231. Sundararaman, A.; Ray, M.; Ravindra, P.V.; Halami, P.M. Role of Probiotics to Combat Viral Infections with Emphasis on COVID-19. *Appl. Microbiol. Biotechnol.* **2020**, *104*, 8089–8104. [CrossRef] [PubMed]
232. Zhang, Y.-G.; Wu, S.; Sun, J. Vitamin D, Vitamin D Receptor, and Tissue Barriers. *Tissue Barriers* **2013**, *1*, e23118. [CrossRef]
233. Battistini, C.; Ballan, R.; Herkenhoff, M.E.; Saad, S.M.I.; Sun, J. Vitamin D Modulates Intestinal Microbiota in Inflammatory Bowel Diseases. *Int. J. Mol. Sci.* **2021**, *22*, 362. [CrossRef]
234. Zhang, Y.-G.; Lu, R.; Xia, Y.; Zhou, D.; Petrof, E.; Claud, E.C.; Sun, J. Lack of Vitamin D Receptor Leads to Hyperfunction of Claudin-2 in Intestinal Inflammatory Responses. *Inflamm. Bowel Dis.* **2019**, *25*, 97–110. [CrossRef]
235. Wang, J.; Thingholm, L.B.; Skiecevičienė, J.; Rausch, P.; Kummen, M.; Hov, J.R.; Degenhardt, F.; Heinsen, F.-A.; Rühlemann, M.C.; Szymczak, S.; et al. Genome-Wide Association Analysis Identifies Variation in Vitamin D Receptor and Other Host Factors Influencing the Gut Microbiota. *Nat. Genet.* **2016**, *48*, 1396–1406. [CrossRef]
236. Rigby, W.F.; Denome, S.; Fanger, M.W. Regulation of Lymphokine Production and Human T Lymphocyte Activation by 1,25-Dihydroxyvitamin D3. Specific Inhibition at the Level of Messenger RNA. *J. Clin. Investig.* **1987**, *79*, 1659–1664. [CrossRef] [PubMed]
237. Lim, W.-C.; Hanauer, S.B.; Li, Y.C. Mechanisms of Disease: Vitamin D and Inflammatory Bowel Disease. *Nat. Rev. Gastroenterol. Hepatol.* **2005**, *2*, 308–315. [CrossRef] [PubMed]
238. Chen, S.; Sims, G.P.; Chen, X.X.; Gu, Y.Y.; Chen, S.; Lipsky, P.E. Modulatory Effects of 1,25-Dihydroxyvitamin D3 on Human B Cell Differentiation. *J. Immunol.* **2007**, *179*, 1634–1647. [CrossRef]
239. Gammoh, N.Z.; Rink, L. Zinc in Infection and Inflammation. *Nutrients* **2017**, *9*, 624. [CrossRef] [PubMed]
240. National Institute of Health Office of Dietary Supplements. Zinc. Available online: https://ods.od.nih.gov/factsheets/Zinc-HealthProfessional/ (accessed on 4 July 2022).
241. Liu, M.-J.; Bao, S.; Bolin, E.R.; Burris, D.L.; Xu, X.; Sun, Q.; Killilea, D.W.; Shen, Q.; Ziouzenkova, O.; Belury, M.A.; et al. Zinc Deficiency Augments Leptin Production and Exacerbates Macrophage Infiltration into Adipose Tissue in Mice Fed a High-Fat Diet123. *J. Nutr.* **2013**, *143*, 1036–1045. [CrossRef]
242. Siva, S.; Rubin, D.T.; Gulotta, G.; Wroblewski, K.; Pekow, J. Zinc Deficiency Is Associated with Poor Clinical Outcomes in Patients with Inflammatory Bowel Disease. *Inflamm. Bowel Dis.* **2017**, *23*, 152–157. [CrossRef]
243. Read, S.A.; Obeid, S.; Ahlenstiel, C.; Ahlenstiel, G. The Role of Zinc in Antiviral Immunity. *Adv. Nutr.* **2019**, *10*, 696–710. [CrossRef]
244. World Health Organization. The World Health Report 2002. *Midwifery* **2003**, *19*, 72–73. [CrossRef]
245. Wessels, I.; Rolles, B.; Rink, L. The Potential Impact of Zinc Supplementation on COVID-19 Pathogenesis. *Front. Immunol.* **2020**, *11*, 1712. [CrossRef] [PubMed]
246. de Almeida Brasiel, P.G. The Key Role of Zinc in Elderly Immunity: A Possible Approach in the COVID-19 Crisis. *Clin. Nutr. ESPEN* **2020**, *38*, 65–66. [CrossRef] [PubMed]
247. Ibs, K.-H.; Rink, L. Zinc-Altered Immune Function. *J. Nutr.* **2003**, *133*, 1452S–1456S. [CrossRef] [PubMed]
248. Skrovanek, S.; DiGuilio, K.; Bailey, R.; Huntington, W.; Urbas, R.; Mayilvaganan, B.; Mercogliano, G.; Mullin, J.M. Zinc and Gastrointestinal Disease. *World J. Gastrointest. Pathophysiol.* **2014**, *5*, 496–513. [CrossRef]
249. Finamore, A.; Massimi, M.; Conti Devirgiliis, L.; Mengheri, E. Zinc Deficiency Induces Membrane Barrier Damage and Increases Neutrophil Transmigration in Caco-2 Cells. *J. Nutr.* **2008**, *138*, 1664–1670. [CrossRef]
250. Baum, M.K.; Lai, S.; Sales, S.; Page, J.B.; Campa, A. Randomized Controlled Clinical Trial of Zinc Supplementation to Prevent Immunological Failure in HIV-Positive Adults. *Clin. Infect. Dis.* **2010**, *50*, 1653–1660. [CrossRef]
251. Fenstermacher, K.J.; DeStefano, J.J. Mechanism of HIV Reverse Transcriptase Inhibition by Zinc. *J. Biol. Chem.* **2011**, *286*, 40433–40442. [CrossRef]
252. te Velthuis, A.J.W.; van den Worm, S.H.E.; Sims, A.C.; Baric, R.S.; Snijder, E.J.; van Hemert, M.J. Zn(2+) Inhibits Coronavirus and Arterivirus RNA Polymerase Activity in Vitro and Zinc Ionophores Block the Replication of These Viruses in Cell Culture. *PLoS Pathog.* **2010**, *6*, e1001176. [CrossRef]
253. Haase, H.; Rink, L. Zinc Signals and Immune Function. *BioFactors* **2014**, *40*, 27–40. [CrossRef]
254. Hasegawa, H.; Suzuki, K.; Suzuki, K.; Nakaji, S.; Sugawara, K. Effects of Zinc on the Reactive Oxygen Species Generating Capacity of Human Neutrophils and on the Serum Opsonic Activity in Vitro. *Luminescence* **2000**, *15*, 321–327. [CrossRef] [PubMed]
255. Skalny, A.V.; Rink, L.; Ajsuvakova, O.P.; Aschner, M.; Gritsenko, V.A.; Alekseenko, S.I.; Svistunov, A.A.; Petrakis, D.; Spandidos, D.A.; Aaseth, J.; et al. Zinc and Respiratory Tract Infections: Perspectives for COVID-19 (Review). *Int. J. Mol. Med.* **2020**, *46*, 17–26. [CrossRef]

56. Wessels, I.; Rink, L. Micronutrients in Autoimmune Diseases: Possible Therapeutic Benefits of Zinc and Vitamin D. *J. Nutr. Biochem.* **2020**, *77*, 108240. [CrossRef] [PubMed]
57. Guan, W.; Ni, Z.; Hu, Y.; Liang, W.; Ou, C.; He, J.; Liu, L.; Shan, H.; Lei, C.; Hui, D.S.C.; et al. Clinical Characteristics of Coronavirus Disease 2019 in China. *N. Engl. J. Med.* **2020**, *382*, 1708–1720. [CrossRef]
58. Iñigo-Figueroa, G.; Maldonado-Fonllem, G.; Quihui-Cota, L.; Mendez-Estrada, R.O.; Velasquez-Contreras, C.; Canett-Romero, R.; Rascon-Duran, L.; Garibay-Escobar, A.; Robles-Zepeda, R.; Astiazaran-Garcia, H. The Effect of Dietary Zinc Level over the IgG Response in a Murine Model of Giardiasis. *FASEB J.* **2012**, *26*, 1027.12. [CrossRef]
59. Kieliszek, M.; Błażejak, S. Selenium: Significance, and Outlook for Supplementation. *Nutrition* **2013**, *29*, 713–718. [CrossRef]
60. Ross, A.C.; Caballero, B.H.; Cousins, R.J.; Tucker, K.L.; Ziegler, T.R. *Modern Nutrition in Health and Disease*, 11th ed.; Wolters Kluwer Health Adis (ESP): Waltham, MA, USA, 2012; ISBN 978-1-60547-461-8.
61. Majeed, M.; Nagabhushanam, K.; Gowda, S.; Mundkur, L. An Exploratory Study of Selenium Status in Healthy Individuals and in Patients with COVID-19 in a South Indian Population: The Case for Adequate Selenium Status. *Nutrition* **2021**, *82*, 111053. [CrossRef]
62. Rayman, M.P. Selenium and Human Health. *Lancet* **2012**, *379*, 1256–1268. [CrossRef]
63. Speckmann, B.; Steinbrenner, H. Selenium and Selenoproteins in Inflammatory Bowel Diseases and Experimental Colitis. *Inflamm. Bowel Dis.* **2014**, *20*, 1110–1119. [CrossRef]
64. Wang, Y.; Gao, X.; Pedram, P.; Shahidi, M.; Du, J.; Yi, Y.; Gulliver, W.; Zhang, H.; Sun, G. Significant Beneficial Association of High Dietary Selenium Intake with Reduced Body Fat in the CODING Study. *Nutrients* **2016**, *8*, 24. [CrossRef]
65. Liu, K.; Zhao, Y.; Chen, F.; Gu, Z.; Bu, G. Enhanced Glutathione Peroxidases (GPx) Activity in Young Barley Seedlings Enriched with Selenium. *Afr. J. Biotechnol.* **2011**, *10*, 11482–11487. [CrossRef]
66. Hrdina, J.; Banning, A.; Kipp, A.; Loh, G.; Blaut, M.; Brigelius-Flohé, R. The Gastrointestinal Microbiota Affects the Selenium Status and Selenoprotein Expression in Mice. *J. Nutr. Biochem.* **2009**, *20*, 638–648. [CrossRef]
67. Zhai, Q.; Cen, S.; Li, P.; Tian, F.; Zhao, J.; Zhang, H.; Chen, W. Effects of Dietary Selenium Supplementation on Intestinal Barrier and Immune Responses Associated with Its Modulation of Gut Microbiota. *Environ. Sci. Technol. Lett.* **2018**, *5*, 724–730. [CrossRef]
68. Kasaikina, M.V.; Kravtsova, M.A.; Cheon Lee, B.; Seravalli, J.; Peterson, D.A.; Walter, J.; Legge, R.; Benson, A.K.; Hatfield, D.L.; Gladyshev, V.N. Dietary Selenium Affects Host Selenoproteome Expression by Influencing the Gut Microbiota. *FASEB J.* **2011**, *25*, 2492–2499. [CrossRef] [PubMed]
69. Ribière, C.; Peyret, P.; Parisot, N.; Darcha, C.; Déchelotte, P.J.; Barnich, N.; Peyretaillade, E.; Boucher, D. Oral Exposure to Environmental Pollutant Benzo[a]Pyrene Impacts the Intestinal Epithelium and Induces Gut Microbial Shifts in Murine Model. *Sci. Rep.* **2016**, *6*, 31027. [CrossRef] [PubMed]
70. Saulnier, D.M.; Riehle, K.; Mistretta, T.; Diaz, M.; Mandal, D.; Raza, S.; Weidler, E.M.; Qin, X.; Coarfa, C.; Milosavljevic, A.; et al. Gastrointestinal Microbiome Signatures of Pediatric Patients With Irritable Bowel Syndrome. *Gastroenterology* **2011**, *141*, 1782–1791. [CrossRef]
71. Lin, Y.; Jiang, L.-Q. Research Progress on the Immunomodulatory Effect of Trace Element Selenium and Its Effect on Immune-Related Diseases. *Food Ther. Health Care* **2020**, *2*, 86–98. [CrossRef]
72. Martinez, S.S.; Huang, Y.; Acuna, L.; Laverde, E.; Trujillo, D.; Barbieri, M.A.; Tamargo, J.; Campa, A.; Baum, M.K. Role of Selenium in Viral Infections with a Major Focus on SARS-CoV-2. *Int. J. Mol. Sci.* **2021**, *23*, 280. [CrossRef]
73. Lubos, E.; Kelly, N.J.; Oldebeken, S.R.; Leopold, J.A.; Zhang, Y.-Y.; Loscalzo, J.; Handy, D.E. Glutathione Peroxidase-1 Deficiency Augments Proinflammatory Cytokine-Induced Redox Signaling and Human Endothelial Cell Activation. *J. Biol. Chem.* **2011**, *286*, 35407–35417. [CrossRef]
74. Guillin, O.M.; Vindry, C.; Ohlmann, T.; Chavatte, L. Selenium, Selenoproteins and Viral Infection. *Nutrients* **2019**, *11*, E2101. [CrossRef]
75. Stone, C.A.; Kawai, K.; Kupka, R.; Fawzi, W.W. The Role of Selenium in HIV Infection Cosby A Stone, Kosuke Kawai, Roland Kupka, Wafaie W Fawzi Harvard School of Public Health. *Nutr. Rev.* **2010**, *68*, 671–681. [CrossRef]
76. Khan, M.S.; Dilawar, S.; Ali, I.; Rauf, N. The Possible Role of Selenium Concentration in Hepatitis B and C Patients. *Saudi J. Gastroenterol.* **2012**, *18*, 106–110. [CrossRef]
77. Kieliszek, M.; Lipinski, B. Selenium Supplementation in the Prevention of Coronavirus Infections (COVID-19). *Med. Hypotheses* **2020**, *143*, 109878. [CrossRef] [PubMed]
78. Diwaker, D.; Mishra, K.P.; Ganju, L. Potential Roles of Protein Disulphide Isomerase in Viral Infections. *Acta Virol.* **2013**, *57*, 293–304. [PubMed]
79. Zhang, J.; Taylor, E.W.; Bennett, K.; Saad, R.; Rayman, M.P. Association between Regional Selenium Status and Reported Outcome of COVID-19 Cases in China. *Am. J. Clin. Nutr.* **2020**, *111*, 1297–1299. [CrossRef] [PubMed]
80. Moghaddam, A.; Heller, R.A.; Sun, Q.; Seelig, J.; Cherkezov, A.; Seibert, L.; Hackler, J.; Seemann, P.; Diegmann, J.; Pilz, M.; et al. Selenium Deficiency Is Associated with Mortality Risk from COVID-19. *Nutrients* **2020**, *12*, 2098. [CrossRef]
81. Hirano, T.; Murakami, M. COVID-19: A New Virus, but a Familiar Receptor and Cytokine Release Syndrome. *Immunity* **2020**, *52*, 731–733. [CrossRef]
82. Hiffler, L.; Rakotoambinina, B. Selenium and RNA Virus Interactions: Potential Implications for SARS-CoV-2 Infection (COVID-19). *Front. Nutr.* **2020**, *7*, 164. [CrossRef]

283. Khoso, P.A.; Yang, Z.; Liu, C.; Li, S. Selenium Deficiency Downregulates Selenoproteins and Suppresses Immune Function in Chicken Thymus. *Biol. Trace Elem. Res.* **2015**, *167*, 48–55. [CrossRef]
284. Zhang, Z.; Gao, X.; Cao, Y.; Jiang, H.; Wang, T.; Song, X.; Guo, M.; Zhang, N. Selenium Deficiency Facilitates Inflammation Through the Regulation of TLR4 and TLR4-Related Signaling Pathways in the Mice Uterus. *Inflammation* **2015**, *38*, 1347–1356. [CrossRef]
285. Kaushal, N.; Kudva, A.K.; Patterson, A.D.; Chiaro, C.; Kennett, M.J.; Desai, D.; Amin, S.; Carlson, B.A.; Cantorna, M.T.; Prabhu, K.S. Crucial Role of Macrophage Selenoproteins in Experimental Colitis. *J. Immunol.* **2014**, *193*, 3683–3692. [CrossRef] [PubMed]

Disclaimer/Publisher's Note: The statements, opinions and data contained in all publications are solely those of the individual author(s) and contributor(s) and not of MDPI and/or the editor(s). MDPI and/or the editor(s) disclaim responsibility for any injury to people or property resulting from any ideas, methods, instructions or products referred to in the content.

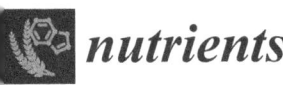

Review

The Role of Diet and Nutrition in Allergic Diseases

Ping Zhang

Center for Integrative Conservation, Yunnan Key Laboratory for the Conservation of Tropical Rainforests and Asian Elephants, Xishuangbanna Tropical Botanical Garden, Chinese Academy of Sciences, Xishuangbanna 6663030, China; zhangping@xtbg.org.cn

Abstract: Allergic diseases are a set of chronic inflammatory disorders of lung, skin, and nose epithelium characterized by aberrant IgE and Th2 cytokine-mediated immune responses to exposed allergens. The prevalence of allergic diseases, including asthma, allergic rhinitis, and atopic dermatitis, has increased dramatically worldwide in the past several decades. Evidence suggests that diet and nutrition play a key role in the development and severity of allergic diseases. Dietary components can differentially regulate allergic inflammation pathways through host and gut microbiota-derived metabolites, therefore influencing allergy outcomes in positive or negative ways. A broad range of nutrients and dietary components (vitamins A, D, and E, minerals Zn, Iron, and Se, dietary fiber, fatty acids, and phytochemicals) are found to be effective in the prevention or treatment of allergic diseases through the suppression of type 2 inflammation. This paper aims to review recent advances in the role of diet and nutrition in the etiology of allergies, nutritional regulation of allergic inflammation, and clinical findings about nutrient supplementation in treating allergic diseases. The current literature suggests the potential efficacy of plant-based diets in reducing allergic symptoms. Further clinical trials are warranted to examine the potential beneficial effects of plant-based diets and anti-allergic nutrients in the prevention and management of allergic diseases.

Keywords: allergy; allergic inflammation; asthma; allergic rhinitis; atopic dermatitis; dietary lipids; dietary fiber; dietary flavonoids; micronutrients

Citation: Zhang, P. The Role of Diet and Nutrition in Allergic Diseases. *Nutrients* 2023, *15*, 3683. https://doi.org/10.3390/nu15173683

Academic Editor: Jon A. Vanderhoof

Received: 30 July 2023
Revised: 17 August 2023
Accepted: 20 August 2023
Published: 22 August 2023

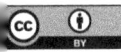

Copyright: © 2023 by the author. Licensee MDPI, Basel, Switzerland. This article is an open access article distributed under the terms and conditions of the Creative Commons Attribution (CC BY) license (https://creativecommons.org/licenses/by/4.0/).

1. Introduction

Allergic diseases are a set of disorders caused by aberrant IgE-mediated immune responses to exposed allergens, resulting in clinical symptoms such as red itchy eyes, sneezing, nasal congestion, rhinorrhea, coughing, and itchy swollen skin [1]. The prevalence of allergic diseases, including asthma, allergic rhinitis (AR), and atopic dermatitis (AD), is high in developed countries [2–4], and the dramatically increased incidence of allergic diseases in developing countries may be due to a shift in lifestyle towards Western customs [5,6]. In allergic diseases, a complex interaction between genetic and environmental factors leads to abnormal immune responses at barrier sites in the body [2–4]. The Western diet is recognized as an environmental risk factor for developing allergic diseases [4–6], whereas the Mediterranean diet has been found to be protective [5,7,8]. Therefore, due to the opposite effects in allergic reactions conferred by different dietary components, diets with different nutrient compositions and varied amounts of specific nutrients either promote sensitization and exacerbate disease severity or protect against allergic diseases and attenuate disease progression. There has been growing interest in dissecting the connection between nutrients, their metabolites, and immune tolerance in allergic conditions.

Apart from diet and nutrition, gut microbiota has recently been linked with allergic diseases [9,10]. Diet and food components play critical roles in shaping the gut microbiota, which is essential in maintaining the integrity of the gut epithelial barrier and gut immune homeostasis [11,12]. Moreover, nutrients and their endogenous or bacterial metabolites can regulate allergic inflammation in distant organs beyond the gut, such as the lung and skin through the gut–lung and gut–skin axes [13,14]. Among bacterial metabolites, short-chain fatty acids (SCFAs), bile acid conjugates, and tryptophan metabolites are the most studied compounds with the ability to modify allergic reactions [8,13,14]. Multiple cells including epithelial cells, stromal cells, sensory nerve cells, and various immune cells are involved in a typical allergic reaction with a signature Th2 cytokine profile and allergic inflammatory mediators including histamines, prostaglandins, and leukotrienes [2–4]. Nutrients and their metabolites can regulate the metabolism and function of both structural cells and various immune cells in all stages of allergic inflammation by altering the membrane lipid composition, key signal transduction pathways related to inflammation and metabolism, and gene expression at the transcriptional level through epigenetic regulation. The impacts of dietary components on allergic reactions are illustrated in Figure 1.

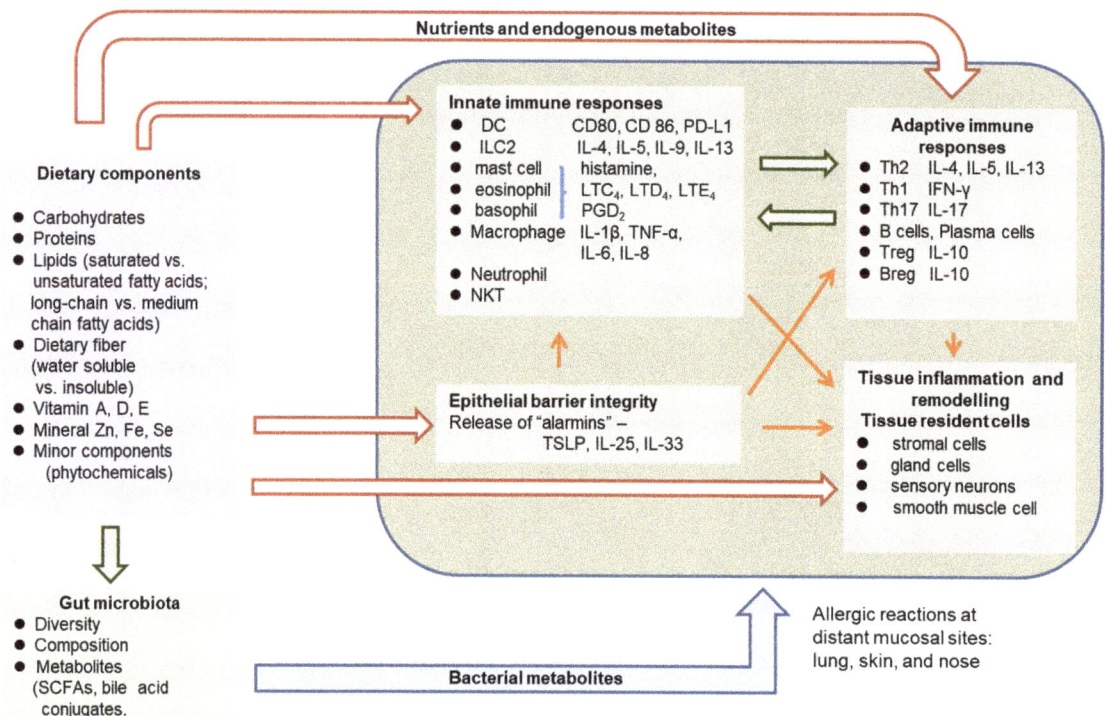

Figure 1. The impact of diet and nutrition on allergic reactions in the lungs, skin, and nose. The arrows indicate regulation. Red arrows represent nutrients and endogenous metabolites and blue arrow represents bacterial metabolites. Food components and endogenous metabolites can affect all stages of an allergic reaction by influencing the epithelial barrier and the release of alarmins, by interacting with innate and adaptive immune cells though special receptors to either promote immune activation or induce tolerance, and by directly acting on tissue epithelium and resident cells to regulate tissue inflammation and remodeling. Diet plays a critical role in determining the ecology of the gut microbiota including diversity, composition, and metabolism. Bacterial metabolites can also reach distant organs and regulate all these processes through multiple mechanisms. DC: dendritic cells; ILC2, type 2 innate lymphoid cells; TSLP, thymic stromal lymphopoietin; SCFAs: short-chain fatty acids; LTC$_4$, leukotriene C$_4$; LTD$_4$, leukotriene D$_4$; LTE$_4$, leukotriene E$_4$.; PGD$_2$, prostaglandin D$_2$; NKT: natural killer T cells; Treg, T regulatory cells; Breg, B regulatory cells.

Accumulating evidence has shown that a broad range of nutrients and dietary components (vitamins A, D, and E, minerals Zn and iron, dietary fiber, fatty acids, and phytochemicals) play critical roles in the prevention or treatment of allergic disease through host and gut microbiota-derived metabolites. The purpose of this paper is to review recent advances in the understanding of diet and food components as contributing factors in the etiology of allergies, molecular targets of nutrient regulation of immune cells and structural cells involved in allergy, and clinical findings about nutrition intervention in treating allergic diseases.

2. Materials and Methods

A systematic literature search was conducted for reports in English from January 2013 to August 2023 using PubMed and Web of Science databases. The following key words were used individually or in combination: allergy, asthma, allergic rhinitis, atopic dermatitis, dietary fiber, dietary lipids, dietary protein, dietary flavonoids, micronutrients, obesity, and plant-based diet. Relevant articles were reviewed, and the most recent ones were preferably cited. Additional reports were identified from selected papers in the reference list. In general, priority was given to original research and review articles based on animal studies and clinical trials.

3. Pathophysiology of Allergic Diseases

All allergic diseases involve type 2 inflammatory allergic responses to various allergens. The prototypical allergic reaction includes a sensitization and memory phase and an effector phase [15]. Common environmental allergens include dust mites, fungi, pets, and pollens [3]. During the sensitization phase, allergens entering through the epithelial barrier, where damage is caused by viruses or other environmental factors, are captured by dendritic cells and presented to naïve CD4$^+$ T cells, leading to the generation of allergen-specific CD4$^+$ Th2 cells which produce IL-4, IL-5, IL-9, and IL-13 [3,15]. Epithelial cells sense the danger and release three cytokines, TSLP, IL-33, and IL-25, which create a cytokine milieu to promote the generation of Th2 cells [16]. Besides epithelial cells, stromal cells can also sense changes in metabolite levels and secrete IL-33 in response to abnormal metabolite profiles [13,17]. High-level IL-4 and IL-13 induce IgE isotype class-switching in B cells, which will produce large amounts of IgE when matured into antigen-specific plasma cells. IgE binds through high-affinity FcεRI receptors on the surface of specific innate effector cells (mast cells and basophils). At this stage, a memory pool of antigen-specific Th2 cells and B cells is generated [3,15]. During the acute effector phase, an encounter with the allergen induces the cross-linking of the IgE on the surface of sensitized effector cells, triggering activation of effector cells and the release of mediators including preformed histamine and tryptase, and de novo synthesized prostaglandin D$_2$ (PGD$_2$) and leukotrienes C$_4$ (LTC$_4$), LTD$_4$, and LTE$_4$ [2,3]. These mediators interact with sensory nerve cells, glandular cells, and epithelial cells to generate acute symptoms such as itching, sneezing, coughing, and diarrhea in mucosal tissues [3]. In the later effector phase, accumulation of the above mediators released by innate immune cells, together with cytokines IL-4, IL-5, IL-9, and IL-13 produced by Th2 cells and type 2 innate lymphoid cells (ILC2s), as well as epithelial cell-derived cytokines, maintain high antigen-specific IgE levels and recruit more inflammatory cells including eosinophils and basophils into inflamed tissue, resulting in tissue damage and chronic inflammation in a type I hypersensitivity reaction.

Epithelial cell-derived TSLP, IL-33, and IL-25 are critical initiators of type 2 immunity; however, their function is beyond merely sending an alarm signal [16]. They regulate a broad range of immune cells including the activation of dendritic cells to present antigens to naïve T cells, promoting Th2 cell development, stimulating neuron cells, activating ILCs, and enhancing memory Th2 cells [16]. Therefore, targeting these alarmins may be effective in lowering susceptibility and decreasing exacerbations in all allergic conditions. In fact, diet can influence the production of alarmins. For example, a high-fat diet promotes serum TSLP [18] and a high inulin fiber diet upregulates IL-33 from stromal cells through gut microbiota-derived bile acids [13]. In contrast, dietary fish oil or fermented fish oil (both are enriched with long-chain unsaturated fatty acids EPA (eicosapentaenoic acid) and DHA (docosahexaenoic)) lowers TSLP expression in mouse ear tissue with AD [19], and a natural flavonoid quercetin lowers TSLP levels in an in vitro AD model using human keratinocytes [20].

Innate lymphoid cells (ILCs) are tissue-resident innate immune cells that regulate tissue-specific immunity through interactions with epithelial cells, neurons, stromal cells, and other tissue-resident cells [21]. ILC2 cells are highly enriched in mucosal sites such as the lung, skin, and gut and are essential in type 2 inflammation. They are rapidly activated by TSLP, IL-33, and IL25 and produce high levels of the classical Th2 cytokines IL-4, IL-5, IL-9, and IL-13, therefore driving the pathogenesis of allergic diseases such as asthma, AR, and AD. Some dietary metabolites, such as retinoic acid in carrots and indole-3-carbinol contained in cabbage and broccoli [22,23], can restrain ILC2 responses through the activation of the aryl hydrocarbon receptor (AhR). The benefits of consuming these vegetables in the prevention of allergic diseases are likely due to these AhR ligands. Dietary factors can affect ILC2 cells through other mechanisms besides acting as AhR ligands. For example, dietary fiber metabolite butyrate can inhibit ILC2 proliferation and inhibit IL-13 and IL-5 production from ILC2 cells through histone deacetylase (HDAC) inhibition. Therefore, systemic administration of butyrate through drinking water or intranasal administration can attenuate ILC2-driven airway inflammation and airway hypersensitivity [24].

Allergen-specific regulatory T cells (Tregs) and regulatory B cells (Bregs) play essential roles in the induction of immune tolerance to allergens and restoring immune homeostasis in allergen-specific immunotherapy [15]. $CD4^+FOXP3^+CD25^+$ Tregs can suppress ongoing allergic inflammation by inhibiting DCs, effector Th (Th1, Th2, and Th17) cells, granulocytes (mast cells, basophils, and eosinophils), B cells, as well as tissue-resident cells, either through secreted inhibitory cytokines (IL-10, TGF-β) or through cell contact-dependent mechanisms [15]. Bregs also play a key role in maintaining tolerance to allergens through the production of anti-inflammatory IgG4 antibodies and by secretion of suppressive cytokines IL-10, TGF-β, and IL-35 which promote Treg generation, inhibit T cell activation, and induce tolerogenic DCs [15]. Nutrient metabolism can influence Treg or Breg generation and function. For example, indoleamine 2, 3-dioxygenase (IDO), a key enzyme responsible for catabolizing dietary tryptophan to kynurenines, is highly expressed in dendritic cells in nose-draining lymph nodes and is essential to immune tolerance of inhaled allergens. A blockade of IDO impairs Treg differentiation during intranasal allergen challenge, which leads to the abrogation of allergen-specific immune tolerance [25]. A lower IDO level is associated with atopy in humans [26]. Moreover, maternal tryptophan metabolism can influence the development of allergic diseases in offspring [27]. Decreased numbers of regulatory B cells or functional changes in them are also observed in patients with allergic disorders including AR, asthma, and AD [28–30]. In patients with AR, decreased IL-10-secreting Bregs are linked to altered glutamine metabolism [31]. Both retinoic acid metabolized from vitamin A [32] and 1, 25-dihydroxyvitamin D_3 metabolized from vitamin D_3 [33] promote $Foxp3^+$ Treg differentiation and immune suppression of T helper cells. Deficiency of dietary vitamin A or vitamin D induces high levels of Th2 cytokines and IgE responses to allergens [34,35]. Fermented fish oil suppresses allergic inflammation in the skin, at least partly through enhancing TGF-β and IL-10 expression, which might lead to tissue-specific $Foxp3^+$ Tregs [19]. The trace mineral Zn also promotes Treg differentiation [36,37] and therefore is essential to immune tolerance of allergens. AhR is highly expressed on various antigen-presenting cells [38,39], and activation of AhR has been shown to promote Treg generation through induction of tolerogenic DC [38,40] or promote IL-10-producing Breg differentiation and function [41]. Recent studies in mice showed dietary supplements of whey-protein-derived β-lactoglobulin complexed with quercetin-iron or catechine-iron to be effective for reducing allergic symptoms [42,43]. Activation of AhR by quercetin or catechine, along with increased Tregs, are associated with the observed beneficial effects [42,43].

Allergic rhinitis (AR) is an inflammation of the nasal mucosa associated with an IgE-mediated response to environmental allergens and characterized by nasal itching, sneezing, rhinorrhea, and nasal congestion. AR is often co-morbid with asthma and conjunctivitis [3]. It is one of the most common chronic inflammatory conditions and a global health problem affecting over 500 million people worldwide [44]. In Europe, the prevalence of AR in some European countries can be as high as 50% of the population [3]. In China, the prevalence of AR ranged from 6.2% to 7.2% in adults living in rural and urban areas, respectively, in 2015 [45]. In Taiwan, the prevalence of AR was much higher, with 28.6% and 19.5% in men and women in 1995 [6]. A higher average income in Taiwan, as opposed to mainland China, could be a contributing factor. According to a recent survey in the city of Uruguaiana, southern Brazil, the prevalence of AR was 31.7% in adults and 28% in adolescents [46]. Although not life-threatening, AR impairs the patient's quality of life, lowers work performance and sleep quality, and therefore can result in substantial economic costs [3]. In AR, initial allergen exposure leads to damage in the nasal epithelial cells and the generation of allergen-specific IgE antibodies and Th2 memory cells. Upon re-exposure to the allergen, crosslinking of IgE on mast cells and basophils results in degranulation and the release of mediators of hypersensitivity which produce immediate nasal symptoms within minutes [47]. The late-phase nasal symptoms, such as nasal blockage and nasal discharge, happen within hours and are mainly caused by recruited eosinophils [47]. $CD4^+$ Th2 cells, B cells, mast cells, neutrophils, and macrophages are observed in the nasal lining infiltrate [47]. Many epidemiological and clinical studies supported the role of diet and nutrition in the etiology, prevention, and treatment of AR [6,46,48–51].

Allergic asthma is the most common inflammatory disease of the lungs, with respiratory symptoms such as wheezing, shortness of breath, chest tightness and coughing, and airway hyper-responsiveness to inhaled allergens [2]. The prevalence of asthma in Western countries plateaued at 10% in recent decades. In contrast, the prevalence of asthma in countries with low and medium gross domestic product (GDP) has had a sharp increase in recent years [2] in contrast to previously much lower incidence statistics, making asthma a worldwide inflammatory disease. With eosinophils as the main airway infiltrate cell type, other cells including mast cells, basophils, neutrophils, monocytes, and macrophages can also be found [2]. Apart from airway inflammation, airway remodeling is another feature of asthma that involves structural changes such as subepithelial basement membrane thickening, subepithelial fibrosis, goblet cell hyperplasia and hypertrophy, and muscle hyperplasia [2]. Airway remodeling parallels disease development and leads to lung function decline. None of the current drug therapies can alter the natural history of asthma [2]. The impact of diet on asthma has been described [5] and most studies in the past were focused on the relationship between nutrients and airway inflammation. However, recent studies show evidence that dietary phytochemicals such as resveratrol [52] and kaempferol [53] can modify airway inflammation as well as airway remodeling, suggesting potential therapeutic value in treating allergic asthma. Some in vitro studies also showed that vitamin D is likely to play a role in airway remodeling in asthma [54].

Atopic dermatitis (AD) is a chronic inflammatory skin disease characterized by intense itching and eczematous lesions. Although recognized as an early onset disease as the first step of the so-called atopic march, it can start later in life and is quite common in adults [4]. It is one of the most common chronic inflammatory diseases, affecting 10–20% of the population in developed countries and its prevalence in developing countries continues to rise [4]. Although originally thought to be a typical allergic disorder, skin barrier dysfunction is discovered to be a key driver of AD [4,55,56]. Current research emphasis shifts from focusing on immune mechanisms to epidermal barrier dysfunction. Abnormal skin structure and altered lipid composition, inherited filaggrin deficiency, and environmental factors such as detergent use and mite allergens all contribute to skin barrier dysfunction in AD [4,55,56]. Skin infiltration of inflammatory cells mainly consists of Th2, Th22, and Th17 cells, together with ILC2 cells [4]. Nutrition plays critical roles in the etiology, prevention, and treatment of AD [57]. For example, a high-fat diet exacerbates AD through upregulation of TSLP [18]. A sufficient level of Vitamin D is essential for the maintenance of a normal skin barrier and vitamin D supplements are considered an alternative strategy for controlling skin barrier dysfunction in AD and the atopic march [55]. The role of dietary fiber in the prevention of AD recently emerged from a preclinical study in a mouse model of AD [14]. A high-fiber diet, or a low-fiber diet with orally administered SCFAs, protected against allergen-induced skin inflammation and allergen sensitization [14]. The underlying mechanism lies in gut-derived SCFAs, particularly butyrate, which promote skin barrier integrity by modulating keratinocyte metabolism and differentiation [14].

4. The Role of Diet and Nutritional Status in Allergy

Dietary factors not only affect the development of allergic diseases [5,6,46,50] but also influence disease course and severity [50,58]. Different dietary components are related to differential allergy outcomes. The intake of high energy, high saturated fat, high protein, and low fiber increases the risks of asthma and AR [6,46]. In contrast, high consumption of vegetables and fruits, olive oil, and fish, characteristic of a Mediterranean diet, has been linked with lower risks of asthma and AR [5,7,8,46,59]. Recent evidence suggests that higher dietary fiber intake is associated with fewer asthma symptoms [58]. Moreover, adequate intake of micronutrients is associated with a lower risk of atopic diseases and reduction of symptoms [50]. The identified diet and nutritional risk factors for allergy are shown in Box 1.

Box 1. Diet and Nutritional Risk Factors for Allergy.

High energy
High protein
High saturated fat, *n*-6 fatty acids, medium-chain fatty acids, cholesterol
Low total dietary fiber
Low vegetables and fruits
High simple sugar and processed foods
Low level of Zn, Fe, Vitamins A, D, E

There is a close connection between nutrient metabolism and allergic diseases. Broad changes in energy, amino acids, and lipid metabolism are found in patients with pollinosis [60]. Patients with AR are shown to have at least 10 elevated metabolites in serum which belong to three pathways, namely, porphyrin and chlorophyll, arachidonic acid, and purine metabolism [61]. More and more cellular and molecular mechanisms are being elucidated concerning the regulation of allergic inflammation by individual dietary components or specific nutrients (Figure 2). The pro-allergic nutrients, such as saturated fatty acids and cholesterol, promote the release of TSLP, IL-25, and IL-33 from epithelial and stromal cells, and activate ILC2 cells to produce IL-4, IL-5, IL-9, and IL-13, therefore producing a cytokine milieu for allergic inflammation. By contrast, anti-allergic nutrients, including phytochemicals, micronutrients, and dietary fiber, can suppress allergic inflammation through inhibition of type 2 cytokine production in ILC2 cells via activation of AhR, promotion of the generation of tolerogenic dendritic cells, anti-inflammatory macrophages, and Tregs, and suppression of the release of histamine, prostaglandins, and leukotrienes from granulocytes.

4.1. Dietary protein, Amino Acids, and Energy

A high-protein diet is associated with an increased risk for type 1 allergy in OVA-sensitized mice, as indicated by increased B cells, total and antigen-specific IgE, and a skewed Th1/Th2 balance towards Th2 dominance [62]. In these mice, moderate protein deficiency without energy restriction results in similar total IgE as a normal protein diet [62], suggesting that energy is critical in regulating IgE production and limiting energy supply is important in controlling high IgE response during the exacerbation period in allergic diseases. Indeed, 40% dietary energy restriction delayed the onset of spontaneous dermatitis in NC/Nga (Nagogy University mice) mice whichs resemble human AD [63]. Moreover, dietary restriction suppressed the progression of dermatitis in these mice and was associated with reduced serum IgE, with much fewer numbers of infiltrating inflammatory cells (lymphocytes and eosinophils) in the skin and decreased dermal IL-4 and IL-5 production [63]. The effects of energy or protein restriction on other allergic diseases remain to be investigated.

Pro-allergic foods/nutrients

- High calorie, animal foods, animal fat and protein
- Saturated fatty acids, cholesterol
- Medium-chain fatty acids

Epithelial cell and stromal cell
TSLP, IL-25, IL-33 high level

ILC2 cell
IL-4, IL-5, IL-9, IL-13 high

Dendritic cell
CD80, CD86, PD-L1 high

Macrophage
M2 pro-inflammatory phenotype
CD163 high; ferritin high; labile iron low

B cell
IgE production high

T cell
- Antigen-specific proliferation high
- Treg differentiation low; IL-10 low
- Th2 differentiation high; IL-4, IL-5, IL-13 high
- Th17 differentiation high; IL-17 high
- Th1 differentiation low; IFN-γ low

Mast cell, basophil, eosinophil
Degranulation; histamine, PGD$_2$, LTC$_4$, LTD$_4$, LTE$_4$ high

Anti-allergic foods/nutrients

- Fruits and vegetables, cereal and legumes
- Dietary fiber, n-3 fatty acids,
- Dietary flavonoids
- Vitamins A, D, E, minerals Zn, Fe

Epithelial cell and stromal cell
TSLP, IL-25, IL-33 low level; HDAC inhibition

ILC2 cell
IL-4, IL-5, IL-9, IL-13 low; AhR activation; HDAC inhibition

Dendritic cell
CD80, CD86, PD-L1 low

Macrophage
M1 anti-inflammatory phenotype
CD163 low; ferritin low; labile iron high

B cell
Mainly IgG; IgE production low

T cell
- Antigen-specific proliferation inhibited
- Treg differentiation normal; IL-10 high
- Th2 differentiation low; IL-4, IL-5, IL-13 low
- Th17 differentiation low; IL-17 low
- Th1 differentiation normal; IFN-γ high

Mast cell, basophil, eosinophil
Intact granules; histamine, PGD$_2$, LTC$_4$, LTD$_4$, LTE$_4$ low

Figure 2. The roles of nutrients and foods in allergic inflammation. Epidemiological, clinical, and animal studies have demonstrated that the Western diet promotes allergy and exacerbates symptoms of allergic diseases, whereas nutritionally balanced plant-based diets protect from allergy and reduce the severity of allergic diseases. The pro-allergic nutrients associated with a Western diet promote the production and release of TSLP, IL-25, and IL-33 from epithelial cells and stromal cells and activate ILC2 cells to produce large amounts of IL-4, IL-5, IL-9, and IL-13, therefore producing a cytokine milieu for type 2 allergic inflammation reactions characterized by aberrant IgE and type 2 cytokines. By contrast, plant-based diets contain high amounts of anti-allergic nutrients which can suppress type 2 allergic inflammation through inhibition of type 2 cytokine production in ILC2 cells via activation of AhR, promotion of the generation of tolerogenic dendritic cells, anti-inflammatory macrophages, and Tregs, and suppression of the release of histamine, prostaglandins, and leukotrienes from granulocytes. AhR, aryl hydrocarbon receptor; ILC2, innate lymphoid cells; Treg, T regulatory cell; TSLP, thymic stromal lymphopoietin; PGD$_2$, prostaglandin D$_2$; LTC$_4$, leukotriene C$_4$; LTD$_4$, leukotriene D$_4$; LTE$_4$, leukotriene E$_4$. HDAC, histone deacetylase.

The essential amino acid tryptophan is a key regulator of immune tolerance. Tryptophan is metabolized to kynurenine by IDO (indolamin 2, 3-dioxygenase) in DCs and binds to AhR on naïve CD4[+] T cells to generate FoxP3[+] Treg cells [25]. Expression of IDO is much higher in nose-draining lymph nodes, i.e., cervical lymph nodes, compared with peripheral lymph nodes [25]. In a mouse model of OVA-induced delayed hypersensitivity, inhibition of IDO during intranasal OVA administration results in the loss of immune tolerance as indicated by the increase in ear thickness [25]. IDO blockade was associated with dysfunctional Tregs which failed to suppress DTH (delayed type hypersensitivity) responses upon transfer to naïve animals [25]. Therefore, IDO expression in DCs in the nose-draining lymph nodes is essential for immune tolerance to inhaled antigens.

Tryptophan metabolism is altered in many allergic conditions and the IDO pathway plays a central role. Higher serum tryptophan concentrations are found in patients with seasonal AR [64] and asthmatic children [65]. Higher tryptophan and kynurenine levels are found in children with asthma and AR [26]. Low IDO activity has been found in asthma and AR patients [26,66]. IDO activity is induced by IFN-γ and is considered a Th1 cell activation marker [67]. During Th2 allergic inflammation, an elevated level of nitric oxide inhibits IDO activity by binding to the heme group of the enzyme. Therefore, the rationale of antioxidants as an anti-allergic therapy lies in their ability to block inducible nitric oxide synthase [67] and rescue the IDO activity which is essential to generate Tregs.

L-glutamine is another amino acid that plays a critical role in immune cell function. Although not an essential amino acid, L-glutamine is the primary fuel for immune cells and is essential for basic immune cell functions such as lymphocyte proliferation and cytokine production [68]. A recent study showed that abnormal glutamine metabolism is associated with allergic diseases [31]. IL-10-secreting B cells are a type of B regulatory cell that suppresses allergic reactions. Decreased numbers of regulatory B cells or functional changes in them are observed in patients with allergic disorders including AR, asthma, and AD [28–30]. The underlying mechanism of the defects in Bregs is the altered glutamine metabolism. In normal cells, glutamine is transported into the cells by a cell surface transporter called ASCT2 (alanine, serine, cysteine-preferring transporter 2), to be metabolized in a process called glutaminolysis [69]. B cells from patients with AR express low levels of ASCT2 and generate less IL-10[+] regulatory B cells under IL-10-inducing culture conditions [31].

4.2. Dietary Lipids

The amount of dietary lipids and type of fatty acids influence allergic inflammation. High total fat, animal fat, saturated fatty acids (SFAs), cholesterol, n-6 polyunsaturated fatty acids (PUFAs), and medium-chain fatty acids (MCFs) are risk factors, whereas monounsaturated fatty acids (MUFAs) and n-3 PUFAs have protective properties. High animal fat and SFAs are associated with allergic rhinitis in human adults while high MUFA intake is associated with a lower risk for asthma [46,59]. In humans, high consumption of olive oil, a rich source of MUFAs, is associated with reduced risk for asthma in Italian adults [59] and teenagers in Taiwan [70].

A high-fat diet (60% Kcal from saturated fat) has been shown to increase serum TSLP in C57BL/6 mice and exacerbate dermatitis in mice through upregulation of TSLP in NC/Nga mice that develop AD spontaneously [18]. The high-fat diet increased TSLP in dorsal skin, infiltration of inflammatory cells, and epidermal thickening in NC/Nga mice compared with a low-fat diet. Dermatitis score was much lower in high-fat-fed NC-TSLP-KO mice, suggesting TSLP mediates a high-fat-diet-induced increase in dorsal skin inflammation [18]. Long-term feeding (10 months since weaning) of a Western diet (21.2% fat, 34% sucrose, and 0.2% cholesterol) also substantially increased spontaneously developed dermatitis in aged C57BL/6 mice, as compared with a control diet (5.2% fat, 12% sucrose, and 0.01% cholesterol) [71]. The Western diet-fed mice had increased epidermal thickness in their dorsal skin and much more epidermal hyperplasia in the lesion skin, with hypergranulosis and spongiosis typical of AD [71]. The Western diet leads to increased total bile acids, altered bile acid profiles, and elevated bile acid signaling through two bile acid receptors

TGR5 (transmembrane G-protein-coupled receptor-5) and S1PR2 (sphingosine-1-phosphate receptor-2) in the lesion skin [71]. Lowering serum cholesterol with a bile acid sequestrant cholestyramine reduced epidermal hyperplasia and decreased Th2 and Th17 cytokines [71]. Therefore, dysregulated bile acid metabolites, induced by the Western diet, are the main contributors to the dermatitis lesion.

Besides saturated fatty acids and cholesterol, medium-chain fatty acids (MCFs) contained in coconut oil or palm oil also prove to be a dietary risk factor for allergy [5]. In a mouse model of peanut allergy, compared with n-6 PUFAs from peanut oil, MCFs decreased dietary peanut or OVA antigen absorption into the circulation and increased antigen in the Peyer's patches, which resulted in a significant increase in activated DC cells [72]. Single feeding of peanut protein with MCFs resulted in increased serum IgE, anti-peanut IgG, and IL-13 production from splenocytes. MCFs promoted allergic sensitization through the upregulation of mRNA of TSLP, IL25, and IL-33 from jejunum epithelium and promoted Th2 cytokines in splenocytes in OVA-challenged mice. Moreover, MCFs also exacerbated orally challenged antigen-induced anaphylaxis compared with n-6 PUFAs.

The phospholipids isolated from asparagus (*Asparagus officinalis* L.) are demonstrated to have anti-allergic properties. Oral administration of these phospholipids suppressed serum total IgE and OVA-specific IgE in OVA-challenged mice and ameliorated clinical scores of AD induced by picryl chloride in NC/Nga mice [73]. Phospholipid and glycolipid fractions from asparagus also potently inhibited β-hexosaminidase release from cultured RBL-2H3 (rat basophilic leukemia-histamine-releasing cell line) cells, indicating a direct effect on degranulation in allergic responses [73].

Although conflicting results are generated from human studies about the effects of long-chain PUFA supplementation on asthma, AR, and AD [74], animal studies provide clear evidence of the protection of dietary n-3 PUFA in these allergic conditions. Dietary n-3 fatty acid α-linolenic acid shows beneficial effects in allergic inflammation by improving skin barrier function in AD mice [75] and attenuating symptoms in OVA-induced AR in mice, as compared with n-6 fatty acid linoleic acid [76]. Dietary linseed oil (enriched with α-linolenic acid) increases EPA-derived metabolite 15-HEPE (hydroxyeicosapentaenoic acid in eosinophils) in eosinophils in the nasal passage, which inhibits mast cell degranulation by binding to PPAR (peroxisome proliferator-activated receptor) γ [76]. In human mast cells, both EPA and DHA suppress IL-4 and IL-13 [77], suggesting their possible protective roles in type 2 inflammation. In contrast, long-chain n-6 fatty acid-derived arachidonic acid increases TNF-α and PGD$_2$ in human mast cells [77], supporting the concept that an increased n-6/n-3 fatty acid ratio in the Western diet is pro-inflammatory and likely to promote type 2 inflammation. In the DNCB-induced AD mouse model, both dietary fish oil and fermented fish oil significantly alleviated scratching behavior, decreased epidermal thickness, and infiltration of cell infiltration in skin lesions, suppressed TSLP protein expression in ear tissue and serum histamine and IgE [19], with fermented fish oil having a better effect. Compared with natural fish oil, fermented fish oil resulted in higher TGF-β and IL-10 mRNA expression and a stronger suppressive effect on IL-13 and IFN-γ in the ear tissue due to higher content of EPA and DHA, known to be incorporated into the skin tissue. The suppressive effect on Th2 cytokines by fish oil and fermented fish oil may not be a direct effect on Th2 cells, but rather through the indirect effect of Tregs because fish oil does not affect Th2 differentiation [19]. Fermented fish oil did not increase Tregs in the spleens of these mice. However, increased Foxp3 expression in CD4$^+$ T cells from fermented fish-oil-supplemented mice is observed upon anti-CD3/anti-CD28 activation, suggesting fermented fish oil alters the cytokine milieu to promote Treg differentiation. Additional research is needed to investigate the mechanisms of how EPA and DHA affect structural cells and innate immune cells to reduce type 2 allergic inflammation. Indeed, orally administered EPA was shown to markedly ameliorate special diet-induced AD-like symptoms in hairless mice accompanied by attenuated TSLP, IL-4, and IL-5, along with improved skin barrier function [78]. Analysis of the composition of lipids covalently bound to corneocytes revealed that dietary EPA significantly increased covalently bound ceramides in the stratum corneum [78].

Olive oil, as a major component of the Mediterranean diet, has many health benefits. Olive oil is enriched with monosaturated n-9 fatty acids. Recently, it was shown that olive oil confers protection again food allergies by improving gut mucosal barrier integrity [79]. Olive oil also enhances oral tolerance to dietary allergens by decreasing serum antigen-specific IgE, antigen-specific IgG, and histamine [80]. Increased IL-10 and decreased IL-4 associated with olive oil feeding indicate that Tregs and Bregs are induced. Detailed mechanisms warrant further investigation. Altered gut microbiota is also associated with an olive oil diet, and the polyphenols and other phytochemicals in olive oil may be the contributing factors. For example, uvaol, a triterpene in olive oil, exhibits anti-inflammatory activity in two murine models of allergic inflammation [81].

4.3. Dietary Fiber

Recent animal studies show that dietary fiber protects against AD or allergic asthma through its bacterial metabolites short-chain fatty acids, particularly butyrate [14,82,83]. Gut microbiota fermentation of dietary fiber into SCFAs is the key to the gut–skin axis or gut–lung regulation of allergic reactions in the skin and lungs. Consistent with animal studies, dysbiosis characterized by the enrichment of *Faecalibacterium prausnitzii* and a reduced capacity for butyrate fermentation in the human gut microbiome has been found in patients with AD [84]. Gut microbiota-derived butyrate has been found to be inversely associated with mite-specific IgE levels in childhood asthma [85]. Furthermore, infants who develop allergies in childhood have reduced bacterial enzymes for carbohydrate breakdown and butyrate production in their gut microbiome [86]. A recent clinical study in Japan showed that gut microbial factors are associated with AR [48]. The relative abundance of *Prevotella* was lower and the relative abundance of Escherichia was higher in AR patients compared with healthy controls [48]. *Prevotella* abundance reflects the intake level of dietary fiber and is linked to a diet based on plant foods. Decreased relative abundance of *Prevotella* is associated with the Western diet [87,88]. Increased abundance of *Escherichia* is linked to a high-protein diet [89]. A higher abundance of *Escherichia* is also found in children with asthma and rhinitis [90]. Despite observed alterations in the gut microbiota in allergic individuals, the efficacy of probiotic treatment remains unclear [91]. A more comprehensive approach, which restores the overall health of the gut microbiome through dietary approaches, might have better effects than the use of a single probiotic species. There is some evidence from human studies that a higher dietary fiber intake has protective effects on the clinical outcome of asthma [58,92,93].

Short-chain fatty acids, particularly butyrate, regulate type 2 inflammation mainly through the inhibition of HDAC (histone deacetylase) on various immune cells and structural cells. Vancomycin treatment in mice results in dramatic alterations in the gut microbiome characterized by decreased richness, diversity, and decreased abundance of butyrate-producing families, leading to increased susceptibility to allergic inflammation [83]. A supplement of SCFA in drinking water attenuated OVA or papain-induced allergic asthma by suppression of DC activation and trafficking, therefore restraining Th2 cell development in Peyer's patches [83]. Butyrate also directly regulates ILC2 cells by suppressing IL-33-induced IL-13 and IL-5 production in cultured ILC2 lung cells from Rag2$^{-/-}$ (recombination-activating gene 2 deficient) mice who lack T cells [24]. When administered either through drinking water or through an intranasal route, butyrate ameliorated ILC2 cell-driven lung inflammation. The inhibitory effect of butyrate on ILC2 cell proliferation was due to histone deacetylase (HDAC) inhibition [24]. In a mouse model of AR, intranasal administration of sodium butyrate improved clinical symptoms and nasal mucosal epithelial morphology, accompanied by decreased serum levels of Th2 cytokines and increased Th1 cytokines [94]. Butyrate attenuates TSLP protein expression level in stromal cells in nasal mucosa by working as an inhibitor of HDAC1 and HDAC3 [94]. Dietary fiber can influence asthma through epigenetic mechanisms by inhibiting HDAC enzymes [10].

Mouse studies showed that pups from pregnant mothers on a high-fiber diet or acetate are protected from house dust mite (HDM)-induced asthma [95]. Besides epigenetic regulation of HDAC, dietary fiber also affects the metabolism and function of structural cells at the barrier sites, which are critical for the initiation of an allergic reaction. For example, in a mouse model of HDM-induced AD, high-fiber (inulin, a highly fermentable dietary fiber) intake or butyrate protects animals from developing skin inflammation [14]. A lower disease severity is accompanied by an improved skin barrier, decreased epidermal thickening, less inflammatory cell infiltration, and decreased antigen-specific IgE. Butyrate feeding results in the enrichment of pathways related to immune and barrier function in skin transcriptome [14]. Surprisingly, butyrate does not modify skin immune cells before allergy exposure and does not affect skin Tregs. Butyrate blunts immune responses to HDM through enhancing mitochondria fatty acid β-oxidation and long chain fatty acid synthesis and promoting epidermal keratinocyte differentiation, therefore strengthening the skin barrier at the baseline and following HDM exposure [14].

Both the amount and type of dietary fiber affect susceptibility to allergic airway inflammation and the severity of the inflammation. A low-fiber diet (<0.3%) increases susceptibility to HDM-induced allergic airway inflammation in mice compared with the standard 4% chow diet [14]. Besides increased eosinophils and lymphocytes in the lung, elevated total IgE and HDM-specific IgG_1 were observed in mice on a low-fiber diet compared with a normal-level fiber diet, suggesting that the low-fiber diet promotes systematic allergic inflammatory responses. The low-fiber diet also results in a more activated phenotype of dendritic cells, as indicated by increased surface expression of CD40, CD80, PD-L1, and PD-L2. A high-pectin (a water-soluble and highly fermentable dietary fiber) diet decreases susceptibility to allergic airway inflammation, as compared with a high-cellulose (a water-insoluble dietary fiber which is not fermented by the gut microbes) diet, indicating the gut fermentation process of pectin to SCFA, particularly propionate, is the key for this beneficial effect [14]. Nonetheless, even the high-pectin diet does not increase SCFA levels in the lung. High pectin intake leads to increased propionate in the circulation which enhances bone marrow hematopoiesis and generation of DC precursors, which express low levels of MHCII and CD40 and have an impaired ability to promote Th2 cell responses.

Highly fermentable fibers other than pectin also influence allergic inflammation, an effect dependent on the gut microbiota fermentation process. Compared with a high-fiber diet composed of cellulose, a high-inulin or high-psyllium diet induces increased serum bile acids and triggers eosinophilia in the colon and lungs [13]. Increased bile acids bind to farnesoid X receptors on stromal cells and epithelial cells and trigger the release of IL-33, which acts on ILC2 cells to produce IL-5, therefore promoting allergen-induced type 2 barrier inflammations in the lungs [13]. This effect of inulin is dependent on intestinal bacterial bile salt hydrolase (BSH) expressed on *Bacteroides ovatus* which hydrolases conjugated bile acids into unconjugated bile acids. Inulin promoted the growth of *Bacteroides ovatus*, therefore leading to increased serum bile acids.

4.4. Dietary Flavonoids and Other Phytochemicals

Flavonoids are a major type of phytochemicals in the diet and are naturally occurring phenolic compounds which are commonly found in fruits, vegetables, herbs and spices, legumes, tea, and vinegar [96,97]. There are six subclasses of dietary flavonoids based on their chemical structures, namely flavanols, flavones, isoflavones, flavanones, flavonols, and anthocyanidin [96,97]. Accumulating evidence has shown the anti-allergic effect of dietary flavonoids. The effects of dietary flavonoids in AR, AD, and asthma are summarized in Table 1.

As a major dietary flavonol-type flavonoid, quercetin is found in many fruits and vegetables including onions, shallots, apples, berries, tea, tomatoes, grapes, nuts, and seeds. The anti-inflammatory effect of quercetin is well documented in various animal models of allergy [98]. Quercetin is effective in reducing allergic symptoms by decreasing serum

IgE and Th2-related cytokines, reducing eosinophil, neutrophil, and mast cell infiltration into local tissue, reducing epithelial thickness in the lung and hyperkeratosis, and suppressing epithelial cell-derived cytokines IL-25, IL-33, and TSLP [98]. However, in most in vivo animal studies, quercetin is administered through i.p. injection. As quercetin is a glycone (namely, carbohydrate conjugate), how dietary quercetin is metabolized by the gut microbiota and the subsequent effects on allergic inflammation remain to be explored. In a recent study, oral administration of quercetin was shown to attenuate nasal symptoms of OVA-induced AR in BALB/c (Halsey J Bagg albino mice strain c) mice by suppressing angiogenic factors and proinflammatory cytokines TNF-α, IL-6, and IL-8 in nasal lavage fluids [99]. The minimum effective dose for the above in vivo inhibition is similar to the maximum daily recommended dosage for dietary quercetin supplements. Furthermore, in IgE-sensitized mouse peritoneal mast cells, quercetin at concentrations comparable to physiological blood concentrations achieved by recommended dietary quercetin supplement intake dosage completely inhibited VEGF (vascular epithelial growth factor) and bEGF (basic fibroblast growth factor) at mRNA level and potently suppressed TNF-α, IL-6, and IL-8 at mRNA level [99]. In human keratinocytes treated with a cytokine cocktail that induces TSLP production, quercetin suppressed TSLP production and MMP mRNA expression [20]. Quercetin also increased protein expressions of epithelial junction protein E-cadherin, Occludin, and two proteins related to tissue repair: Twist and Snail [20], indicating quercetin's ability to promote wound repair. Notably, quercetin also highly upregulated IL-10 mRNA and further increased IL-10 following proinflammatory cytokine cocktail treatment, indicating that quercetin affects the cytokine milieu in the tissue to promote IL-10 T or B regulatory cells under inflammatory conditions. Baicalin, a flavone-type flavonoid present in lettuce and cantaloupe, also regulates IL-10/IL-17 and is able to attenuate symptoms in a mouse model of AR [100].

Table 1. Beneficial effects of dietary phytochemicals in allergic diseases.

Flavonoids	Experimental Models	Results	Reference
Quercetin	OVA-induced AR in BALB/c mice 25 mg/kg dosage 5 d during challenge	Inhibited sneeze and nasal rubs Suppressed angiogenic factors and TNF-α, IL-6, IL-8	[99]
Quercetin	Human HaCaT keratinocytes	Promoted wound repair ↑ E-cadherin, Occludin, Twist, Snail ↑ IL-10 at basal level ↓ MMP1, MMP2, MMP9, ↓ TSLP	[20]
Kaempferol	DNCB/mite extract induced dermatitis in BALB/c mice ear 15, 50 mg/kg 5 d on/2 d off for 4 wks following 2nd DNCB Jurkat cells	↓ ear thickness ↓ Dermal and epidermal thickness ↓ Mast cell infiltration ↓ Serum IgE ↓ mRNA of IL-4, IL-13, IFNγ IL-17a, IL-6, IL-31, TSLP in ear tissue ↓ αCD3/CD28, PMA/A23187 stimulated IL-2 production ↓ AICD Inhibited MRP-1 activity Suppressed JNK phosphorylation	[101]
Kaempferol	OVA-induced allergic asthma in BALB/c mice 10, 20 mg/kg for 3 days during challenge	↓ TGF-β production in the lung ↑ E-cadherin and epithelial thickening ↓ α-SMA, ↓ Collagen IV, ↓ MT1-MMP ↓ Lung fibrosis ↓ PAR1 signaling	[53]

Table 1. Cont.

Flavonoids	Experimental Models	Results	Reference
Naringenin	OVA-induced AR in Sprague Dawley rats 100 mg/kg 7 d during challenge	Reduced nasal scratching and number of sneezing Decreased serum IL-4, IL-5	[102]
Diosmetin	DNCB-induced AD in SKH-1 hairless mice 5 mg/kg for 14 d during challenging period	↑ Skin barrier function ↓ Skin swelling, erythema ↓ Skin erosion and dryness ↓ Epidermal thickness ↓ Mast cell infiltration in skin ↓ Serum IgE and IL-4	[103]
Baicalin	OVA-induced AR in BALB/c mice L-Baicalin 50 mg/kg H-Baicalin 200 mg/kg 10 d following sensitization and 4 d before challenge	Reduced inflammatory cells in nasal lavage fluid ↓ Nasal symptoms ↓ Thickness of nasal epithelium ↓ Nasal mucus production ↓ IL-17, ↑ IL-10 in nasal discharge ↓ OVA-specific IgE, IgG1 antibodies Inhibited autophagy in nasal mucosa	[100]
Baicalin	DNTB-induced AD in BALB/c mice 50, 100, 200 mg/kg 14-d following DNTB stimulation	↓ Dorsal skin thickness ↓ Trans-dermal water loss ↓ Epidermal thickness ↑ Skin barrier function, ↓ TSLP ↓ NF-κB signaling pathway in skin ↓ JAK, STAT signaling pathway ↑ Actinobacteria	[104]
Licoricidin	DNCB/mite induced atopic dermatitis in ear tissue in BALB/c mice 50 mg/kg 5 d on/2 d off following the 2nd DNCB for 4 wks	↓ Epidermal and dermal tissue ↓ Infiltrating mast cells ↓ Serum IgE, IgG1, IgG2a ↓ mRNA of IL-4, IL-5, IL-6, IL-13 in ear tissue ↓ Size and weight of draining lymph nodes ↓ T cells and Th2 cytokines in dLNs ↑ T cell PTPN1 phosphorylation in dLNs ↓ DC activation through antagonizing PTPN1	[105]
Resveratrol	3-month repeated OVA exposure induced chronic asthma in BALB/c mice	↓ Airway hyperresponsiveness ↓ Inflammatory cells, IL-4, Il-5, Il-13 in BAL fluid ↓ Lung infiltration of inflammatory cells ↓ Goblet cell number ↓ Peribronchial α-SMA ↓ Collagen amount in lung tissue	[52]
SDG	OVA-induced AR in BALB/c mice 100 mg/kg 3 times a week for 4 wks before initial sensitization	Ameliorated sneezing number Decreased eosinophil and neutrophil infiltration Enhanced β-glucuronidase activity and increased ED levels in nasal passage	[106]

HACAT—cells-human epidermal keratinocyte cell line; MMP—matrix metalloproteinases; DNCB—dinitrochlorbenzene; Jurkat cells–T-lymphocyte cell line; CD—cluster of differentiation; PMA—phorbol-myristate-acetate; AICD—activation-induced cell death; MRP—motility related protein; JNK—c-Jun-N-terminal kinases; TGF—transforming growth factor; MT1-MMP—membrane type 1-matrix-metalloproteinase; OVA—ovalbumin; SDG—secoisolariciresinol diglucoside; ED—enterodiol; PTPN1—protein tyrosine phosphatase-receptor type 1; dLN—draining lymph nodes; alpha SMA—anti-alpha-smooth muscle actin; PAR—protease-activated receptor. ↑, up-regulation; ↓, down-regualtion.

Kaempferol, another flavonol-type flavonoid found in many fruits, vegetables, herbs, teas, and medicinal plants, also exhibits anti-inflammatory, antioxidant, and anti-allergic properties. In cultured lung epithelial BEAS-2B (human broncho-epithelial-alveolar stem cell-derived cells) cells, nontoxic kaempferol suppresses LPS (lipopolysaccharide)-induced TGF-β production, TGF-β-induced myofibroblast formation, LPS-induced collagen, and MT1-MMP, suggesting its ability to suppress the epithelial-to-mesenchymal transition and fibrosis. In a mouse model of asthma, orally administered kaempferol not only suppressed eosinophil infiltration and airway inflammation but also inhibited the airway epithelial-to-mesenchymal transition (EMT) and fibrosis [53]. As fibrotic airway remodeling is characteristic of asthma, leading to lung function deterioration, and is not treated by current drug therapy, kaempferol may be a potential therapy for asthma-related airway construction and is worthy of further clinical studies. Kaempferol also protects mice against AD by suppressing T cell activation though interaction with MRP-1 [101].

Oral administration of naringenin, a flavanone mostly found in citrus peel, was shown to significantly reduce nasal scratching score in rats with OVA-induced AR with improved histology in the nasal epithelium and decreased serum IgE, IL-4, and IL-5 [103]. In addition, naringenin inhibited TSLP production in PMA/Ionophore-activated human mast cells (HMC-1 cells) through inhibition of NF-κB and TSLP-induced mRNA expressions of IL-13, TNF-α, IL-17 receptors, and TSLP receptors in these cells [102]. Therefore, naringenin and many other flavonoids may have a protective role against allergic conditions in allergen-sensitized individuals by regulating TSLP, the key initiator of Th2-driven allergic inflammation. Future clinical studies of naringenin on human allergic conditions are warranted.

The gut microbiota-derived metabolites are critical for the anti-allergic function of some flavonoids. For example, the flavone glycoside diosmin and its aglycone form diometin were shown to diminish DNCB-induced AD symptoms in SKH-1 hairless mice, such as increased trans-epidermal water loss and hydration, epidermal thickness, and infiltration of mast cells [103]. Decreased serum IgE and IL-4 in these mice were observed for both diosmin and diometin; however, in cultured RBL-2H3 cells, only diosmetin and not diosmin showed inhibitory effects on IL-4 production. This suggests that the in vivo anti-allergic effect of diosmin depends on its breakdown into the aglycone form by the gut microbiota. The anti-AD effect of baicalin also depends on the gut microbiota because fecal transplantation from baicalin-treated mice to GF (germ-free) mice resulted in significantly reduced skin thickness and clinical symptoms accompanied by decreased serum IgE and IL-4 [104].

Some dietary phytochemicals other than flavonoids also exhibit strong anti-allergic properties. Licoricidin, a component isolated from licorice (*Glycyrrhiza uralensis*) root which is a commonly used herb in traditional medicine, shows protection against mouse AD by suppression of T cell activation through regulating PTPN1 activity [105]. Resveratrol, the best-studied polyphenol, inhibits mast cell activation and shows potential in treating allergic conditions [107]. A recent study showed that orally administered resveratrol inhibits airway inflammation and remodeling in a murine chronic asthma model [52]. In mice that developed asthma from repeated exposure to OVA over the course of three months, resveratrol effectively inhibited TGF-β production and signaling in the lung tissue and epithelial–mesenchymal transition, therefore improving lung function as measured by airway hyper-responsiveness to methacholine [52]. This suggests the potential of resveratrol as an effective therapy for treating airway remodeling associated with asthma. The nasal metabolism of phytoestrogen is important in the observed anti-allergic property for secoisolariciresinol diglucoside (SDG), a phytoestrogen enriched in flaxseed. Dietary SDG was shown to ameliorate OVA-induced AR symptoms in mice and was associated with less infiltration of neutrophils and eosinophils [106]. SDG did not alter antigen-specific IgE or IgG levels in plasma. Enterodiol (ED), the bacterial metabolite of SDG, is circulated in the blood in the form of EDGlu, but converted to ED aglycone in the nasal passage where it inhibits IgE-mediated degranulation of basophil degranulation in a

GRR (interferon-gamma response region) 30-dependent manner [106]. Host or nasal cavity microbiota-derived β-glucuronidase activity is responsible for generating active phenolic metabolites. The metabolites form many phenolic compounds, including resveratrol, EGCG (epigallocatechin gallate), and curcumin, and are likely able to control the nasal local tissue environment in a similar manner to reduce effector immune cell activation in allergic responses. Several plant extracts show good anti-allergic abilities in several animal studies, although the exact active chemicals in these extracts remain to be determined. For example, the anti-AD effect of celery extract [108], black soybean extract [109], and the anti-AR effects of the extracts of *Musa paradisiaca* L. inflorescence [110], *Piper nigrum* fruit [111], and *Cuminum cyminum* L. seed [112], are recently demonstrated in various animal models. Exploring dietary phytochemicals and their metabolites for anti-allergic potential represents a new direction for basic research and more clinical studies are needed to verify their effects in human patients. The beneficial effects of dietary phytochemicals [51,113] in allergic diseases are supported by the recent clinical intervention studies listed in Table 2. Daily intake of 15 g of a novel barley-based formulation for 14 days proved to significantly reduce all symptoms in patients with AR and, with even better results than fexofenadine in terms of controlling nasal congestion, postnasal drip, and headache [114]. This beneficial effect on the control of allergic symptoms could be due to the phytochemicals and soluble fiber present in the barley drink power.

Table 2. The impact of dietary supplements in allergic diseases.

Year Location	Study Design	Subjects and Intervention	Results	
2022 Tokyo Japan	RCT	Patients ($n = 60$) with eye/nose allergic symptoms Supplementation of 200 mg quercetin for 4 wks vs. the placebo food	Improved allergic symptoms including eye itching, sneezing, nasal discharge, sleep disorder ↓ Nasal discharge ecosipophil Improved life quality	[113]
2022 Chiang Mai Thailand	RCT	AR patients ($n = 16$) Treatment with 10 mg cetirizine for 4 wks plus oral supplement of 3 g shallot capsule vs. the placebo capsule	↑ Overall symptoms in 62.5% in shallot group 37.5% in placebo group ↓ Overall symptom score ↓ Total ocular symptom score	[51]
2022 Tehran, Mashhad Iran	RCT	AR patients ($n = 77$) Treatment with 60 mg Fexofenadine (FX) for 14 d. vs. 15 g dried power of, Ma-al-Shaeer (MS), a barley-based hot-water extracted formulation	Improved all symptoms except cough in both groups MS better in nasal congestion, postnasal drip, and headache ↓ Serum total IgE in both groups	[114]
2022 Vienna, Austria	RCT	Allergic women ($n = 51$) Supplement for 6-month of a lozenge called holoBLG ($n = 25$) containing β-lactoglobulin with iron, polyphenol, retinoic acid, zinc vs. placebo ($n = 26$)	↓ Total nasal symptom score 42% improvement in treated group vs. 13% in placebo group 45%, 31%, 40% improvement in combined symptom score in holoBLG group in birch peak, entire birch season, the entire grass pollen season ↑ Iron levels in circulating CD14$^+$ monocytes ↑ Hematocrit values ↓ Red cell distribution width	[49]

Table 2. Cont.

Year Location	Study Design	Subjects and Intervention	Results	
2018 Mexico City Mexico	RCT	Patients with AD (n = 65) Standard treatment with Vitamin D3 5000 IU/day for 12 wks vs. no extra vitamin	↑ Serum vitamin D level Inverse relationship between final serum vitamin D level and severity of AD Serum vitamin D > 20 ng·/mL with standard therapy is sufficient to reduce AD severity	[115]
2019 Newcastle Australia	RCT	Asthma patients (n = 17) Treated with 7 d inulin (6 g powder twice daily), inulin + probiotic, placebo with a 2 wks run-in and 2 wks wash out periods	Inulin decreased airway eosinophils and HDAC9 expression in sputum cells Inulin improved asthma control in poorly controlled eosinophilic asthmatics	[92]

RCT, randomized controlled trial; HDAC, histone deacetylase; ↑, up-regulation; ↓, down-regualtion.

4.5. Vitamins and Minerals

Vitamins and minerals have long been known for their immunomodulatory roles. Vitamins A, D, and E, and trace elements zinc and iron, are particularly important dietary factors, influencing allergic inflammation and the development of allergic diseases. Sufficient intake of Vitamins A, D, and E is required to control asthma [5]. Supplementation with vitamins E and D alone or in combination improves symptom management of AD [116]. Serum vitamin D level is a determining factor in remission with standard therapy for AD. A serum level of 1, 25(OH)$_2$VD$_3$ higher than 20 ng/mL plus standard therapy is sufficient to reduce the severity of AD [115]. In a randomized, double-blind, placebo-controlled clinical study, an oral supplement of 5000 IU/day vitamin D$_3$ in patients with AD significantly increases the serum level of 1, 25(OH)$_2$VD$_3$ to a much higher level than the placebo group, and this dosage achieved sufficiency in 100% of the patients [115]. Vitamin D also shows potential in managing airway remodeling in asthma, based on a number of in vitro studies showing the inhibitory effects of vitamin D on bronchial smooth muscle cells, human airway smooth muscle cells, human asthmatic bronchial fibroblasts, and human bronchial fibroblasts [54]. Recent studies suggest that deficiencies in iron, zinc, and vitamins contribute to the etiology of atopic diseases in children, and supplementation with micronutrients is considered essential for managing the atopic march [50]. Even in adults, evidence also accumulates to support the role of micronutrients in the etiology or treatment of atopic diseases [117]. At cellular and molecular levels, micronutrients are essential for the proper growth and function of all immune cells. Vitamins A and D are particularly important in maintaining immune tolerance to allergens by promoting Treg induction [5]. Deficiencies in micronutrients mimic pathogen infection and lead to the activation of immune cells, therefore priming the host for a Th2 response when encountering an allergen [50]. For example, iron depletion is related to elevated IgE levels and functional iron deficiency is sufficient to evoke mast cell degranulation [50]. Therefore, adequate intake of micronutrients contributes to immune tolerance by increasing allergic resilience, promoting Tregs, and maintaining Th1/Th2 balance.

Recent evidence suggests that vitamin E plays a role in AR. In a mouse model of OVA-induced AR, oral administration of vitamin E (100 mg/kg/day) at the time of OVA sensitization decreased bronchoalveolar lavage fluid (BALf) IL-33 (more than 50%), IL-25, and Th2 cytokines IL-4, IL-5, and IL-13 [118]. Interestingly, co-administration of selenium resulted in a further decrease in IL-13 production, indicating synergistic effects between vitamin E and selenium on IL-13 production. Vitamin E also decreased serum IgE by more than 50% and histamine by 78% [118]. In a similar mouse model of AR, nasally administered α-Tocopherol before nasal challenge in OVA-sensitized mice suppressed nasal symptoms, with fewer inflammatory lesions and better integrity in nasal tissue [119].

Reduced nasal eosinophils and mast cells, upregulated Th1 cytokine IFN-γ gene expression and downregulated Th2 cytokines IL-4, IL-5, and IL-13 gene expression, and reduced total IgE, specific IgE, IgG, and the PI3K-PKB (phosphatidylinositol 3-kinase-protein kinase) pathway in mast cells were observed in α-Tocopherol-treated mice. These results suggest that vitamin E status (systemic or local) affects both arms of the innate and adaptive immune responses in AR. The molecular mechanisms of how vitamin E affects epithelial cells and ILC cells warrant further research.

The trace element zinc is essential for immune function. Zinc deficiency is often linked to allergies. A zinc supplement is shown to be effective in relieving asthma but not beneficial to AD [50,57]. In an animal asthma model, zinc deficiency is related to greater airway hyper-responsiveness compared with normal zinc intake, whereas zinc supplementation reduces inflammatory cell infiltration and improves clinical symptoms [120]. At the cellular level, the beneficial impact of zinc on allergic immune reactions mainly includes T cell differentiation and antigen-specific T cell proliferation. In cultured human PBMCs (peripheral blood mononuclear cells), zinc deficiency increases Th17 differentiation [121]. On the other hand, the zinc supplement in the cell culture of allergen-stimulated PBMCs alters the Th1/Th2 ratio and decreases the proportion of Th17 [122]. Zinc supplementation also enhances Treg differentiation either in allergen-stimulated PBMCs from atopic patients [37] or in TGF-β treated PBMCs and mixed lymphocyte cultures [36]. Moreover, in vitro, a supplement of zinc suppresses allergen-stimulated proliferation of atopic PBMCs [37].

Iron is another trace element that has been linked to the etiology of atopic diseases [123]. As the most common nutritional disorder, iron deficiency is associated with half anemia which affects about a third of the world's population [124]. Iron deficiency can be present either as low hemoglobin levels in the blood or with low levels of metabolically active iron despite normal ferritin iron storage in the body [123]. While the majority of the iron requirement in the human body is met by recycling from senescent red blood cells by splenic macrophages and redistribution to other cells, dietary intake of iron provides only about one-tenth of the daily requirement [123]. Therefore, the macrophage regulation of the iron pool and metabolism is highly important, which determines the activation state of the immune system. When iron mobilization is blocked under various conditions, iron deficiency in immune cells is perceived as a danger signal and leads to abnormal activation such as mast cell degranulation [123]. Hepcidin, an acute-phase protein induced by inflammation, affects the iron level in the circulation by blocking iron absorption and iron mobilization from macrophages, thereby leading to functional iron deficiency in atopic patients [123]. Raw milk whey-protein-derived β-lactoglobumin, as a carrier of iron flavonoid complexes, has been shown to be effective in delivering iron to human monocytic cells and impairing antigen presentation of allergens [43]. The so-called holo β-lactoglobulin complexed with ligands is able to reduce allergic symptoms in mice by decreasing lymphocytic and B cell proliferation and promoting Treg induction [42]. Consistent with preclinical observations, in a randomized, double-blind, placebo-controlled study (n = 51), a 6-month course of supplementation with a β-lactoglobulin-based micronutrients lozenge formula (iron, polyphenol, retinoic acid, and zinc) in grass/birch pollen allergic women resulted in more improvement in nasal symptoms, as compared with the placebo group (42% vs. 13%) in an allergen-independent manner [49]. Dietary intervention with the lozenge significantly improved iron status in myeloid cells, as indicated by increased hematocrit levels and reduced width of red cell distribution, and increased iron levels in CD14$^+$ monocytes, but not in T lymphocytes. This study highlights the importance of iron deficiency in allergy development, and correcting micronutrient deficiency in immune cells as an effective therapy for allergy treatment.

Copper is closely related to iron metabolism. The copper-containing ferroxidase ceruloplasmin is involved with iron mobilization during acute inflammation, and its elevation indicates iron deficiency [117,123]. A recent clinical study in Japan showed that multiple nutritional and gut microbial factors are associated with AR [48]. Four nutrients (retinol, vitamin A, cryptoxanthin, and copper) were negatively associated with AR [48]. In a cohort study in Poland ($n = 80$), the plasma level of Cu was found to be associated with AR in children aged 9–12 [125].

Selenium is an essential trace element that is very important for optimal immune function. Populations from China, the UK, and Scandinavia generally tend to have reduced Se levels [126]. While Se deficiency leads to impaired immune responses, Se supplements boost immune competence. Selenium is an essential component of glutathione peroxidase (GSH-Px), a key antioxidant enzyme that functions to reduce peroxides, therefore protecting against inflammation-induced, excessive oxidative stress-related membrane damage [127]. While a lower serum level of selenium is reported to be associated with an increased risk of asthma in human studies [128,129], an animal study demonstrated that a lower level of selenium is associated with a lower asthma outcome. Although adequate dietary intake of selenium does not protect against the development of allergic asthma in mice, dietary selenium supplements have a synergistic anti-asthma effect with vitamin E in reducing airway inflammation and Th2-related cytokines [118]. In a mouse model of OVA-induced AR, co-administration of selenium with vitamin E resulted in a further decrease in IL-13 levels, as compared with supplementation with selenium or vitamin E alone [118], indicating that selenium and vitamin E affect different pathways of IL-13 production.

5. Obesity and Allergy

Due to the increasing prevalence of obesity and allergic diseases worldwide in recent decades, the link between obesity and individual allergic disease is of great interest. Obesity is a proven risk factor for asthma [130–132] and negatively impacts asthma outcomes [133]. Previously, no clear association was made between obesity and allergic rhinitis [130,131]; however, a recent meta-analysis study showed that obesity is perhaps associated with a higher risk of allergic rhinitis in children [134]. Moreover, obesity can contribute to the exacerbation of inflammation in severe persistent allergic rhinitis through increased IL-1β and leptin levels [135]. A growing body of evidence suggests a link between obesity and atopic dermatitis [136]. Although the prevalence of atopic dermatitis is higher in obese children and adults, the association between obesity and the severity of atopic dermatitis varies with age and gender [136]. The proposed underlying mechanisms for the link between obesity and allergy include pro-inflammatory adipokines (leptin, IL-6, TNF-α) released from adipose tissue [133], pro-inflammatory Th1 cells and Th17 cells associated with adipose tissue from obese individuals [5], and the ILC2–eosinophil–macrophage axis [5] in adipose tissue.

Dietary interventions producing weight loss in obese patients have been shown to be effective in improving asthma control [137]. Randomized controlled trials on dietary intervention showed that weight loss through restrictive diets with low energy is effective in improving asthma outcomes [138] and reducing airway inflammation in obese patients [139]. Even a normal caloric diet with a reduced content of fat, particularly saturated fat, was associated with reduced body weight and improvement of asthma-related quality of life in obese pubertal adolescents [140]. Although there are very limited studies, weight loss is associated with improved symptoms in atopic dermatitis. In a case report, weight loss through combined dietary control and exercise treatment improved skin lesions and normalized IgE and eosinophil counts in an obese patient who did not respond to standard cyclosporine treatment [141]. A randomized controlled study showed that weight reduction in obese patients with atopic dermatitis was associated with significant improvements in symptoms of atopic dermatitis, measured by eczema area and severity index score and decreased dosage of cyclosporine [142]. There has been no study on the effect of dietary intervention-induced weight loss on allergic rhinitis.

Plant-based diets are effective for weight loss [143–145] and can be an effective strategy for weight control, as well as in the treatment of obesity [145]. A plant-based vegan diet excludes all animal products, mainly consisting of grains, legumes, and vegetables and fruits; while in comparison, a vegetarian diet does not eliminate all animal products but emphasizes the consumption of fruits, vegetables, and nuts [145]. The weight reduction effect of such diets may be attributed to reduced calories and low fat intake [145]. Plant protein, as part of a plant-based diet, has recently been shown to be a contributing factor for weight control in overweight individuals [143]. An increased intake of protein and a decreased intake of animal protein are associated with a decrease in body fat mass. Plant-based diets are nutritionally adequate if planned well [144]. However, nutrient intake in the long term can be a concern, as revealed in a study of the weight-loss effects of a vegan diet in overweight postmenopausal women. The adoption of a low-fat vegan diet for 14 weeks leads to changes in macronutrients such as decreased intake of total fat, saturated fat and cholesterol, protein, and increased carbohydrate and fiber intake [144]. In terms of micronutrients, the vegan diet increased intakes of total vitamin A, β-carotene, thiamine, vitamin B6, folic acid, vitamin C, magnesium, and potassium, but decreased intakes of vitamin D, vitamin B12, calcium, phosphorous, selenium, and zinc [144]. Fortified food or supplements may help those following a vegan diet to meet the requirements of micronutrient intakes.

Despite limited data being available, plant-based diets appear to be remarkably effective in improving asthma [146] and atopic dermatitis [147]. According to a report from Sweden, a vegan diet therapy has a pronounced favorable effect on bronchial asthma [146]. After following the diet therapy for one year, patients became more tolerant of various environmental stimuli, such as dust, smoke, and flowers [146]. A significant decrease in asthma symptoms and improvement in clinical variables resulted in reduced needs for medication [146]. Similar striking results show that a two-month course of treatment with a customized vegetarian diet strongly inhibited the severity of atopic dermatitis [147]. A sharp reduction in the number of peripheral eosinophils and of PGE_2 (prostaglandin E_2) synthesis by monocytes was associated with this treatment [147]. Body weight-independent mechanisms with these diets may contribute to the observed beneficial effects on allergy outcomes, in addition to efficacy in body weight loss. In contrast to the Western diet which contains high amounts of pro-inflammatory nutrients, plant-based diets are enriched with micronutrients and dietary flavonoids associated with potent anti-inflammatory and anti-allergy effects (Figure 2). A plant-based diet may be particularly useful for the treatment of severe allergic diseases associated with obesity. Further clinical studies are required to validate the speculation.

6. Conclusions

In conclusion, diet and nutrition play a key role in the development and severity of allergic diseases by regulating tissue and immune homeostasis. Excessive calories, high intake of protein and saturated fatty acids, or lack of dietary fiber and micronutrients can trigger the defense mechanism in the immune system and prime the host for allergic reactions. Therefore, calorie restriction, coupled with sufficient dietary fiber and adequate macronutrient intake, will be essential for maintaining immune tolerance to allergens. The plant-based diets, which emphasize the high consumption of fruits and vegetables, grains, and legumes while avoiding or reducing animal foods, are associated with the reduction of inflammation and weight loss. Further dietary intervention studies are warranted to explore the potential beneficial effects of plant-based diets and the specific nutrients related to such diets on allergic outcomes. As basic research efforts identify more novel dietary components with anti-allergic properties, randomized placebo-controlled trials are also needed to verify their efficacy in human patients. Nutritional therapy holds great promise in reducing allergy symptoms, either as primary therapy and treatment or in support of drug therapy. Assessment of nutritional status and anthropometric characteristics of the patients, and analysis of host and gut microbiota by the multi-omics approach, will be important in future clinical trials to identify novel mechanisms linking nutrition and allergy.

Funding: This research received no external funding.

Institutional Review Board Statement: Not applicable.

Informed Consent Statement: Not applicable.

Data Availability Statement: Data sharing is not applicable to this article. No new data were created in this study.

Conflicts of Interest: The author declares no conflict of interest.

References

1. Undem, B.J.; Taylor-Clark, T. Mechanisms underlying the neuronal-based symptoms of allergy. *J. Allergy Clin. Immunol.* **2014**, *133*, 1521–1534. [CrossRef]
2. Holgate, S.T.; Wenzel, S.; Postma, D.S.; Weiss, S.T.; Renz, H.; Sly, P.D. Asthma. *Nat. Rev. Dis. Primers* **2015**, *1*, 15025. [CrossRef] [PubMed]
3. Bousquet, J.; Anto, J.M.; Bachert, C.; Baiardini, I.; Bosnic-Anticevich, S.; Canonica, C.W.; Melén, E.; Palomares, O.; Scadding, G.K.; Togias, A.; et al. Allergic rhinitis. *Nat. Rev. Dis. Primers* **2020**, *6*, 95. [CrossRef]
4. Weidinger, S.; Novak, N. Atopic dermatitis. *Lancet* **2016**, *387*, 1109–1122. [CrossRef] [PubMed]
5. Julia, V.; Macia, L.; Dombrowicz, D. The impact of diet on asthma and allergic diseases. *Nature* **2015**, *15*, 308–322. [CrossRef] [PubMed]
6. Lin, Y.P.; Kao, Y.C.; Pan, W.H.; Yang, Y.H.; Chen, Y.C.; Lee, Y.L. Associations between respiratory diseases and dietary patterns derived by factors analysis and reduced rank regression. *Ann. Nutr. Metab.* **2016**, *68*, 306–314. [CrossRef]
7. Netting, M.J.; Middleton, P.F.; Markrides, M. Does maternal diet during pregnancy and lactation affect outcomes in offspring? A systemic review of food-based approaches. *Nutrition* **2014**, *30*, 1225–1241. [CrossRef]
8. Thorburn, A.N.; Macia, L.; Mackay, C.R. Diet, metabolites, and "Western-lifestyle" inflammatory diseases. *Immunity* **2014**, *40*, 833–842.
9. Pascal, M.; Perez-Gordo, M.; Caballero, T.; Escribese, M.M.; Longo, M.N.L.; Luerigo, O.; Manso, L.; Matheu, V.; Seoane, E.; Zamorano, M.; et al. Microbiome and allergic diseases. *Front. Immunol.* **2018**, *9*, 1584. [CrossRef]
10. McKenzie, C.; Tan, J.; Macia, L.; Mackay, C.R. The nutrition-gut microbiome-physiology axis and allergic diseases. *Immunol. Rev.* **2017**, *278*, 277–295.
11. Sugihara, K.; Kamada, N. Diet-microbiota interactions in inflammatory bowel disease. *Nutrients* **2021**, *13*, 1533. [CrossRef]
12. Zhang, P. Influence of foods and nutrition on the gut microbiome and implications for intestinal health. *Int. J. Mol. Sci.* **2022**, *23*, 9588. [CrossRef]
13. Arifuzzaman, M.; Won, T.H.; Li, T.T.; Yano, H.; Digumarthi, S.; Heras, A.F.; Zhang, W.; Parkhurst, C.N.; Kashyap, S.; Jin, W.B.; et al. Inulin fiber promotes microbiota-derived bile acids and type 2 inflammation. *Nature* **2022**, *611*, 578–584. [CrossRef] [PubMed]
14. Trompette, A.; Pernot, J.; Perdijk, O.; Alqahtani, R.A.A.; Domingo, J.S.; Camacho-Muñoz, D.; Wong, N.C.; Kendall, A.C.; Wiederkehr, A.; Nicod, L.P.; et al. Gut-derived short-chain fatty acids modulate skin barrier integrity by promoting keratinocyte metabolism and differentiation. *Mucosal Immunol.* **2022**, *15*, 908–926. [CrossRef] [PubMed]
15. Palomares, O.; Akdis, M.; Martin-Frontecha, M.; Akdis, C.A. Mechanisms of immune regulation in allergic diseases: The role of regulatory T and B cells. *Immunol. Rev.* **2017**, *278*, 219–236.
16. Roan, F.; Obata-Ninomiya, K.; Ziegler, S.F. Epithelial cell-derived cytokines: More than just signaling the alarm. *J. Clin. Investig.* **2019**, *129*, 1441–1451. [PubMed]
17. Dahlgren, M.W.; Jones, S.W.; Cautivo, K.M.; Dubinin, A.; Oritiz-Carpena, J.F.; Farhat, S.; Yu, K.S.; Lee, K.; Wang, C.Q.; Molofsky, A.V.; et al. Adventitial stromal cells define group 2 innate lymphoid cell tissue niches. *Immunity* **2019**, *50*, 702–722. [CrossRef]
18. Moon, P.D.; Han, N.R.; Kim, H.M.; Jeong, H.J. High-fat diet exacerbates dermatitis through up-regulation of TSLP. *J. Investig. Dermatol.* **2019**, *139*, 1198–1201. [CrossRef]
19. Han, S.C.; Kang, G.J.; Ko, Y.J.; Kang, H.K.; Moon, S.W.; Ann, Y.S.; Yoo, E.S. Fermented fish oil suppresses T helper 1/2 cell response in a mouse model of AD via generation of CD4+CD25+Foxp3+ T cells. *BMC Immunol.* **2012**, *13*, 44. [CrossRef]
20. Beken, B.; Serttas, R.; Yazicioglu, M.; Turkekul, K.; Erdogan, S. Quercetin improves inflammation, oxidative stress, and impaired would healing in AD model of human keratinocytes. *Pediatr. Allergy Immunol. Pulmonol.* **2020**, *33*, 69–79. [CrossRef]
21. Klose, C.S.N.; Artis, D. Innate lymphoid cells control signaling circuits to regulate tissue-specific immunity. *Cell Res.* **2020**, *30*, 475–491.
22. Kiss, E.A.; Vonarbourg, C.; Kopfmann, S.; Hobeika, E.; Finke, D.; Esser, C.; Diefenbach, A. Natural aryl hydrocarbon receptor ligands control organogenesis of intestinal lymphoid follicles. *Science* **2011**, *334*, 1561–1565. [CrossRef] [PubMed]
23. Li, S.; Bostick, J.W.; Ye, J.; Qiu, J.; Zhang, B.; Urban, J.F.; Auram, D.; Zhou, L. Aryl hydrocarbon receptor signaling cell intrinsically inhibits intestinal group 2 innate lymphoid cell function. *Immunity* **2018**, *49*, 915–928. [CrossRef] [PubMed]
24. Thio, C.L.P.; Chi, P.Y.; Lai, A.C.Y.; Chang, Y.J. Regulation of type 2 innate lymphoid cell-dependent airway hyperreactivity by butyrate. *J. Allergy Clin. Immunol.* **2018**, *142*, 1867–1883.
25. Van der Marel, A.P.J.; Samsom, J.N.; Greuter, M.; van Berkel, L.A.; O'Toole, T.; Kraal, G.; Mebius, R.E. Blockade of IDO inhibits nasal tolerance induction. *J. Immunol.* **2007**, *179*, 894–900. [CrossRef]

26. Ünüvar, S.; Erge, D.; Kiliçarslan, B.; Bağ, H.G.G.; Çatal, F.; Girgin, G.; Baydar, T. Neopterin levels and indoleamine 2,3-dioxygenase activity as biomarkers of immune system activation and childhood allergic diseases. *Ann. Lab. Med.* **2019**, *39*, 284–290. [PubMed]
27. Lau, H.X.; El-Heis, S.; Yap, Q.V.; Chan, Y.H.; Tan, C.P.T.; Karnani, N.; Tan, K.M.L.; Tham, E.H.; Goh, A.E.N.; Teoh, O.H.; et al. Role of maternal tryptophan metabolism in allergic diseases in the offspring. *Clin. Exp. Allergy* **2021**, *51*, 1346–1360. [CrossRef] [PubMed]
28. Kim, A.S.; Doherty, T.A.; Karta, M.R.; Das, S.; Baum, R.; Rosenthal, P.; Beppu, A.; Miller, M.; Kurten, R.; Broide, D.H. Regulatory B cells and T follicular helper cells are reduced in AR. *J. Allergy Clin. Immunol.* **2016**, *138*, 1192–1195. [CrossRef] [PubMed]
29. Wiest, M.; Upchurch, K.; Hasan, M.M.; Cardenas, J.; Lanier, B.; Millard, M.; Turner, J.; Oh, S.; Joo, H. Phenotypic and functional alterations of regulatory B cell subsets in adult asthma patients. *Clin. Exp. Allergy* **2019**, *49*, 1214–1224. [CrossRef]
30. Yoshihara, Y.; Ishiuji, Y.; Yoshizaki, A.; Kurita, M.; Hayashi, M.; Ishiji, T.; Nakagawa, H.; Asahina, A.; Yanaba, K. IL-10-producing regulatory B cells are decreased in patients with AD. *J. Investig. Dermatol.* **2019**, *139*, 475–478. [CrossRef]
31. Liu, J.Q.; Geng, X.R.; Hu, T.Y.; Mo, L.M.; Luo, X.Q.; Qiu, S.Y.; Liu, D.B.; Liu, Z.G.; Shao, J.B.; Liu, Z.Q.; et al. Glutaminolysis is required in maintaining immune regulatory functions in B cells. *Mucosal Immunol.* **2022**, *15*, 268–278. [PubMed]
32. Mucida, D.; Park, Y.; Kim, G.; Turovskaya, O.; Scott, I.; Kronenberg, M.; Cheroutre, H. Reciprocal Th17 and regulatory T cell differentiation mediated by retinoic acid. *Science* **2007**, *317*, 256–260. [CrossRef] [PubMed]
33. Kang, S.W.; Kim, S.H.; Lee, N.; Lee, W.W.; Hwang, K.A.; Shin, M.S.; Lee, S.H.; Kim, W.U.; Kang, I. 1,25-dihydroxyvitamin D-3 promotes foxp3 expression via binding to vitamin D response elements in its conserved sequence region. *J. Immunol.* **2012**, *188*, 5276–5282. [CrossRef]
34. Yokota-Nakatsuma, A.; Takeuchi, H.; Ohoka, Y.; Kato, C.; Song, S.Y.; Hoshino, T.; Yagita, H.; Ohteki, T.; Iwata, M. Retinoic acid prevents mesenteric lymph node dendritic cells from inducing IL-13-producing inflammatory Th2 cells. *Mucosal Immunol.* **2014**, *7*, 786–801. [CrossRef] [PubMed]
35. Vasiliou, J.E.; Lui, S.; Walker, S.A.; Chohan, V.; Xystrkis, E.; Bush, A.; Hawrylowicz, C.M.; Saglani, S.; Lloyd, C.M. Vitamin D deficiency induces Th2 skewing and eosiphilia in neonatal allergic airway disease. *Allergy* **2014**, *69*, 1380–1389. [CrossRef]
36. Maywald, M.; Meurer, S.K.; Weiskirchen, R.; Rink, L. Zinc supplementation augments TGF-β1-depedent regulatory T cell induction. *Mol. Nutr. Food Res.* **2017**, *61*, 1600493. [CrossRef]
37. Rosenkranz, E.; Hilgers, R.D.; Uciechowski, P.; Petersen, A.; Plümäkers, B.; Rink, L. Zinc enhances the number of regulatory T cells in allergen-stimulated cells from atopic subjects. *Eur. J. Nutr.* **2017**, *56*, 557–567. [CrossRef]
38. Vaidyanathan, B.; Chaudhy, A.; Yewdell, W.T.; Angeletti, D.; Yen, W.F.; Wheatley, A.K.; Bradfield, C.A.; McDermott, A.B.; Yewdell, J.W.; Rudensky, A.Y.; et al. The aryl hydrocarbon receptor controls cell-fate decisions in B cells. *J. Exp. Med.* **2017**, *214*, 197–208. [CrossRef]
39. Barroso, A.; Mahler, J.V.; Fonseca-Castro, P.H.; Quintana, F.J. Therapeutic induction of tolerogenic dendritic cells via aryl hydrocarbon receptor signaling. *Curr. Opin. Immunol.* **2021**, *70*, 33–39. [CrossRef]
40. Ye, J.; Qiu, J.; Bostick, J.W.; Ueda, A.; Schjerven, H.; Li, S.Y.; Jobin, C.; Chen, Z.M.E.; Zhou, L. The aryl hydrocarbon receptor preferentially marks and promotes gut regulatory T cells. *Cell Rep.* **2017**, *21*, 2277–2290. [CrossRef]
41. Piper, C.J.M.; Rosser, E.C.; Oleinika, K.; Nistala, K.; Krausgruber, T.; Rendeiro, A.P.F.; Banos, A.; Drozdov, I.; Villa, M.; Thomson, S.; et al. Aryl Hydrocarbon Receptor Contributes to the Transcriptional Program of IL-10-Producing Regulatory B Cells. *Cell Rep.* **2019**, *29*, 1878–1892. [CrossRef]
42. Afify, S.M.; Regner, A.; Pacios, L.F.; Blokhuis, B.R.; Jensen, S.A.; Redegeld, F.A.; Pali-Schöll, I.; Hufnagl, K.; Bianchini, R.; Guethoff, S.; et al. Micronutritional supplementation with a holoBLG-based FSMP (food for special medical purposes)-lozenge alleviates allergic symptoms in BALB/c mice: Imitating the protective farm effect. *Clin. Exp. Allergy* **2022**, *52*, 426–441. [CrossRef] [PubMed]
43. Roth-Walter, F.; Afify, S.M.; Pacios, L.F.; Blokhuis, B.R.; Redegeld, F.; Regner, A.; Petje, L.M.; Flocchi, A.; Untersmayr, E.; Dvorak, Z.; et al. Cow's milk protein β-lactoglobulin confers resilience against allergy by targeting complexed iron into immune cells. *J. Allergy Clin. Immunol.* **2021**, *147*, 321–334. [CrossRef] [PubMed]
44. Bousquet, J.; Khaltaev, N.; Cruz, A.A.; Denburg, J.; Fokkens, W.J.; Togias, A.; Zuberbier, T.; Baena-Cagnani, C.E.; Canonica, G.W.; van Weel, C.; et al. AR and its impact on asthma (ARIA) 2008 update. *Allergy* **2008**, *63* (Suppl. S86), 8–160. [PubMed]
45. Zheng, M.; Wang, X.; Bo, M.; Wang, K.; Zhao, Y.; He, F.; Cao, F.; Zhang, L.; Bachert, C. Prevalence of AR among Adults in Urban and Rural Areas of China: A Population-Based Cross-Sectional Survey. *Allergy Asthma Immunol. Res.* **2015**, *7*, 148–157. [CrossRef]
46. Urrutia-Pereira, M.; Mocelin, L.P.; Ellwood, P.; Garcia-Marcos, L.; Simon, L.; Rinelli, P.; Chong-Neto, H.J.; Solé, D. Prevalence of rhinitis and associated factors in adolescents and adults: A global asthma network study. *Rev. Paul. Pediatr.* **2023**, *41*, e2021400. [CrossRef]
47. Eifan, A.O.; Durham, S.R. Pathogenesis of rhinitis. *Clin. Exp. Allergy* **2016**, *46*, 1139–1151. [CrossRef]
48. Sahoyama, Y.; Hamazato, F.; Shiozawa, M.; Nakagawa, T.; Suda, W.; Ogata, Y.; Hachiya, T.; Kawakami, E.; Hattori, M. Multiple nutritional and gut microbial factors associated with AR: The Hitachi Health Study. *Sci. Rep.* **2022**, *12*, 3359. [CrossRef]
49. Bartosik, T.; Jensen, S.A.; Afify, S.M.; Bianchini, R.; Hufnagl, K.; Hofstetter, G.; Berger, M.; Bastl, M.; Berger, U.; Rivelles, E.; et al. Ameliorating atopy by compensating micronutrioal deficiencies in immune cells: A double-blinded placebo-controlled pilot study. *J. Allergy Clin. Immunol.* **2022**, *10*, 1889–1902. [CrossRef]
50. Peroni, D.G.; Hufnagl, K.; Comberiati, P.; Roth-Walter, F. Lack of iron, zinc, and vitamins as contributor to the etiology of atopic diseases. *Front. Nutr.* **2023**, *9*, 1032481. [CrossRef]
51. Arpornchayanon, W.; Klinprung, S.; Chansakaow, S.; Hanprasertpong, N.; Chaiyasate, S.; Tokuda, M.; Tamura, H. Antiallergic activities of shallot (*Allium ascalonicum* L.) and its therapeutic effects in AR. *Asian Pac. J. Allergy Immunol.* **2022**, *40*, 393–400.

52. Lee, H.Y.; Kim, I.K.; Yoon, H.K.; Kwon, S.S.; Rhee, C.K.; Lee, S.Y. Inhibitory effects of resveratrol on airway remodeling by transforming growth factor-β/smad signaling pathway in chronic asthma model. *Allergy Asthma Immunol. Res.* **2017**, *9*, 25–34. [CrossRef] [PubMed]
53. Gong, J.H.; Cho, I.H.; Shin, D.; Han, S.Y.; Park, S.H.; Kang, Y.H. Inhibition of airway epithelial-to-mesenchymal transition and fibrosis in endotoxin-induced epithelial cells and ovalbumin-sensitized mice. *Lab. Investig.* **2014**, *94*, 297–308.
54. The role of vitamin D supplementation on airway remodeling in asthma: A systemic review. *Nutrients* **2023**, *15*, 2477. [CrossRef]
55. Leung, D.Y.M.; Berdyshev, E.; Gloeva, E. Cutaneous barrier dysfunction in allergic diseases. *J. Allergy Clin. Immnol.* **2020**, *145*, 1485–1497.
56. Kraft, M.T.; Prince, B.T. AD is a barrier issue, not an allergy issue. *Immunol. Allergy Clin. N. Am.* **2019**, *39*, 507–519. [CrossRef]
57. Khan, A.; Adalsteinsson, J.; Whitaker-Worth, D.L. AD and nutrition. *Clin. Dermatol.* **2022**, *40*, 135–144. [CrossRef]
58. Andrianasolo, R.M.; Hercberg, S.; Kesse-Guyot, E.; Druesne-Pecollo, N.; Touvier, M.; Galan, P.; Varraso, R. Association between dietary fiber intake and asthma (symptoms and control) results from the French national e-cohort NutriNet-Santé. *Brit. J. Nutr.* **2019**, *122*, 1040–1051. [CrossRef] [PubMed]
59. Cazzoletti, L.; Zanolin, M.E.; Speita, F.; Bono, R.; Chamitava, L.; Cerveri, I.; Garcia-Larsen, V.; Grosso, A.; Mattioli, V.; Pirina, P.; et al. Dietary fats, olive oil and respiratory diseases in Italian adults: A population-based study. *Clin. Exp. Allergy* **2019**, *49*, 799–807. [CrossRef]
60. Zhou, Y.J.; Li, L.S.; Sun, J.L.; Guan, K.; Wei, J.F. 1H NMR-based metabolomics study of metabolic profiling for pollinosis. *World Allergy Org. J.* **2019**, *12*, 100005. [CrossRef]
61. Ma, G.C.; Wang, T.S.; Wang, J.; Ma, Z.J.; Pu, S.B. Serum metabolomics of patients with AR. *Biomed. Chromatogr.* **2020**, *34*, e4739. [CrossRef]
62. Yoshino, K.; Sakai, K.; Okada, H.; Sakai, T.; Yamamoto, S. IgE responses in mice fed moderate protein deficient and high protein diets. *J. Nutr. Sci. Vitaminol.* **2003**, *49*, 172–178. [CrossRef]
63. Fan, W.Y.; Kouda, K.; Nakamura, H.; Takeuchi, H. Effects of dietary restriction on spontaneous dermatitis in NC/Nga mice. *Exp. Biol. Med.* **2001**, *226*, 1045–1050. [CrossRef] [PubMed]
64. Kositz, C.; Schroecksnadel, K.; Grander, G.; Schennach, H.; Kofler, H.; Fuchs, D. Serum tryptophan concentration in patients predicts outcome of specific immunotherapy with pollen extracts. *Int. Arch. Allergy Immunol.* **2008**, *147*, 35–40. [CrossRef] [PubMed]
65. Licari, A.; Fuchs, D.; Marseglia, G.; Ciprandi, G. Tryptophan metabolic pathway and neopterin in asthmatic children in clinical practice. *Ital. J. Pediatr.* **2019**, *45*, 11. [CrossRef] [PubMed]
66. Luukkainen, A.; Karjalainen, J.; Hurme, M.; Paavonen, T.; Toppila-salmi, S. Relationships of indoleamine 2,3-dioxygenase activity and cofactors with asthma and nasal polyps. *Am. J. Rhinil. Allergy* **2014**, *28*, e5–e10. [CrossRef] [PubMed]
67. Gostner, J.M.; Becker, K.; Kofler, H.; Strasser, B.; Fuchs, D. Tryptophan metabolism in allergic disorders. *Int. Arch. Allergy Immunol.* **2016**, *169*, 203–215. [CrossRef] [PubMed]
68. Cruzat, V.; Rogero, M.M.; Keane, K.N.; Curi, R.; Newshoime, P. Glutamine: Metabolism and immune function, supplementation and clinical transition. *Nutrients* **2018**, *10*, 1564. [CrossRef] [PubMed]
69. Nakaya, M.; Xiao, Y.C.; Zhou, X.F.; Chang, J.H.; Chang, M.; Cheng, X.H.; Blonska, M.; Lin, X.; Sun, S.C. Inflammatory T cell responses rely on amino acid transporter ASCT2 facilitation of glutamine uptake and mTORC1 kinase activation. *Immunity* **2014**, *40*, 692–705. [CrossRef]
70. Huang, S.L.; Pan, W.H. Dietary fats and asthma in teenagers: Analyses of the first nutrition and health survey in Taiwan (NAHSIT). *Clin. Exp. Allergy* **2001**, *31*, 1875–1880. [CrossRef]
71. Jena, P.K.; Sheng, L.; McNeil, K.; Chau, T.Q.; Yu, S.; Kiuru, M.; Fung, M.A.; Hwang, S.T.; Wan, Y.J.Y. Long-term western diet intake leads to dysregulated bile acid signaling and dermatitis with Th2 and Th17 pathway features in mice. *J. Dermatol. Sci.* **2019**, *95*, 13–20. [CrossRef] [PubMed]
72. Li, J.; Wang, Y.; Tang, L.; de Villiers, W.J.S.; Cohen, D.; Woodward, J.; Finkelman, F.D.; Eckhardt, E.R.M. Dietary medium-chain triglycerides promote oral allergic sensitization and orally induced anaphylaxis to peanut protein in mice. *J. Allergy Clin. Immunol.* **2013**, *131*, 442–450. [CrossRef]
73. Iwamoto, A.; Hamajima, H.; Tsuge, K.; Tsuruta, Y.; Nagata, Y.; Yotsumoto, H.; Yanagita, T. Inhibitory effects of green asparagus extract, especially phospholipids, on allergic responses in vitro and in vivo. *J. Agric. Food Chem.* **2020**, *68*, 15199–15207. [CrossRef] [PubMed]
74. Radzikowska, U.; Rinaldi, A.O.; Sözener, Z.Ç.; Karaguzel, D.; Wojcik, M.; Cypryk, K.; Akdis, M.; Akdis, C.A.; Sokolowska, M. The influence of dietary fatty acids on immune responses. *Nutrients* **2019**, *11*, 2990. [CrossRef]
75. Fujii, M.; Nakashima, J.; Tomozawa, J.; Shimazaki, Y.; Ohyanagi, N.; Kawaguchi, S.; Ohya, S.; Kohno, S.; Nabe, T. Deficiency of n-6 polyunsaturated fatty acids is mainly responsible for AD-like pruritic skin inflammation in special diet-fed hairless mice. *Exp. Dermatol.* **2013**, *22*, 272–277. [CrossRef]
76. Sawane, K.; Nagatake, T.; Hosomi, K.; Hirata, S.; Adachi, J.; Abe, Y.; Isoyama, J.; Suzuki, H.; Matsunaga, A.; Kunisawa, J.; et al. Dietary omega-3 fatty acid dampens AR via eosinophilic production of the anti-allergic lipid mediator 15-hydroxyeicosapentaenoic acid in mice. *Nutrients* **2019**, *11*, 2868. [CrossRef]

77. Van den Elsen, L.W.; Nusse, Y.; Balvers, M.; Redegeld, F.A.; Knol, E.F.; Garssen, J.; Willemsen, L.E.M. n-3 long-chain PUFA reduce allergy-related mediator release by human mast cells in vitro via inhibition of reactive oxygen species. *Br. J. Nutr.* **2013**, *109*, 1821–1831. [CrossRef] [PubMed]
78. Fujii, M.; Ohyanagi, C.; Kawaguchi, N.; Matsuda, H.; Miyamoto, Y.; Ohya, S.; Nabe, T. Eicosapentaenoic acid ethyl ester ameliorates AD-like symptoms in special diet-fed hairless mice, partly by restoring covalently bound ceramides in the stratum corneum. *Exp. Dermatol.* **2018**, *27*, 837–840. [CrossRef]
79. Ma, Y.; Liu, M.; Li, D.; Li, J.; Guo, Z.; Liu, Y.; Wan, S.; Liu, Y. Olive oil ameliorate allergic response in ovalbumin-induced food allergy mouse by promoting intestinal mucosal immunity. *Food Sci. Hum. Wellness* **2023**, *12*, 801–808. [CrossRef]
80. Ma, Y.; Li, J.; Guo, Y.; Ma, L.; Liu, Y.; Kuang, H.; Han, B.; Xiao, Y.; Wang, Y. Dietary olive oil enhances the oral tolerance of the food allergen ovalbumin in mice by regulating intestinal microecological homeostatis. *J. Food Biochem.* **2022**, *46*, e14297. [CrossRef] [PubMed]
81. Agra, L.C.; Lins, M.P.; da Silva Marques, P.; Smaniotto, S.; de Melo, C.B.; Lagente, V.; Barreto, E. Uvaol attenuates pleuritis and eosinophilic inflammation in ovalbumin-induced allergy in mice. *Eur. J. Pharmacol.* **2016**, *780*, 232–242.
82. Trompette, A.; Gollwitzer, E.S.; Yadava, K.; Sichelstiel, A.K.; Sprenger, N.; Ngom-Bru, C.; Blanchard, C.; Junt, T.; Harris, N.L.; Marsland, B.J.; et al. Gut microbiota metabolism of dietary fiber influences allergic airway disease and hematopoiesis. *Nat. Med.* **2014**, *20*, 159–166. [PubMed]
83. Cait, A.; Huges, M.R.; Antignano, F.; Cait, T.; Dimitriu, P.A.; Maas, K.R.; Reynolds, L.A.; Hacker, L.; Mohr, J.; Finlay, B.B.; et al. Microbiome-driven allergic lung inflammation is ameliorated by short-chain fatty acids. *Mucosal Immunol.* **2018**, *11*, 785–795. [CrossRef] [PubMed]
84. Song, H.; Yoo, Y.; Hwang, J.; Na, Y.C.; Kim, H.S. Faecalibacterium prausnitzii subspecies-level dysbiosis in the human gut microbiome underlying AD. *J. Allergy Clin. Immunol.* **2016**, *137*, 852–860. [CrossRef]
85. Chiu, C.Y.; Cheng, M.L.; Chiang, M.H.; Kuo, Y.L.; Tsai, M.H.; Chiu, C.C.; Lin, G. gut microbial-derived butyrate is inversely associated with IgE responses to allergens in childhood asthma. *Pediatr. Allergy Immunol.* **2019**, *30*, 689–697. [CrossRef]
86. Cait, A.; Cardenas, E.; Dimitriu, P.A.; Amenyogbe, N.; Dai, D.; Cait, J.; Sbihi, H.; Stiemsma, L.; Subbarao, P.; Mandhane, P.J.; et al. Reduced genetic potential for butyrate fermentation in the gut microbiome of infants who develop allergic sensitization. *J. Allergy Clin. Immunol.* **2019**, *144*, 1638–1647.
87. Rinninella, E.; Cintoni, M.; Raoul, P.; Lopetuso, L.R.; Scaldafferri, F.; Pulcini, G.; Miggiano, G.A.D.; Gasbarrini, A.; Mele, G.P. Food components and dietary habits: Keys for a healthy gut microbiota composition. *Nutrients* **2019**, *11*, 2393.
88. Li, X.; Guo, J.; Ji, K.; Zhang, P. Bamboo shoot fiber prevents obesity in mice by modulating the gut microbiota. *Sci. Rep.* **2016**, *6*, 32953. [CrossRef]
89. Beaumont, M.; Portune, K.J.; Steuer, N.; Lan, A.; Cerrudo, V.; Audebert, M.; Dumont, F.; Mancano, G.; Khodorova, N.; Andriamihaja, M.; et al. Quantity and source of dietary protein influence metabolic production by gut microbiota and rectal mucosa gene expression: A randomized, parallel, double-blind trail in overweight humans. *Am. J. Clin. Nutr.* **2017**, *106*, 1005–1019. [PubMed]
90. Chiu, C.Y.; Chan, Y.L.; Tsai, M.T.; Wang, C.J.; Chiang, M.H.; Chiu, C.C. Gut microbial dysbiosis is associated with allergen-specific IgE responses in young children with airway allergies. *World Allergy Organ. J.* **2019**, *12*, 100021. [CrossRef]
91. Anand, S.; Mande, S.S. Diet, Microbiota and gut-lung connection. *Front. Microbiol.* **2018**, *9*, 2147. [CrossRef] [PubMed]
92. McLoughlin, R.; Berthon, B.S.; Rogers, G.B.; Baines, K.J.; Leong, L.E.X.; Gibson, P.G.; Williams, E.J.; Wood, L.G. soluble fiber supplementation with and without a probiotic in adults with asthma: A 7-day randomized, double-blind, three way cross-over trial. *eBioMedicine* **2019**, *46*, 473–485. [CrossRef] [PubMed]
93. Venter, C.; Meyer, R.W.; Greenhawt, M.; Pali-Schöll, I.; Nwaru, B.; Roduit, C.; Untersmayr, E.; Adel-Patient, K.; Agache, I.; Agostoni, C.; et al. Role of dietary fiber in promoting immune health-an EAACI position paper. *Allergy* **2022**, *77*, 3185–3198. [CrossRef]
94. Wang, J.; Wen, L.; Wang, Y.; Chen, F. Therapeutic effect of histone deacetylase inhibitor, sodium butyrate, on AR in vivo. *DNA Cell Biol.* **2016**, *35*, 203–208. [CrossRef]
95. Geraghty, A.A.; Lindsay, K.L.; Alberdi, G.; McAuliffe, F.M.; Gibney, E.R. Nutrition during pregnancy impacts offspring's epigenetic status-evidence from human and animal studies. *Nutr. Metab. Insights* **2015**, *8* (Suppl. S1), 41–47. [CrossRef]
96. Rakha, A.; Umar, N.; Rabail, R.; Butt, M.S.; Kieliszek, M.; Hassoun, A.; Aadil, R.M. Anti-inflammatory and anti-allergic potential of dietary flavonoids. *Biomed. Pharmacother.* **2022**, *156*, 113945. [CrossRef] [PubMed]
97. Maleki, S.J.; Crespo, J.F.; Cabanillas, B. Anti-inflammatory effects of flavonoids. *Food Chem.* **2019**, *299*, 125124. [CrossRef]
98. Jafarinia, M.; Hosseini, M.S.; Kasiri, N.; Fazel, N.; Fathi, F.; Hakemi, M.G.; Eskandari, N. Quercetin with the potential on allergic diseases. *Allergy Asthma Clin. Immunol.* **2020**, *16*, 36. [CrossRef]
99. Okumo, T.; Furuta, A.; Kimura, T.; Yusa, K.; Asano, K.; Sunagawa, M. Inhibition of angiogenic factor productions by quercetin in vitro and in vivo. *Medicines* **2021**, *8*, 22. [CrossRef]
100. Li, J.; Lin, X.; Liu, X.; Ma, Z.; Li, Y. Baicalin regulates Treg/Th17 cell imbalance by inhibiting autophagy in AR. *Mol. Immunol.* **2020**, *125*, 162–171. [CrossRef]
101. Lee, H.S.; Jeong, G.S. Therapeutic effect of kaempferol on AD by attenuation of T cell activity via interaction with multidrug-associated protein. *Br. J. Pharmacol.* **2021**, *178*, 1772–1788. [CrossRef]

102. Sahin, A.; Sakat, M.S.; Kilic, K.; Aktan, B.; Yildirim, S.; Kandemir, F.M.; Dortbudak, M.B.; Kucukler, S. The protective effect of naringenin against ovalbumin-induced AR in rats. *Eur. Arch. Oto-Rhino-Laryngol.* **2021**, *278*, 4839–4846. [CrossRef] [PubMed]
103. Park, S.; Bong, S.K.; Lee, J.W.; Park, N.J.; Choi, Y.; Kim, S.M.; Yang, M.H.; Kim, Y.K.; Kim, S.N. Diosmetin and its glycoside, diosmin, improves AD-like lesions in 2,4-dinitrochlorobenzene-induced murine models. *Biomol. Ther.* **2020**, *28*, 542–548. [CrossRef] [PubMed]
104. Wang, L.; Xian, Y.F.; Loo, S.K.F.; Ip, S.P.; Yang, W.; Chan, W.Y.; Lin, Z.X.; Wu, J.C.Y. Baicalin ameliorates 2, 4-dinitrochlorobenzene-induced AD-like skin lesions in mice through modulating skin barrier function, gut microbiota and JAK/STAT pathway. *Bioorg. Chem.* **2022**, *119*, 105538. [CrossRef]
105. Lee, H.S.; Kim, J.; Choi, H.G.; Kim, E.K.; Jun, C.D. Licoricidin abrogates T-cell activation by modulating PTPN1 activity and attenuates AD in vivo. *J. Investig. Dermatol.* **2021**, *141*, 2490–2498. [CrossRef]
106. Sawane, K.; Nagatake, T.; Hosomi, K.; Kunisawa, J. Anti-allergic property of dietary phytoestrogen secoisolariciresinol diglucoside through microbial and β-glucuronidase-mediated metabolism. *J. Nutr. Biochem.* **2023**, *112*, 109219. [CrossRef] [PubMed]
107. Civelek, M.; Bilotta, S.; Lorentz, A. Resveratrol attenuates mast cell mediated allergic reactions: Potential for use as a nutraceutical in allergic diseases. *Mol. Nutr. Food Res.* **2022**, *66*, 2200170. [CrossRef] [PubMed]
108. Che, D.N.; Cho, B.O.; Shin, J.Y.; Kang, H.J.; Kim, J.; Choi, J.; Jang, S. Anti-AD effects of hydrolyzed celery extract in mice. *J. Food Biochem.* **2020**, *44*, e13198. [CrossRef]
109. Dorjsemble, B.; Nho, C.W.; Choi, Y.; Kim, J.C. Extract from black soybean cultivar A63 extract ameliorates AD-like skin inflammation in an oxazolone-induced murine model. *Molecules* **2022**, *27*, 2751. [CrossRef]
110. Gadelha, F.A.A.F.; Cavalcanti, R.F.P.; Vieira, G.C.; Ferrira, L.K.D.P.; de Sousa, G.R.; Filho, J.M.B.; Barbosa, M.A.; dos Santos, S.G.; Piuvezam, M.R. Immunomodulatory properties of *Musa papadisiaca* L. inflorescence in combined AR and asthma syndrome (CARAS) model towards NFκB pathway inhibiton. *J. Funct. Food* **2021**, *83*, 104540. [CrossRef]
111. Bui, T.T.; Piao, C.H.; Hyeon, E.; Fan, Y.; Nguyen, T.V.; Jung, S.Y.; Choi, D.W.; Lee, S.; Shin, H.S.; Song, C.H.; et al. The protective role of Piper nigrun fruit extract in an ovalbumin-induced AR by targeting of NFκBp65 and STAT3 signaling. *Biomed. Pharmacother.* **2019**, *109*, 1015–1923. [CrossRef] [PubMed]
112. Ishida, M.; Miyagawa, F.; Nishi, R.; Sugahara, T. Aqueous extract from Cuminum cyminum L. seed alleviates ovalbumin-induced AR in mouse via balancing of helper T cells. *Foods* **2022**, *11*, 3224. [CrossRef] [PubMed]
113. Yamada, S.; Shirai, M.; Inaba, Y.; Takara, T. Effects of repeated oral intake of a quercetin-containing supplement on allergic reaction: A randomized, placebo-controlled, double-blind parallel-group study. *Eur. Rev. Med. Pharmacol.* **2022**, *26*, 4331–4345.
114. Derakhshan, A.; Khodadoost, M.; Ghanei, M.; Gachkar, L.; Hajimahdipour, H.; Taghipour, A.; Yousefi, J.; Khoshkhui, M.; Azad, F.J. Effects of a novel barley-based formulation on AR: A randomized controlled trial. *Endocr. Metab. Immune Disord. Drug Targets* **2019**, *19*, 1224–1231. [CrossRef]
115. Sanchez-Armendariz, K.; Garcia-Gil, A.; Romero, C.A.; Contreras-Ruiz, J.; Karam-Orante, M.; Balcazar-Antonio, D.; Dominguez-Cherit, J. Oral vitamin D3 5000 IU/day as an adjuvant in the treatment of AD: A randomized control trial. *Int. J. Dermatol.* **2018**, *57*, 1516–1520. [CrossRef]
116. Reynolds, K.A.; Juhasz, M.L.W.; Mesinkovska, N.A. The role of oral vitamins and supplements in the management of AD: A systematic review. *Int. J. Dermatol.* **2019**, *58*, 1371–1376. [CrossRef] [PubMed]
117. Petje, L.M.; Jensen, S.A.; Szikora, S.; Sulzbacher, M.; Bartosik, T.; Pjevac, P.; Hausmann, B.; Hufnagi, K.; Untersmayr, E.; Fischer, L.; et al. Functional iron-deficiency in women with AR is associated with symptoms after nasal provocation and lack of iron-sequestering microbes. *Allergy* **2021**, *76*, 2882–2923. [CrossRef]
118. Jiang, J.; Nasab, E.M.; Athari, S.M.; Athari, S.S. Effects of vitamin E and selenium on AR and asthma pathophysiology. *Respir. Physiol. Neurobiol.* **2021**, *286*, 103614. [CrossRef]
119. Wu, G.; Zhu, H.; Wu, X.; Liu, L.; Ma, X.; Yuan, Y.; Fu, X.; Zhang, L.; Lv, Y.; Li, D.; et al. Anti-allergic function of α-Tocopherol is mediated by suppression of PI3K-PKB activity in mast cells in mouse model of AR. *Allergol. Immnopathol.* **2020**, *48*, 395–400. [CrossRef]
120. Truong-Tran, A.Q.; Ruffin, R.E.; Foster, P.S.; Koskinen, A.M.; Coyle, P.; Philox, J.C.; Rofe, A.M.; Zalewski, P.D. Altered zinc homeostasis and caspase-3 activity in murine allergic airway inflammation. *Am. J. Respir. Cell Mol. Biol.* **2002**, *27*, 286–296. [CrossRef]
121. Kulik, L.; Maywald, M.; Kloubert, V.; Wessels, I.; Rink, L. Zinc deficiency drives Th17 polarization and promotes loss of Treg cell function. *J. Nutr. Biochem.* **2019**, *63*, 11–18. [CrossRef]
122. Tsai, Y.L.; Ko, W.S.; Hsino, J.L.; Pan, H.H.; Chiou, Y.L. zinc sulfate improved the unbalanced T cell profiles in Der p-allergic asthma: An ex vivo study. *Clin. Respir. J.* **2018**, *12*, 563–571. [CrossRef] [PubMed]
123. Roth-Walter, F. Iron-deficiency in atopic diseases: Innate immune priming by allergens and siderophores. *Front. Allergy* **2022**, *3*, 859922. [CrossRef]
124. Camaschella, C. Iron deficiency. *Blood* **2019**, *133*, 30–39. [CrossRef] [PubMed]
125. Podlecka, D.; Jerzynska, J.; Sanad, K.; Polanska, K.; Bobrow-Korzeniowska, M.; Stelmach, I.; Brzozowska, A. Micronutrients and the risks of allergic diseases in school children. *Intl. J. Environ. Res. Public Health* **2022**, *19*, 12187. [CrossRef] [PubMed]
126. Norton, R.L.; Hoffmann, P.R. Selenium and Asthma. *Mol. Asp. Med.* **2012**, *33*, 98–106. [CrossRef]
127. Gozzi-Silva, S.C.; Teixeira, F.M.E.; Duarte, A.J.S.; Sato, M.N.; de Oliveira, L.M. Immunomodulatory role of nutrients: How can pulmonary dysfunctions improve? *Front. Nutr.* **2021**, *8*, 674258. [CrossRef]

128. Chen, M.; Sun, Y.; Wu, Y.L. Lower circulating zinc and selenium levels are associated with an increased risk of asthma: Evidence from a meta-analysis. *Public Health Nutr.* **2019**, *23*, 1555–1562. [CrossRef]
129. Kuti, B.P.; Kuti, D.K.K.; Smith, O.S. Serum zinc, selenium and total antioxidant contents of Nigerian children with asthma: Association with disease severity and symptoms control. *J. Trop. Pediatr.* **2020**, *66*, 395–402. [CrossRef]
130. Baumann, S.; Lorentz, A. Obesity—A promoter of allergy? *Int. Arch. Allergy Immunol.* **2013**, *162*, 205–213. [CrossRef]
131. Sybilski, A.J.; Raciborski, F.; Lipiec, A.; Tomaszewska, A.; Lusawa, A.; Furmańczyk, K.; Krzych-Fałta, E.; Komorowski, J.; Samoliński, B. Obesity—A risk factor for asthma, but not for atopic dermatitis, allergic rhinitis and sensitization. *Public Health Nutr.* **2015**, *18*, 530–536. [CrossRef]
132. Chang, C.L.; Ali, G.B.; Pham, J.; Dharmage, S.C.; Lodge, C.J.; Tang, M.K.; Lowe, A.J. Childhood body mass index trajectories and asthma and allergies: A sysmatic review. *Clin. Exp. Allergy* **2023**, 1–19. [CrossRef] [PubMed]
133. Sharma, V.; Cowan, D.C. Obesity, Inflammation, and Severe Asthma: An Update. *Curr. Allergy Asthma Rep.* **2021**, *21*, 46. [CrossRef]
134. Zhou, J.; Luo, F.; Han, Y.; Lou, H.; Tang, X.; Zhang, L. Obesity/overweight and risk of allergic rhinitis: A meta-analysis of observational studies. *Allergy* **2020**, *75*, 1272–1275. [CrossRef]
135. Han, M.W.; Kim, S.H.; Oh, I.; Kim, Y.H.; Lee, J. Obesity can contribute to severe persistent allergic rhinitis in children through leptin and interleukin-1 beta. *Int. Arch. Allergy. Immunol.* **2021**, *18*, 546–552. [CrossRef] [PubMed]
136. Yang, S.; Zhu, T.; Wakefield, J.S.; Mauro, T.M.; Elias, P.M.; Man, M.Q. Link between obesity and atopic dermatitis: Does obesity predispose to atopic dermatitis, or vice versa? *Exp. Dermatol.* **2023**, *2*, 975–985. [CrossRef] [PubMed]
137. Alwarith, J.; Kahleova, H.; Crosby, L.; Brooks, A.; Brandon, L.; Levin, S.M.; Barnard, N.D. The role of nutrition in asthma prevention and treatment. *Nutr. Rev.* **2020**, *78*, 928–938. [CrossRef]
138. Jensen, M.E.; Gibson, P.G.; Collins, C.E.; Hilton, J.M.; Wood, L.G. Diet-induced weight loss in obese children with asthma: A randomized controlled trial. *Clin. Exp. Allergy* **2013**, *43*, 775–784. [CrossRef] [PubMed]
139. Scott, H.A.; Gibson, P.G.; Garg, M.L.; Pretto, J.J.; Morgan, P.J.; Callister, R.; Wood, L.G. Dietary restriction and exercise improve airway inflammation and clinical outcomes in overweight and obese asthma: A randomized trial. *Clin. Exp. Allergy* **2013**, *43*, 36–49. [CrossRef]
140. Luna-Pech, J.A.; Torres-Mendoza, B.M.; Luna-Pech, J.A.; Garcia-Cobas, C.Y.; Navarrete-Navarro, S.; Elizalde-Lozano, A.M. Normocaloric diet improves asthma-related quality of life in obese pubertal adolescents. *Int. Arch. Allergy Immunol.* **2014**, *163*, 252–258. [CrossRef]
141. Son, J.H.; Chung, B.Y.; Jung, M.J.; Choi, Y.W.; Kim, H.O.; Park, C.W. Influence of Weight Loss on Severity of Atopic Dermatitis in a 20-Year-Old Female with Atopic Dermatitis. *Ann. Dermatol.* **2018**, *30*, 626–628. [CrossRef] [PubMed]
142. Jung, M.J.; Kim, H.R.; Kang, S.Y.; Kim, H.O.; Chung, B.Y.; Park, C.W. Effect of Weight Reduction on Treatment Outcomes for Patients with Atopic Dermatitis. *Ann. Dermatol.* **2020**, *32*, 319–326. [CrossRef] [PubMed]
143. Kahleova, H.; Dort, S.; Holubkov, R.; Barnard, N.D. A Plant-Based High-Carbohydrate, Low-Fat Diet in Overweight Individuals in a 16-Week Randomized Clinical Trial: The Role of Carbohydrates. *Nutrients* **2018**, *8*, 58. [CrossRef] [PubMed]
144. Turner-McGrievy, G.; Barnard, N.D.; Scialli, A.R.; Lanou, A.J. Effects of a low-fat vegan diet and a Step II diet on macro- and micronutrient intakes in overweight postmenopausal women. *Nutrition* **2004**, *20*, 738–746.
145. Ivanova, S.; Delattre, C.; Karcheva-Bahchevanska, D.; Benbasat, N.; Nalbantova, V.; Ivanov, K. Plant-Based Diet as a Strategy for Weight Control. *Foods* **2021**, *10*, 3052. [CrossRef]
146. Lindahl, O.; Lindwall, L.; Spångberg, A.; Stenram, A.; Ockerman, P.A. Vegan regimen with reduced medication in the treatment of bronchial asthma. *J. Asthma* **1985**, *22*, 45–55. [CrossRef]
147. Tanaka, T.; Kouda, K.; Kotani, M.; Takeuchi, A.; Tabei, T.; Masamoto, Y.; Nakamura, H.; Takigawa, M.; Suemura, M.; Takeuchi, H.; et al. Vegetarian diet ameliorates symptoms of atopic dermatitis through reduction of the number of peripheral eosinophils and of PGE2 synthesis by monocytes. *J. Physiol. Anthropol. Appl. Hum. Sci.* **2001**, *20*, 353–361. [CrossRef]

Disclaimer/Publisher's Note: The statements, opinions and data contained in all publications are solely those of the individual author(s) and contributor(s) and not of MDPI and/or the editor(s). MDPI and/or the editor(s) disclaim responsibility for any injury to people or property resulting from any ideas, methods, instructions or products referred to in the content.

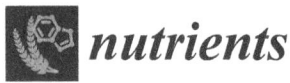

Review

Potential of Dietary HDAC2i in Breast Cancer Patients Receiving PD-1/PD-L1 Inhibitors

Yuqian Wang [1,2], Lingeng Lu [3,4,5], Changquan Ling [1,2], Ping Zhang [6] and Rui Han [1,2,3,4,5,7,*]

1. Department of Chinese Medicine Oncology, The First Affiliated Hospital of Naval Medical University, Shanghai 200433, China
2. Department of Chinese Medicine, Naval Medical University, Shanghai 200433, China
3. Department of Chronic Disease Epidemiology, Yale School of Public Health, Yale University, 60 College Street, New Haven, CT 06520, USA
4. School of Medicine, Center for Biomedical Data Science, Yale University, 60 College Street, New Haven, CT 06520, USA
5. Yale Cancer Center, Yale University, 60 College Street, New Haven, CT 06520, USA
6. Center for Integrative Conservation, Yunnan Key Laboratory for the Conservation of Tropical Rainforests and Asian Elephants, Xishuangbanna Tropical Botanical Garden, Xishuangbanna 666303, China
7. Department of Oncology, The First Hospital Affiliated to Guangzhou University of Chinese Medicine, Guangzhou 510405, China
* Correspondence: dianxiqiao@foxmail.com

Abstract: Breast cancer (BC) is a lethal malignancy with high morbidity and mortality but lacks effective treatments thus far. Despite the introduction of immune checkpoint inhibitors (ICIs) (including PD-1/PD-L1 inhibitors), durable and optimal clinical benefits still remain elusive for a considerable number of BC patients. To break through such a dilemma, novel ICI-based combination therapy has been explored for enhancing the therapeutic effect. Recent evidence has just pointed out that the HDAC2 inhibitor (HDAC2i), which has been proven to exhibit an anti-cancer effect, can act as a sensitizer for ICIs therapy. Simultaneously, dietary intervention, as a crucial supportive therapy, has been reported to provide ingredients containing HDAC2 inhibitory activity. Thus, the novel integration of dietary intervention with ICIs therapy may offer promising possibilities for improving treatment outcomes. In this study, we first conducted the differential expression and prognostic analyses of HDAC2 and BC patients using the GENT2 and Kaplan–Meier plotter platform. Then, we summarized the potential diet candidates for such an integrated therapeutic strategy. This article not only provides a whole new therapeutic strategy for an HDAC2i-containing diet combined with PD-1/PD-L1 inhibitors for BC treatment, but also aims to ignite enthusiasm for exploring this field.

Keywords: dietotherapy; breast carcinoma; HDAC2 suppression; immune checkpoint inhibitor; immunotherapy sensitizer

Citation: Wang, Y.; Lu, L.; Ling, C.; Zhang, P.; Han, R. Potential of Dietary HDAC2i in Breast Cancer Patients Receiving PD-1/PD-L1 Inhibitors. *Nutrients* 2023, 15, 3984. https://doi.org/10.3390/nu15183984

Academic Editor: Francisco J. Pérez-Cano

Received: 2 August 2023
Revised: 9 September 2023
Accepted: 12 September 2023
Published: 14 September 2023

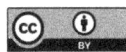

Copyright: © 2023 by the authors. Licensee MDPI, Basel, Switzerland. This article is an open access article distributed under the terms and conditions of the Creative Commons Attribution (CC BY) license (https://creativecommons.org/licenses/by/4.0/).

1. Introduction

Breast cancer is one of the most common malignancies in women worldwide, which can occur in both men and women, and ranks as the second cancer-related cause of death worldwide [1,2]. Its development has been reported to be significantly associated with dietary habits (such as alcohol consumption, high intake of total fat, and low consumption of dietary fiber, etc.) [3]. Five molecular subtypes are classified based on the expression levels of the estrogen receptor (ER), progestogen receptor (PR), human epidermal growth factor receptor 2 (HER2) and Ki-67: Luminal A (ER positive and/or PR positive, HER2 negative, Ki-67 < 20%); Luminal B (HER2 negative/B1: ER positive and/or PR < 20%, HER2 negative, Ki-67 ≥ 20%; HER2 positive/B2: ER positive and/or PR positive, HER2 overexpression); HER2 positive type (HER2 positive, ER negative, PR negative); triple-negative (HER2 negative, ER negative, and PR negative) (TNBC); and other special types [1,2]. The recurrence and/or metastasis of breast cancer significantly contributes to breast cancer-specific mortality, as recurrent tumors tend to be more aggressive and often show resistance to currently available treatments [4]. Thus, to improve treatment outcomes, including overall survival (OS) and disease control, endocrine-, chemo-, targeted- and immuno-therapy alone or in combination have been studied extensively [5]. Immune checkpoint inhibitors (ICIs), which reactivate exhausted CD8+ T cells to kill tumor cells [6], have especially made significant progress in the clinical application of breast cancer treatment [5]. However, the benefit population of breast cancer from ICI monotherapy is limited, making the combined regimen a new research hotspot [5].

The usage of ICIs is to harness the body's immune system to recognize and attack cancer cells more effectively. For instance, by blocking the interaction between immune checkpoints, such as programmed cell death protein 1 (PD-1) and its ligand (PD-L1), the "brakes" on the immune system could be released, allowing immune effector cells to recognize and attack cancer cells more effectively [5]. Fortunately, ICIs have demonstrated a certain efficacy in combination with chemotherapy in the treatment of both early- and late-stage triple-negative breast cancer (TNBC) [7]. The KEYNOTE-355 trial evaluated the efficacy of PD-1 antibody pembrolizumab in combination with chemotherapy for patients with metastatic TNBC. In the context of early-stage disease, the KEYNOTE-522 study demonstrated significant benefits by adding pembrolizumab to chemotherapy, irrespective of the PD-L1 status [7–9]. Furthermore, ongoing studies are currently exploring the application of ICI therapy for hormone receptor-positive and HER2-positive breast cancer [7]. Additionally, novel ICIs are being investigated for their potential across all breast cancer subtypes [7].

Despite these advancements, there are still important unresolved issues. For instance, determining the optimal partners for ICIs to mitigate ICI side effects, and predictive biomarkers to identify who benefit from ICI therapy [7,10]. Another issue that cannot be ignored is that ICIs caused loss of appetite, consequently reducing the patient's nutritional intake [11], and aggravating the patient's already damaged physique and immunity, forming a vicious circle.

Histone deacetylases 2 (HDAC2), as a member of HDACs, is a special protease involved in the tightening of the chromatin structure and suppression of gene transcription. Its expression level was significantly in positive correlation with the poor overall survival of patients with BC or hepatocellular carcinoma (HCC) and with the potential adverse effect of patients to PD-1 antibody therapy [12–15]. Moreover, breast cancer tissues show significantly higher HDAC2 expression than normal breast tissue [13–15]. HDAC2 inhibition is a potential anti-cancer agent against breast cancer [16–18]. HDAC2 inhibitors can exert a synergistic effect with ICIs [18,19]. Given that short-chain fatty acids (SCFA, e.g., butyric acid) are the fermentation products of dietary fibers, dietary intervention may provide a superior safety profile improving immunotherapy by functioning as HDAC2i [20]. Furthermore, SCFA-producer *Lachnoclostridium* in tumors was positively associated with infiltrating CD8+ T cells and chemokines of CXCL9 and CXCL10, as well as better survival in melanoma cancer [21].

Healthy eating is recommended for cancer patient survivors according to guidelines. Besides providing nutrition and energy intake, dietary intervention has been found to improve the body's immunity and anti-cancer activity [22]. Therefore, based on our previous study and the latest findings, this review, for the first time, brings out a novel dietary intervention with potential synergistic effects for ICIs therapy by adding HDAC2i containing food, aiming to ignite enthusiasm to explore the potential application of an HDAC2i-containing diet combined with ICI for BC patients, and to eventually improve the clinical benefits for patients.

2. Materials and Methods

A comprehensive search of the literature was conducted to identify relevant reports from 2000 to 2023, using the PubMed and Web of Science databases. The search utilized various keywords, either individually or in combinations, including PD1, PDL1, breast cancer, HDAC2 inhibitor, immune checkpoint inhibitors, dietary intervention, herbal remedy, neoadjuvant, and immunotherapy sensitizer. The identified articles were thoroughly reviewed, with preference given to the most recent ones. Additional sources were extracted from the reference lists of selected papers. Priority was primarily assigned to original research and review articles based on animal studies and clinical trials.

Differential expression and prognostic analysis. The differential expression analysis of HDAC2 across cancer and normal tissues were obtained from the GENT2 platform (http://gent2.appex.kr/gent2/, accessed on 11 July 2023). The prognostic analysis was performed by applying the Kaplan–Meier plotter platform (https://kmplot.com/analysis/index.php?p=background, accessed on 11 July 2023). BC patients with high or low HDAC2 protein (or gene) expression were divided by median expression level or by best cutoff value. Cutoff values used in analysis for HDAC2 gene and protein were 1568 and 3, respectively. The total amount of samples for analyzing the HDAC2 gene figure was 4929 (high 2465 vs. low 2464), its counterpart for HDAC2 protein was 65 (high 47 vs. low 18).

3. Results

The HDAC2 expression profile across cancer and normal tissues was detected by using the GENT2 platform. Significant difference in HDAC2 expression was displayed between breast cancer tissue and normal breast tissue ($p < 0.001$, Log2FC, 0.122) (Figure 1A). (Significant test results by Two-sample t-test for the HDAC2 expression profile is displayed in Supplementary Materials). As shown in Kaplan–Meier survival curves (Figure 1B,C), BC Patients with a high expression of the HDAC2 gene [hazard ratio (HR), 1.65; $p < 1 \times 10^{-16}$; Figure 1B] or high expression level of the HDAC2 protein (HR, 2; $p = 0.059$; Figure 1C) exhibited a less favorable prognosis compared with patients with low expression levels. However, a significant difference has not been detected in the group of HDAC2 proteins.

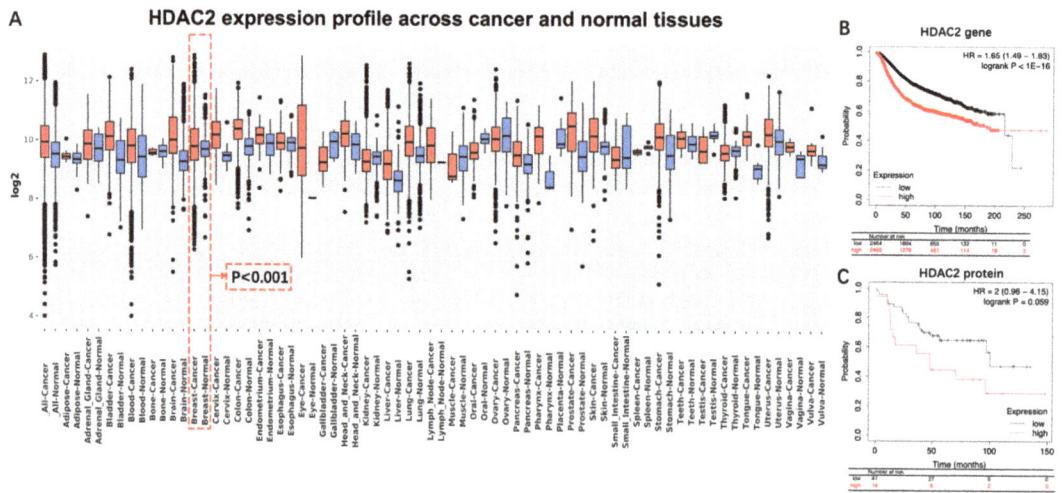

Figure 1. Differential expression and prognostic significance of HDAC2 in breast cancer. (**A**) Significant difference existed between normal breast tissue and breast cancer tissue ($p < 0.001$, Log2FC = 0.122): (**B**) BC patients with either high HDAC2 level of gene, or (**C**) high HDAC2 level of protein exhibited unfavorable overall survival. HR, hazard ratio; BC, breast cancer.

4. Discussion

4.1. HDAC2: A Potential Index of Aggressiveness and a Therapeutic Target against BC

HDAC2 is an enzyme involved in the tightening of the chromatin structure and suppression of gene transcription. Evidence has indicated that HDAC2 is overexpressed in breast cancer cells compared to normal breast tissue. Higher levels of HDAC2 have also been associated with more aggressive tumor characteristics, such as increased cell proliferation, invasion, and metastasis [12–15]. For instance, a clinical study that included 226 BC patients reported that expression of HDAC2 protein is significantly higher in breast cancer than in benign tumors and indicates that HDAC2 may be involved in invasion, metastasis, anthracyclines therapy resistance, and poor prognosis of sporadic breast cancer (Table 1) [14]. Another study, conducted by Afroditi Nonni's group, also examined the expression of HDAC2 in 118 deceased sporadic BC patients and its correlation with clinicopathological characteristics of the tumor and the prognosis of the patient. It was found that high expression of the HDAC2 protein is associated with higher histological grade, stage of disease, and worse prognosis (Table 1) [12]. As for the expression of the HDAC2 gene, evidence has also reported that HDAC2 is one of the most commonly amplified genes in aggressive basal-like breast cancer. Additionally, overexpression of HDAC2 was significantly correlated with high tumor grade, positive lymph node status, and poor prognosis [13]. Those results are also consistent with the outcomes of our analysis. For instance, our results indicated that expression of HDAC2 in BC tissue was significantly higher than that in breast normal tissue ($p < 0.001$) (Figure 1). Moreover, the trend can be observed that BC patients with high expression of HDAC2 gained worse prognosis than those without (Figure 1C). However, a significant difference was been detected ($p = 0.059$) (Figure 1). We speculated that the reason may be due to an insufficient sample size (n = 75).

Table 1. Correlation between HDAC2 protein expression and breast cancer.

Measurement	Sample Size	Patient Selection Criteria	Outcomes	Year	Refs
IHC	226	sporadic breast cancer patients who underwent surgery; All patients did not undergo radiation therapy and chemotherapy before surgery	High expression of HDAC2 was associated with: 1. advanced clinical stages ($p = 0.016$); 2. lymphatic metastasis ($p = 0.02$); 3. high histological grade ($p = 0.001$); 4. shorter OS of BC patients ($p = 0.035$); 5. shorter OS in multidrug resistance protein-positive patients ($p = 0.034$); 6. shorter survival in patients who received chemotherapy containing anthracyclines (OS, $p = 0.041$; disease-free survival, $p = 0.084$).	2016	[15]
IHC	118	Tumor size < 20 mm; Stage I, II and III; No preoperative anticancer therapy; Deceased from BC	High expression of HDAC2 was associated with: 1. BC in stage III ($p < 0.001$); 2. BC with histological grade 3 ($p = 0.013$).	2022	[13]
IHC	300	Invasive ductal carcinoma patients who underwent curative surgery	High expression of HDAC2 was correlated with improved OS in ER-negative BC patients ($p = 0.048$).	2014	[23]
IHC	212	patients with primary invasive breast cancer	High expression of HDAC2 was associated with: 1. overexpression of HER2 ($p = 0.005$); 2. lymphatic metastasis ($p = 0.04$).	2013	[24]

Abbreviations: BC, breast cancer; OS, overall survival; IHC, immunohistochemistry; DFS, disease-free survival.

4.2. HDAC2 Inhibition for Treating Breast Cancer

HDAC2 has been identified as a crucial regulator of epigenetic control in BC and HDAC2 suppression has been further proved to be an effective approach to treating BC by numerous studies [24–26]. For instance, HDAC2 inhibition has been observed to inhibit cellular proliferation in a p53-dependent manner in BC cells [27]. MiR-155 can also decrease the expression of erythroblastic oncogene B by targeting HDAC2 [28]. Moreover, evidence has indicated that PELP1 (proline, glutamate, and leucine-rich protein 1) can bind to miR-

200a and miR-141 promoter sequences and modulate the expression of these miRNAs by recruiting HDAC2; therefore, regulating tumorigenic and metastatic potential of BC cells [29]. Thus, a molecular network involving HDAC2 has been considered to serve as a target for developing anti-cancer drugs [29].

Inhibition of HDAC2 has also been found to exert a synergistic effect in BC treatment. For instance, evidence indicates that depleting HDAC2 can sensitize breast cancer cells to apoptosis induced by epirubicin. This finding highlighted the potential of HDAC2 as a therapeutic target and a biomarker in treating breast cancer [30]. Moreover, the modulation of estrogen receptor (ER) signaling is a promising therapeutic approach in ER-expressing breast cancers, and the progesterone receptor (PR) also plays a critical role in this process [31]. Interestingly, selective inhibition of HDAC2, has been found to enhance the apoptotic effects of tamoxifen (a commonly used drug for ER/PR-positive breast cancer) and has demonstrated significant antitumor activity [31]. Additionally, HDAC2 inhibition has also been found to strongly restrain the multidrug-resistance of BC cells induced by the SRGN (serglycin)–YAP (YES-associated protein) axis, therefore enhancing the therapeutic effect of chemotherapy [32].

Taken together, these findings suggested that HDAC2-targeting intervention could represent an effective approach for breast cancer control.

4.3. HDAC2 Inhibition Enhances the Therapeutic Effect of ICIs in BC Treatment

The emergence of immune checkpoint inhibitors (ICI) has revolutionized the treatment of breast cancer [33–40]. Adjuvant or neoadjuvant immune checkpoint blockades are used for metastatic breast cancer [34]. Despite ICI therapy being promising, breast cancer cells often find ways to evade the host's immune system, necessitating combination therapies to overcome these limitations. HDAC inhibitors (HDACi) have demonstrated potent immunomodulatory activity, making them a rational choice for cancer immunotherapies.

4.3.1. HDAC2 Regulates PD-L1 Nuclear Translocation

As a ligand of PD-1, high PD-L1 levels indicate tumor progression and are associated with poor prognosis in immunotherapy-treated human cancer [35]. PD-L1 nuclear translocation has been identified as a key mechanism underlying the immune evasion of BC cells, hindering PD-1 inhibitors [36]. Both cytoplasmic and nuclear PD-L1 can exert immunosuppressive functions on BC cells [37]. Nuclear PD-L1 has been linked to various cellular processes, for example, increasing the anti-apoptotic capacity of tumor cells, promoting mTOR activity, and upregulating glycolytic metabolism [36]. A study has shown that the level of nuclear PD-L1 expression was positively correlated with immune response-related transcription factors, such as STAT3, RelA (p65), and c-Jun [19]. Nuclear PD-L1 interacts with transcription factors, such as RelA and the IFN regulatory factor (IRF), influencing antitumor immunity. Inhibition of nuclear PD-L1 expression led to downregulation of genes involved in evading immune surveillance, such as PDCD1LG2 (encoding PD-L2), VSIR (encoding VISTA), and CD276 (encoding B7-H3), which enhance cytotoxic T-lymphocyte depletion and promote tumor aggressiveness, distant metastasis, and resistance to PD-L1/PD-1 blockade therapy [18,19,38] (Figure 2).

Several recent studies have reported that HDAC2-associated deacetylation promotes the nuclear translocation of PD-L1, leading to tumor immune evasion in BC cells [18,19]. HDAC2 decreases the acetylation level of Lys 263 in the C-tail of PD-L1, resulting in PD-L1 nuclear translocation. In contrast, depletion of endogenous HDAC2 using siRNA, shRNA, or CRISPR-Cas9 increases PD-L1 acetylation [19]. Selective HDAC2is, such as Santacruzamate A (SCA) and ACY957, increase the acetylation of PD-L1, blocking the PD-L1 nuclear translocation. Clathrin-dependent endocytosis is involved in PD-L1 nuclear translocation, and HIP1R initiates this process by interacting with PD-L1's C-tail. Lys 263 acetylation directly blocks the interaction between HIP1R and PD-L1. Overall, HDAC2 inhibition disrupts PD-L1 nuclear translocation, potentially enhancing the therapeutic efficacy of immune checkpoint inhibitors and boosting antitumor immune responses for BC [19].

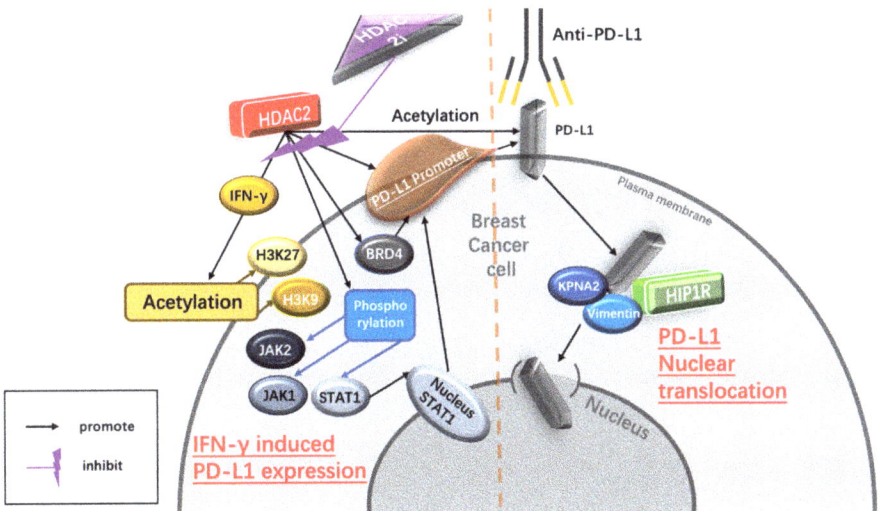

Figure 2. Potential mechanism of HDAC2i enhancing the therapeutic effect of the PD-1/PD-L1 inhibitor. HDAC2i suppresses IFNγ-induced PD-L1 expression regulated by HDAC2, therefore decreasing the immune escape of BC cells mediated by PD-L1. In addition, HDAC2i inhibits the process of PD-L1 nuclear translocation regulated by HDAC2/HIP1R axis, hence enhancing the therapeutic effect of PD-1 blockade treatment. Abbreviations: IFN-γ, interferon-γ; H3K27, histone 3 lysine 2; H3K9, histone 3 lysine 9; JAK2, Janus kinase 2; JAK1, Janus kinase 1; stat1, signal transducer and activator of transcription 1; BRD4, Bromodomain-containing protein 4; KPNA2, karyopherin α-2; HIP-1R, Huntingtin-interacting protein 1-related.

4.3.2. HDAC2 Regulates IFN-γ- Induced PD-L1 Expression

a. IFN-γ upregulates the expression of PD-L1

Evidence has revealed that high expression of PD-L1 is correlated with advanced histology and lymph node metastasis in TNBC and HER2+ subtypes, indicating a poor prognosis biomarker [39]. Moreover, PD-L1 knockdown has been found to inhibit the proliferation and migration of TNBC cells [40]. To date, the clinical trials of immunotherapies based on the PD-1/PD-L1 antagonists have shown a notable and durable response in TNBC patients, indicating PD-L1 as a crucial therapeutic target [41,42].

Interferon-γ (IFN-γ) is a crucial cytokine in both innate and adaptive immunity and should be considered as an important driving force for PD-L1 expression in tumor microenvironment. It is able to induce PD-L1 expression on BC cells and increase the apoptosis of antigen-specific T cells, such a process is referred to as "adaptive resistance" [43]. Depleting IFN-γ receptor 1 has been reported to decrease the expression of PD-L1 expression in BC cells, increase the amount of tumor-infiltrating CD8+ lymphocytes or CTLs, and to inhibit the development of BC cells [44]. In addition, injection of IFN-γ into subcutaneous BC cells induced PD-L1 expression and promoted the growth of BC cells. Inversely, PD-L1 depletion completely abrogated the growth of BC cells induced by IFN-γ injection [44] (Figure 2).

b. HDAC2i affects IFN-γ induced PD-L1

HDAC2 can promote PD-L1 induced via IFN-γ stimulation in BC cells [18,19]. Specifically, IFN-γ can induce gene transcription involving STAT1 binding to the gamma interferon activation site (GAS), recruiting HAT and HDAC for chromatin remodeling [45]. Following IFN-γ stimulation, BRD4 is rapidly recruited to the PD-L1 locus, accompanied by increased H3K27ac and RNA Polymerase II (RNA Pol II) occupancy in cancer cells [45]. A ChIP-qPCR assay confirmed enhanced HDAC2 binding to the PD-L1 promoter after IFN-γ treatment. HDAC2 knockout led to reduced STAT1 occupancy and bromodomain-containing 4 (BRD4) recruitment to the PD-L1 promoter, attenuated H3K27ac and H3K9ac (markers of active transcription in the PD-L1 promoter) upregulation induced by IFN-γ, highlighting HDAC2's role in activating PD-L1 expression through IFN-γ induced signaling pathways [18]. Moreover, upon the binding of IFN-γ to interferon receptors, it transduces signal through Janus kinases (JAKs), signal transducer and activators of transcriptions (STATs) [36]. The JAK/STAT1 pathway activated by IFN-γ positively correlates with PD-L1 expression and plays a critical role in breast cancer immune escape [46]. IFN-γ treatment induces phosphorylation of JAK1, JAK2, and STAT1 in TNBC cells, leading to upregulated STAT1 and PD-L1 expression. However, HDAC2 knockdown inhibits the phosphorylation of JAK1, JAK2, and STAT1, resulting in decreased IFN-γ-induced PD-L1 expression on the TNBC cell surface. HDAC2 knockout also hinders the translocation of STAT1 to the nucleus and inhibits intracellular PD-L1 expression stimulated by IFN-γ, indicating HDAC2's promotion of IFN-γ induced PD-L1 expression in TNBC cells via JAK-STAT1 pathway activation [18] (Figure 2).

4.4. Dietary Intervention Is Important for Breast Cancer Patients Receiving Anti-Cancer Immunotherapy

A healthy diet rich in vitamins, minerals, antioxidants, and phytochemicals, provides essential ingredients for building and strengthening a healthy immune system. Thus, the American Cancer Society (ACS) releases the Nutrition and Physical Activity Guideline for Cancer Survivors, which enhances immune function by supporting essential nutrients [47–50], helping to optimize the effectiveness of immunotherapy and improve treatment outcomes. Moreover, anti-cancer immunotherapy also possesses toxicities and can lead to various adverse effects on breast cancer patients, such as fatigue, nausea, loss of appetite, and gastrointestinal issues [51]. However, proper dietary interventions have been found to help alleviate these side effects by providing proper nutrition, promoting hydration, and supporting gastrointestinal health [52–54]. In addition (Reducing Inflammation), chronic inflammation has been found to be associated with cancer development and progression. Certain foods, such as fruits, vegetables, whole grains, and omega-3 fatty acids, possess anti-inflammatory properties [55–57]. Including these foods in the diet can help reduce inflammation, potentially benefiting breast cancer patients undergoing immunotherapy.

Furthermore (Maintaining Weight and Nutritional Status), cancer and its treatment can lead to weight loss, malnutrition, and muscle wasting, which can further weaken the body and hinder treatment effectiveness [58]. Dietary intervention aims to provide adequate calories, protein, and other essential nutrients to maintain a healthy weight and preserve nutritional status during immunotherapy [59,60]. Additionally, (Enhancing Overall Well-Being), a nutritious diet can contribute to overall well-being by promoting energy levels, reducing fatigue, improving mood, and supporting mental health [61,62]. Breast cancer patients undergoing immunotherapy may experience physical and emotional challenges [63,64] and a healthy diet can play a role in supporting their overall quality of life (Figure 1).

4.5. Dietary HDAC2i

Compared to commonly used anti-cancer therapies, dietary interventions are safer and more cost-effective [65,66]. Even if dietary interventions cannot be considered a replacement for conventional cancer treatments, their role in improving the outcomes of cancer treatment also cannot be ignored [67,68] (Figure 3).

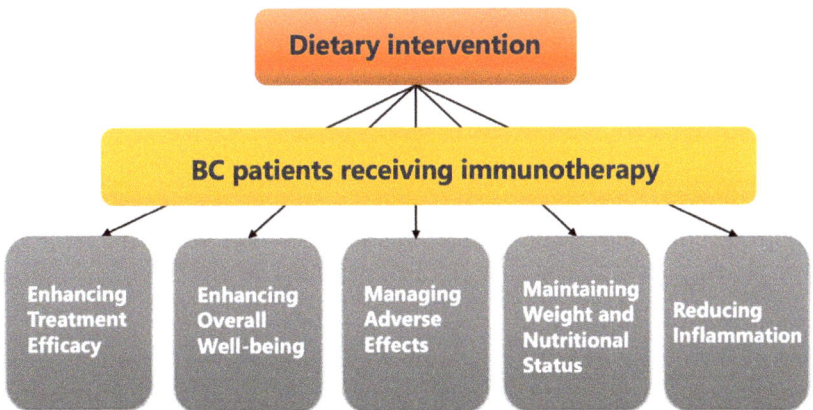

Figure 3. Potential advantages of applying proper dietary intervention in BC patients who receive ICIs treatment.

One advantage of dietary intervention is the minimal side effects compared to anti-cancer therapies [69,70]. Immunotherapy, chemotherapy, and radiation therapy can often cause adverse reactions such as fatigue, arthralgia, rash, pruritus, pneumonitis, acute kidney injury, and also a weakened immune system [71–74]. In contrast, dietary changes usually focus on incorporating natural, nutrient-rich foods, which are less likely to cause significant side effects [70].

Anti-cancer therapies often involve powerful and aggressive drugs that can be toxic to healthy and normal cells in the human body [75]. Such toxicity can lead to additional health complications and adversely affect a patient's well-being [75]. Dietary interventions, on the other hand, prioritize whole foods, fruits, vegetables, and other plant-based sources that provide essential nutrients without the toxic effects associated with some medical treatments [76].

Cancer patients who undergo multiple treatments or take various medications simultaneously will face the increased risk of adverse effects due to drug interactions or unwanted chiral compounds [77]. Dietary interventions generally use natural foods rather than pharmacological compounds, which have both left- and right-hand chiral compounds in balance [78].

Dietary interventions can be customized to suit each individual's needs and medical conditions [60]. This adaptability allows dietary plans to be tailored based on any pre-existing conditions, allergies, or specific dietary restrictions of each patient, ensuring a safer approach [60].

As a long-term lifestyle change, dietary interventions offer the advantage of being sustainable even after the initial treatment period. This sustainable approach helps maintain the patient's overall health and reduces the risk of developing long-term side effects associated with certain anti-cancer therapies [79].

Dietary interventions can complement anti-cancer therapies by providing a supportive role [78]. A healthy diet can help strengthen the immune system, improve overall health, and enhance the body's ability to cope with cancer treatments.

Certain dietary strategies, such as adopting a balanced and nutrient-rich diet, regular physical activity, and weight management, have the potential to reduce the risk of developing cancer [68,80–84]. Prevention is a crucial aspect of cancer management, and dietary interventions can also play a significant role in reducing the occurrence of cancer [78].

4.6. Selected Candidates of HDAC2i

Dietary compounds which possess HDAC2 inhibitory activity offer a new strategy for BC prevention and treatment. These potential candidates may enhance the anti-cancer effect of PD-1 inhibitors (Table 2).

Table 2. Examples of dietary compounds identified as inhibiting HDAC2 activity.

Dietary Component	Food Source	Potential Benefits in Breast Cancer	Diseases	Refs
Genistein (GE)	Soybean products	Anti-cancer effects on breast cancer, modulation of Dnmt3b, Tet3 and HDAC	Breast cancer, cervical cancer,	[85]
Sulforaphane (SFN)	Broccoli sprouts, kale	Cytotoxic effects in breast, colon, and prostate cancer cells, inhibition of HDAC-2 and HDAC-8	Breast cancer, colon cancer, prostate cancer, neurodegenerative diseases, bladder carcinoma,	[86]
Chrysin	Fruits, vegetables, olive oil and red wine	Cytotoxic effects in breast, colon, and prostate cancer cells, inhibition of HDAC-2 and HDAC-8	Breast cancer, melanoma, fibrosarcoma, leukemia	[87–89]
Resveratrol (RSV)	Grapes, apples, blueberries, mulberries, peanuts, pistachios, plums, and red wine	Induced ATP2A3 upregulation correlates with reduced HDAC activity and reduced nuclear HDAC2 expression and occupancy on ATP2A3 promoter	Breast cancer, glioma	[90–93]
Oleuropein (OLE)	Virgin olive oil	Antineoplastic properties, modulation of HDAC2 and HDAC3 in breast cancer cells	Breast cancer, alzheimer,	[94,95]
Curcumin	Turmeric	Inhibited both HDAC activity and the expression of HDACs 1 and 2 in a concentration-dependent manner in cancer cells	Breast Cancer, lung cancer, hematological cancers, inflammation, arthritis, metabolic syndrome,	[96,97]
Valeric acid	Valerian herb	Anti-cancer effects on liver and breast cancer, modulation of HDAC2 and HDAC3	Breast cancer, prostate cancer, liver cancer	[98,99]
Ginsenoside Rh4	Ginseng herb	Inhibition of PD-L1 expression by regulating HDAC2-mediated JAK/STAT pathway in breast cancer cells	Breast cancer, lung adenocarcinoma, colorectal cancer, gastric cancer	[100,101]
Butyrate	Dietary fiber, resistant starch, undigested carbohydrates	Anticancer activity, inhibition of breast cancer cell proliferation, induction of apoptosis	Multiple cancer, cardiovascular disease, and type 2 diabetes	[102–106]
Green tea polyphenols	Green tea	Suppressed cancer progression by regulating circ_MITF/miR-30e-3p/HDAC2 axis	breast cancer, malignant melanoma, prostate cancer,	[107,108]
Rosmarinic acid (RA)	Rosemary tea	Potential pan-HDAC inhibitor, inhibition of nuclear HDAC2 protein levels in breast cancer cells	Breast cancer, prostate cancer	[109]

Table 2. *Cont.*

Dietary Component	Food Source	Potential Benefits in Breast Cancer	Diseases	Refs
Ursolic acid (UA)	Blueberries, cranberries and apple peels	Reduced the expression of epigenetic modifying enzymes, including the DNMT1 and DNMT3a and the histone deacetylases (HDACs) HDAC1, HDAC2, HDAC3, HDAC6 and HDAC7 activity	Skin cancer, breast cancer, colorectal cancer	[110]

4.6.1. Genistein (GE)

GE is the most predominant bioactive isoflavone found mainly in soybean products and other food sources such as lupin, fava beans, kudzu, and psoralea [84]. GE has been reported to act as a potent chemo-preventive and therapeutic agent against various types of cancers including breast, prostate, and lung cancer [85]. For instance, GE suppresses the growth of BC cells in patient-derived tumor xenograft (PDX) [85]. Moreover, GE has been reported to modify the expression levels and activities of key epigenetic-associated genes, including HDAC2, DNA methyltransferases (DNMT3b) and ten-eleven translocation (TET3) methylcytosine dioxygenases. These genes are involved in epigenetic modifications, such as DNA methylation and histone methylation, which can regulate gene expression and impact cellular behavior [85]. By modulating the activities of these epigenetic regulators, GE may influence the epigenetic landscape of breast cancer cells, leading to changes in gene expression patterns that can affect cancer-related pathways.

4.6.2. Sulforaphane (SFN)

SFN is a natural compound and is abundant in cruciferous vegetables such as broccoli sprouts (BSp) and kale [111]. It has gained attention for its potential health benefits, including its ability to inhibit HDAC2 activity [112,113]. In the context of breast cancer, a dietary regimen of genistein and BSp in combination has been shown effective in reducing mammary tumor incidence and delaying tumor latency in a spontaneous breast cancer mouse model [86]. The combination of GE and SFN downregulated HDAC2 protein levels in breast cancer cells. This suggests that the combined action of GE and SFN can influence gene expression in breast cancer cells by modulating HDAC2 activity, thereby affecting immune response [86].

4.6.3. Chrysin and Its Analogues

Chrysin and its analogues are a group of polyphenolic compounds found in various dietary sources such as fruits, vegetables, olive oil, tea, and red wine [114]. The cytotoxic effects of chrysin have been shown against a wide range of cancer cell lines, including BC (MCF-7, MDA-MB-231), colon cancer (Lovo, DLD-1), and prostate cancer cells [87,88]. It is able to induce G1 cell cycle arrest and inhibit the activity of HDACs, specifically HDAC2 [89]. Moreover, polyphenolic compounds could promote the growth of SCFA-producer *Lachnoclostridium* [21], consequently modulating immune response.

4.6.4. Resveratrol (RSV)

RSV is also a polyphenol abundant in grape skin and seeds. It also presents in other food sources such as apples, blueberries, mulberries, peanuts, pistachios, plums, and red wine [90]. RSV has numerous beneficial properties of anti-glycosylation, anti-inflammation, anti-neurodegeneration, and antioxidation in various types of cancer [91]. One intriguing aspect of RSV is its proposed potential as a pan-HDAC inhibitor [92]. Studies have shown that RSV can inhibit the growth of BC cells (MCF-7 and MDA-MB-231) by inhibiting the activity of HDAC2 in a dose-dependent manner [93].

4.6.5. Oleuropein (OLE)

OLE is a polyphenolic compound in virgin olive oil with antineoplastic properties and it is well tolerated by humans [94]. Studies have shown that OLE can reduce progression, invasion, and proliferation of breast cancer cells by suppressing the activity of both HDAC2 and HDAC3 [95]. However, OLE exhibits little negative effect on normal breast epithelial cells, suggesting a potential selectivity towards BC cells and its potential for BC patients receiving ICIs therapy [95].

4.6.6. Curcumin

Curcumin, a lipophilic polyphenol derived from turmeric (Curcuma longa), has been extensively studied for its diverse health-promoting properties, including antioxidant, anti-inflammatory, hepatoprotective, anti-atherosclerotic, and antidiabetic effects [96]. Moreover, curcumin has been investigated for its potential as an HDAC inhibitor in MCF-7 and MDA-MB-231 cells [97], showing inhibitive effects on both HDAC activity and the expression of HDAC 1 and 2 in a dose-dependent manner [97].

4.6.7. Valeric Acid

Valerian (Valeriana officinalis) is a medicated diet that has been commonly used in cooking soup by some ethnic minorities in China for hundreds of years for restoring and balancing body energy [98]. Valeric acid, a major active component of valerian, has been identified as a potential HDAC inhibitor with anti-cancer effects on liver and breast cancer [98]. A study reported that valeric acid significantly decreases HDAC2 activity in treated breast cancer cells and may lead to alterations of DNA methylation [99].

4.6.8. Rh4

Ginseng is also a typical medicated diet item and is commonly used for making cuisine mainly in Asia. It is also a traditional Chinese herb with multiple biological effects. One of its components, Rh4, has been identified as a rare ginsenoside with potential inhibitive effects on the development of various cancers [100]. Rh4 can inhibit the expression of PD-L1 by regulating HDAC2-mediated JAK/STAT in breast cancer cells [101]. In addition, a study of the binding of Rh4 and HDAC2 suggests a high binding affinity existing between Rh4 and HDAC2, indicating the potential of ginseng as a dietary intervention for BC patients [101].

4.6.9. Butyrate (NaB)

NaB, a short-chain fatty acid generated via the fermentation of dietary fiber by the colonic microbiota, has shown anticancer activities mediated through HDACi [102]. NaB is primarily derived from undigested dietary carbohydrates, such as resistant starch and dietary fiber and, to a lesser extent, from dietary and endogenous proteins [103,104]. Studies have demonstrated that treatment with NaB, when combined with retinoids, enhances the inhibition of breast cancer cell proliferation [105]. Furthermore, the combination of butyrate with tumor necrosis factor-α (TNF-α), tumor necrosis factor-related apoptosis-inducing ligand (TRAIL), and anti-Fas agonist has been found to strongly induce apoptosis, leading to a significant decrease in the viability of breast cancer cells [106]. The action of NaB is often mediated through Sp1/Sp3 binding sites (e.g., p21 (Waf1/Cip1)). Both Sp1 and Sp3 were associated with HDAC activity in human breast cancer cells. And Sp1 and Sp3 recruit HDAC1 and HDAC2, with the latter being phosphorylated by protein kinase CK2 [115]. CK2 is upregulated in several cancers including breast cancer, which may promote breast cancer by deregulating key transcription processes [115].

4.6.10. Other Potential Candidates

Some other dietary compounds have also been identified as HDAC2i in other cancer types. For instance, green tea and its bioactive components, especially polyphenols, possess many health-promoting and disease-preventing benefits with anti-inflammatory, antimutagenic, antioxidant, and anticancer properties, but have no significant toxicity on normal cells in vivo. It has the potential as an effective chemotherapeutic agent for cancer prevention and treatment through various cellular, molecular, and biochemical mechanisms [116]. The major polyphenol components of green tea are (-)-epigallocatechin-3-gallate (EGCG), (-)-epigallocatechin (EGC), (-)-epicatechin-3-gallate (ECG) and (-)-epicatechin (EC) [116]. One of the molecular mechanisms underlying the anticancer effects of green tea polyphenols (GTPs) is HDAC2 inhibition [107]. Another study presented GTPs suppressed melanoma via regulating the circ_MITF/miR-30e-3p/HDAC2 axis [108]. Rosmarinic acid (RA), a main phenolic compound in rosemary, presents anti-inflammatory, anti-oxidant, and anti-cancer effects [109]. RA induced cell cycle arrest and apoptosis through modulation of HDAC2 expression in prostate cancer [109]. In addition, ursolic acid (UA) is a well-known natural triterpenoid abundant in apple peels, basil (*Ocimum basilicum*), blueberries (*Vaccinium* spp.), cranberries (*Vaccinium macrocarpon*), heather flowers (*Calluna vulgaris*), Labrador tea (*Ledum groenlandicum* Retzius), olives (*Olea europaea*), pears (*Pyrus pyrifolia*), and rosemary (*Rosmarinus officinalis*). A study reported that UA reduced the expression of epigenetic modifying enzymes, including DNA methyltransferases DNMT1 and DNMT3a and histone deacetylases (HDACs) HDAC1, HDAC2, HDAC3 and HDAC8 (Class I), and HDAC6 and HDAC7 (Class II), and HDAC activity [110]. Given that fungal *Neurospora crassa* contains enriched retinal, and flavin adenine dinucleotide (FAD) or flavin mononucleotide (FMN), showing tumor growth inhibition of breast cancer [117,118], it will be interesting to explore whether *N. crassa* has potential as an adjuvant of ICIs. Overall, these dietary compounds mentioned above can also be considered as potential candidates. However, their HDAC2 inhibitory effects should be further confirmed and evaluated in breast cancer cells.

4.7. Potential Approaches of Taking Bioactive Compound

For enhancing absorption efficiency and therefore improving the potential health benefits and biological activities of certain bioactive compounds, many means of application have been developed [119]. Some of them might provide a better way for BC patients receiving ICIs to gain HDAC2i efficiently. However, it is important to emphasize that thorough exploration in this area is still a pressing necessity.

a. Nutraceuticals and Dietary Supplements

Many bioactive compounds with antioxidant or anti-inflammatory properties, found in certain fruits or vegetables, have been produced as nutraceuticals and dietary supplements for taking them more conveniently and easily [65]. Moreover, nutraceuticals and dietary supplements have been found to maintain excellent safety levels [120]. For instance, anthocyanins from berries, flavonols from dark chocolate, and resveratrol from red grapes have been widely used as consumed nutraceuticals [121]. Hence, dietary HDAC2i can be potentially produced as nutraceuticals and dietary supplements for clinical use.

b. Nanotechnology and Drug Delivery

Bioactive compounds can also be incorporated into well-designed nanoparticles for targeted drug delivery, enhancing drug efficacy and reducing side effects [122]. For instance, theracurmin, a curcumin formulation consisting of dispersed curcumin with colloidal nanoparticles, possesses significantly improved bioavailability and therapeutic efficacy for treating osteoarthritis, compared to turmeric powder monotherapy [123–125]. More specifically, by adding nanoparticles, theracurmin was shown to have greater bioavailability than turmeric powder by 40 fold in rats and 27 fold higher in humans [125], and to have fewer side effects [123]. Moreover, many nanoparticles have already been developed for specific targeted delivery to breast cancer cells with excellent safety, such as Cur-Dox-NPs (selective co-delivery of doxorubicin and curcumin), FeAC-DOX@PC-HCQ NPs, DHAPN, and Opaxio™ [126–128]. Thus, this approach has potential for widespread utilization among BC patients seeking HDAC2 inhibitors. Nevertheless, it is essential to emphasize that substantial research is imperative to substantiate its feasibility and efficacy.

c. Pharmaceuticals and Medicinal Products

Some bioactive compounds can be isolated and developed into pharmaceutical drugs to efficiently improve their therapeutic effect [129]. For instance, curcumin, a bioactive compound that has been found to possess multiple biological regulatory functions, has been successfully isolated from plant curcuma aromatica salisb for treating different types of cancer, including BC [130,131]. Moreover, paclitaxel, an efficient anti-cancer tricyclic diterpenoid compound, was also originally isolated from the plant Taxus brevifolia and subsequently synthesized for cancer treatment [132]. Therefore, plants containing HDAC2i may also be generated as pharmaceuticals and medicinal products.

d. Phytotherapy and Traditional Medicine

Phytotherapy and traditional medicine have been widely applied in treating various of diseases [133,134]. They are natural, with relatively low irritation and side effects on the human body, and can also be utilized in combination with other treatment [135,136]. Moreover, evidence has proven that these therapeutic approaches can help to enhance the therapeutic effect of anti-cancer treatment, such as chemotherapy [137]. Normally, patients can achieve certain active ingredients of nutrients by decocting herbal plants. For instance, valeric acid, the dietary HDAC2i mentioned above can be obtained by a traditional Chinese medicine decoction containing the valerian herb [98,99]. Thus, phytotherapy (or traditional medicine) seems to be a reliable way for patients to take HDAC2i. However, the effectiveness of these methods for absorbing HDAC2i needs more evaluation.

4.8. Nutrients That May Impair the Therapeutic Effect of ICIs

Even some dietary items that contain HDAC2i may improve the efficiency of ICIs, while other nutrients of diets that can potentially hamper the therapeutic effect of such therapy should also be noted [138]. Hence, those nutrients have been summarized below in order to emphasize the potential risks and provoke further exploration on their specific mechanisms and exact interactions.

a. Omega-3 Fatty Acids

Omega-3 fatty acids, commonly present in fish oil and certain plant sources, possess anti-inflammatory properties and are essential for synthesizing hormones and endogenous substances [139]. Natural killer (NK) cells are innate lymphocytes responsible for orchestrating immune responses against tumors and viruses [140]. Fish oil supplementation was found to decrease NK cell activity, which rebounded after supplementation ceased [141]. Notably, the age of individuals might influence the impact of omega-3 supplementation on NK cells [141]. Therefore, excessive consumption of omega-3 fatty acids has been considered to potentially hamper the normal function of immunity, which might further dampen the efficacy of ICIs. Thus, an appropriate amount of omega-3 intake is important for BC patients receiving ICIs. Of course, the exact mechanisms and interactions should be further explored.

b. *Vitamins*

Vitamins are a type of trace organic substance obtained from food that can maintain normal physiological functions in humans [142]. Vitamins participate in the biochemical reactions of the human body and regulate metabolic functions, including immunity [143]. Deficiency or over intake of certain vitamins has been found to impair anti-cancer immunity, therefore affecting the efficiency of ICIs [138]. For instance, vitamin D has shown the ability to elevate the T-regulatory (Treg)/T-helper 17 (Th-17) cell ratio, leading to immune suppression and contributing to the onset of immune-related adverse events (irAEs), indicating its potential risk for patients receiving ICI therapy [144,145]. Moreover, vitamin A has also been reported to suppress the expression of PD-L1 causing cancer resistance to PD-1/PD-L1 blockade therapy [146,147]. In addition, evidence has shown that vitamin B6 can suppress PD-L1 expression and block the PD-1/PD-L1 signaling pathway [148]. Thus, extra attention is required when administrating vitamin supplementation for breast cancer patients receiving ICIs. More research is also indispensable in this field.

c. Probiotics

Probiotics, including bacteria and yeast, are living microorganisms [149,150]. Some of them have been commonly utilized to promote gut health, closely intertwined with immune function [149,150]. Recent evidence has newly pointed out that an excessive immune response in the gut induced by overconsumption of probiotics might constrain the systemic immune reaction necessary for the optimal efficacy of ICIs [151,152]. Briefly, a clinical study involving 46 melanoma patients indicated that taking over-the-counter probiotic supplements (for unrelated conditions) was linked to a 70% reduction in response rate to ICI treatment [152]. Therefore, probiotics should be approached cautiously in BC patients undergoing immunotherapy.

d. High-Fiber Diets

Fiber-rich diets primarily comprise two essential elements: soluble fiber and insoluble fiber. These vital components are found in an array of plant-based foods, including legumes, whole grains, cereals, vegetables, fruits, nuts, and seeds. Dietary fiber is composed of non-starch polysaccharides and various plant constituents like cellulose, resistant starch, and resistant dextrins [153]. High-fiber diets have been considered to modulate the gut microbiota and influence immune responses [154]. While a diverse gut microbiome is generally associated with better health, certain bacterial metabolites produced from high-fiber diets could potentially hamper the efficiency of ICIs [155]. More specifically, evidence has shown that, in non-small cell lung cancer patients, notably increased serum indoleamine-2,3-dioxygenase (IDO) levels, which were potentially produced by high-fiber diets, induced primary resistance to ICI treatment [155]. Thus, such bacterial metabolites might play a pivotal role in ICI resistance [155]. Therefore, the overall benefits of a high-fiber diet should be considered in balance.

e. Ketogenic diet

The ketogenic diet (KD) is characterized by high fat, low to moderate protein, and very low carbohydrate intake [156]. Evidence has shown that KD can lead to a downregulation of CTLA-4 and PD-1 expression on tumor-infiltrating lymphocytes (TILs), as well as PD-L1 expression on glioblastoma cells in animal models [157]. Also, it has been observed that the ketogenic diet KD can lead to the downregulation of cell membrane-associated PD-L1 [158]. Therefore, KD has the potential to reduce the effectiveness of PD-1/PD-L1 blockade therapy and should be avoided by patients using PD-1/PD-L1 inhibitors.

f. Protein-restricted diet

A low-protein diet serves as a therapeutic approach for managing inherited metabolic disorders like phenylketonuria and homocystinuria. Additionally, it can be employed in the treatment of kidney or liver ailments. Furthermore, a reduced intake of protein has been observed to potentially lower the risk of bone fractures, likely due to alterations in calcium [159]. Notably, recent studies have found that the deprivation of glutamine, a building block of proteins, can reduce PD-1 expression, indicating the potential to suppress the efficiency of PD-1 inhibitors [160].

5. Conclusions

According to recent data, the number of new cases of BC has accounted for about 11.7% of all malignant tumors. It has surpassed lung cancer as the most common malignant tumor, and its mortality rate has ranked among the top five of all malignant tumors [118]. In an effort to cure BC patients, ICIs (e.g., PD-1/PD-L1 inhibitors) have been introduced. However, it is still a challenge to provide durable and ideal clinical benefits and cure BC patients. Thus, novel ICI-based therapeutic strategies in combination have been studied to further improve the effect of treatment, such as HDAC2i plus a PD-1/PD-L1 inhibitor.

Dietary intervention, as a supportive therapy, is able to function as an HDAC2i through daily intake for cancer patients. An HDAC2i can suppress IFN-γ-induced PD-L1 expression and inhibit the process of PD-L1 nuclear translocation. Thus, a diet-derived HDAC2i has the potential to improve the clinical outcomes of BC patients, especially for those who are taking PD-1/PD-L1 inhibitors. Furthermore, to the best of our knowledge, there are still no relevant clinical guidelines on the application of an HDAC2i-containing diet for patients, especially for BC patients receiving ICIs. For such a group of patients, this novel dietary therapy can not only provide new dietary options but also may improve their clinical outcomes.

To sum up, multiple anti-cancer and immunomodulatory effects of HDAC2i guarantee future research into investigating such a novel dietary intervention for BC patients receiving ICIs. The potential of diet to enhance the therapeutic effect of ICIs is still to be fully evaluated. Certainly, further research is also required to identify more HDAC2i-containing foods for more dietary choices.

Supplementary Materials: The following supporting information can be downloaded at: https://www.mdpi.com/article/10.3390/nu15183984/s1.

Author Contributions: R.H. independently created the original concept of this paper; R.H. and Y.W. completed the original draft; R.H. conducted the analysis and created the figures; H.R. and Y.W. created the tables; R.H. reviewed and edited the manuscript with the help of L.L., C.L. and P.Z.; visualization, R.H.; supervision, R.H.; project administration, R.H.; funding acquisition, R.H. All authors have read and agreed to the published version of the manuscript.

Funding: This research was supported by the "National Natural Science Foundation of China (Youth foundation) (No.82204864)" project (to Rui Han), and "Basic and Applied Basic Research on Municipal School (College) Joint Funding Projects (Guangzhou municipal science and technology bureau) (No.202201020252)" project (to Rui Han).

Institutional Review Board Statement: Not applicable.

Informed Consent Statement: Not applicable.

Data Availability Statement: Not applicable.

Conflicts of Interest: The authors declare no conflict of interest.

References

1. Tao, X.; Li, T.; Gandomkar, Z.; Brennan, P.C.; Reed, W.M. Incidence, mortality, survival, and disease burden of breast cancer in China compared to other developed countries. *Asia-Pac. J. Clin. Oncol.* **2023**. [CrossRef] [PubMed]
2. Bazzi, T.; Al-Husseini, M.; Saravolatz, L.; Kafri, Z. Trends in Breast Cancer Incidence and Mortality in the United States From 2004-2018: A Surveillance, Epidemiology, and End Results (SEER)-Based Study. *Cureus* **2023**, *15*, e37982. [CrossRef] [PubMed]
3. Pedersini, R.; di Mauro, P.; Bosio, S.; Zanini, B.; Zanini, A.; Amoroso, V.; Turla, A.; Vassalli, L.; Ardine, M.; Monteverdi, S.; et al. Changes in eating habits and food preferences in breast cancer patients undergoing adjuvant chemotherapy. *Sci. Rep.* **2021**, *11*, 12975. [CrossRef] [PubMed]
4. Taylor, C.; McGale, P.; Probert, J.; Broggio, J.; Charman, J.; Darby, S.C.; Kerr, A.J.; Whelan, T.; Cutter, D.J.; Mannu, G.; et al. Breast cancer mortality in 500 000 women with early invasive breast cancer in England, 1993–2015: Population based observational cohort study. *BMJ* **2023**, *381*, e074684. [CrossRef]
5. Bertucci, F.; Gonçalves, A. Immunotherapy in Breast Cancer: The Emerging Role of PD-1 and PD-L1. *Curr. Oncol. Rep.* **2017**, *19*, 64. [CrossRef]
6. Lu, L.; Bai, Y.; Wang, Z. Elevated T cell activation score is associated with improved survival of breast cancer. *Breast Cancer Res. Treat.* **2017**, *164*, 689–696. [CrossRef] [PubMed]
7. Jacob, S.L.; Huppert, L.A.; Rugo, H.S. Role of Immunotherapy in Breast Cancer. *JCO Oncol. Pract.* **2023**, *19*, 167–179. [CrossRef]
8. Hattori, M.; Masuda, N.; Takano, T.; Tsugawa, K.; Inoue, K.; Matsumoto, K.; Ishikawa, T.; Itoh, M.; Yasojima, H.; Tanabe, Y.; et al. Pembrolizumab plus chemotherapy in Japanese patients with triple-negative breast cancer: Results from KEYNOTE-355. *Cancer Med.* **2023**, *12*, 10280–10293. [CrossRef]
9. Downs-Canner, S.; Mittendorf, E.A. Correction: Preoperative Immunotherapy Combined with Chemotherapy for Triple-Negative Breast Cancer: Perspective on the KEYNOTE-522 Study. *Ann. Surg. Oncol.* **2023**, *30*, 3286. [CrossRef]
10. Khalid, A.B.; Calderon, G.; Jalal, S.I.; Durm, G.A. Physician Awareness of Immune-Related Adverse Events of Immune Checkpoint Inhibitors. *Breast Cancer Res. Treat.* **2022**, *20*, 1316–1320. [CrossRef]
11. Gumusay, O.; Callan, J.; Rugo, H.S. Immunotherapy toxicity: Identification and management. *Breast Cancer Res. Treat.* **2022**, *192*, 1–17. [CrossRef] [PubMed]

12. Liu, S.; Zhao, S.; Dong, Y.; Wang, T.; Niu, X.; Zhao, L.; Wang, G. Antitumor activity and mechanism of resistance of the novel HDAC and PI3K dual inhibitor CUDC-907 in pancreatic cancer. *Cancer Chemother. Pharmacol.* **2021**, *87*, 415–423. [CrossRef] [PubMed]
13. Garmpis, N.; Damaskos, C.; Dimitroulis, D.; Kouraklis, G.; Garmpi, A.; Sarantis, P.; Koustas, E.; Patsouras, A.; Psilopatis, I.; Antoniou, E.A.; et al. Clinical Significance of the Histone Deacetylase 2 (HDAC-2) Expression in Human Breast Cancer. *J. Pers. Med.* **2022**, *12*, 1672. [CrossRef] [PubMed]
14. Shan, W.; Jiang, Y.; Yu, H.; Huang, Q.; Liu, L.; Guo, X.; Li, L.; Mi, Q.; Zhang, K.; Yang, Z. HDAC2 overexpression correlates with aggressive clinicopathological features and DNA-damage response pathway of breast cancer. *Am. J. Cancer Res.* **2017**, *7*, 1213–1226.
15. Zhao, H.; Yu, Z.; Zhao, L.; He, M.; Ren, J.; Wu, H.; Chen, Q.; Yao, W.; Wei, M. HDAC2 overexpression is a poor prognostic factor of breast cancer patients with increased multidrug resistance-associated protein expression who received anthracyclines therapy. *Jpn. J. Clin. Oncol.* **2016**, *46*, 893–902. [CrossRef]
16. Maccallini, C.; Ammazzalorso, A.; De Filippis, B.; Fantacuzzi, M.; Giampietro, L.; Amoroso, R. HDAC Inhibitors for the Therapy of Triple Negative Breast Cancer. *Pharmaceuticals* **2022**, *15*, 667. [CrossRef]
17. Li, Y.; Seto, E. HDACs and HDAC Inhibitors in Cancer Development and Therapy. *Cold Spring Harb. Perspect. Med.* **2016**, *6*, a026831. [CrossRef]
18. Xu, P.; Xiong, W.; Lin, Y.; Fan, L.; Pan, H.; Li, Y. Histone deacetylase 2 knockout suppresses immune escape of triple-negative breast cancer cells via downregulating PD-L1 expression. *Cell Death Dis.* **2021**, *12*, 779. [CrossRef]
19. Gao, Y.; Nihira, N.T.; Bu, X.; Chu, C.; Zhang, J.; Kolodziejczyk, A.; Fan, Y.; Chan, N.T.; Ma, L.; Liu, J.; et al. Acetylation-dependent regulation of PD-L1 nuclear translocation dictates the efficacy of anti-PD-1 immunotherapy. *Nat. Cell Biol.* **2020**, *22*, 1064–1075. [CrossRef]
20. Bassett, S.A.; Barnett, M.P.G. The Role of Dietary Histone Deacetylases (HDACs) Inhibitors in Health and Disease. *Nutrients* **2014**, *6*, 4273–4301. [CrossRef]
21. Zhu, G.; Su, H.; Johnson, C.H.; Khan, S.A.; Kluger, H.; Lu, L. Intratumour microbiome associated with the infiltration of cytotoxic CD8+ T cells and patient survival in cutaneous melanoma. *Eur. J. Cancer* **2021**, *151*, 25–34. [CrossRef] [PubMed]
22. Limon-Miro, A.T.; Lopez-Teros, V.; Astiazaran-Garcia, H. Dietary Guidelines for Breast Cancer Patients: A Critical Review. *Adv. Nutr. Int. Rev. J.* **2017**, *8*, 613–623. [CrossRef] [PubMed]
23. Seo, J.; Min, S.K.; Park, H.-R.; Kim, D.H.; Kwon, M.J.; Kim, L.S.; Ju, Y.-S. Expression of Histone Deacetylases HDAC1, HDAC2, HDAC3, and HDAC6 in Invasive Ductal Carcinomas of the Breast. *J. Breast Cancer* **2014**, *17*, 323–331. [CrossRef]
24. Muller, B.M.; Jana, L.; Kasajima, A.; Lehmann, A.; Prinzler, J.; Budczies, J.; Winzer, K.-J.; Dietel, M.; Weichert, W.; Denkert, C. Differential expression of histone deacetylases HDAC1, 2 and 3 in human breast cancer—Overexpression of HDAC2 and HDAC3 is associated with clinicopathological indicators of disease progression. *BMC Cancer* **2013**, *13*, 215. [CrossRef]
25. Long, M.; Hou, W.; Liu, Y.; Hu, T. A Histone Acetylation Modulator Gene Signature for Classification and Prognosis of Breast Cancer. *Curr. Oncol.* **2021**, *28*, 928–939. [CrossRef] [PubMed]
26. Choi, S.R.; Hwang, C.Y.; Lee, J.; Cho, K.-H. Network Analysis Identifies Regulators of Basal-Like Breast Cancer Reprogramming and Endocrine Therapy Vulnerability. *Cancer Res.* **2022**, *82*, 320–333. [CrossRef]
27. Harms, K.L.; Chen, X. Histone Deacetylase 2 Modulates p53 Transcriptional Activities through Regulation of p53-DNA Binding Activity. *Cancer Res.* **2007**, *67*, 3145–3152. [CrossRef]
28. He, X.-H.; Zhu, W.; Yuan, P.; Jiang, S.; Li, D.; Zhang, H.-W.; Liu, M.-F. miR-155 downregulates ErbB2 and suppresses ErbB2-induced malignant transformation of breast epithelial cells. *Oncogene* **2016**, *35*, 6015–6025. [CrossRef]
29. Jo, H.; Shim, K.; Kim, H.-U.; Jung, H.S.; Jeoung, D. HDAC2 as a target for developing anti-cancer drugs. *Comput. Struct. Biotechnol. J.* **2023**, *21*, 2048–2057. [CrossRef]
30. Biçaku, E.; Marchion, D.C.; Schmitt, M.L.; Münster, P.N. Selective Inhibition of Histone Deacetylase 2 Silences Progesterone Receptor–Mediated Signaling. *Cancer Res.* **2008**, *68*, 1513–1519. [CrossRef]
31. Marchion, D.C.; Bicaku, E.; Turner, J.G.; Schmitt, M.L.; Morelli, D.R.; Munster, P.N. HDAC2 regulates chromatin plasticity and enhances DNA vulnerability. *Mol. Cancer Ther.* **2009**, *8*, 794–801. [CrossRef] [PubMed]
32. Zhang, Z.; Qiu, N.; Yin, J.; Zhang, J.; Liu, H.; Guo, W.; Liu, M.; Liu, T.; Chen, D.; Luo, K.; et al. SRGN crosstalks with YAP to maintain chemoresistance and stemness in breast cancer cells by modulating HDAC2 expression. *Theranostics* **2020**, *10*, 4290–4307. [CrossRef] [PubMed]
33. Masoumi, E.; Tahaghoghi-Hajghorbani, S.; Jafarzadeh, L.; Sanaei, M.-J.; Pourbagheri-Sigaroodi, A.; Bashash, D. The application of immune checkpoint blockade in breast cancer and the emerging role of nanoparticle. *J. Control. Release* **2021**, *340*, 168–187. [CrossRef] [PubMed]
34. Isaacs, J.; Anders, C.; McArthur, H.; Force, J. Biomarkers of Immune Checkpoint Blockade Response in Triple-Negative Breast Cancer. *Curr. Treat. Options Oncol.* **2021**, *22*, 38. [CrossRef] [PubMed]
35. Lu, L.; Risch, E.; Halaban, R.; Zhen, P.; Bacchiocchi, A.; Risch, H.A. Dynamic changes of circulating soluble PD-1/PD-L1 and its association with patient survival in immune checkpoint blockade-treated melanoma. *Int. Immunopharmacol.* **2023**, *118*, 110092. [CrossRef] [PubMed]
36. Fan, Z.; Wu, C.; Chen, M.; Jiang, Y.; Wu, Y.; Mao, R.; Fan, Y. The generation of PD-L1 and PD-L2 in cancer cells: From nuclear chromatin reorganization to extracellular presentation. *Acta Pharm. Sin. B* **2022**, *12*, 1041–1053. [CrossRef]

37. Xiong, W.; Gao, Y.; Wei, W.; Zhang, J. Extracellular and nuclear PD-L1 in modulating cancer immunotherapy. *Trends Cancer* **2021**, *7*, 837–846. [CrossRef]
38. Koh, Y.W.; Han, J.-H.; Haam, S.; Lee, H.W. HIP1R Expression and Its Association with PD-1 Pathway Blockade Response in Refractory Advanced NonSmall Cell Lung Cancer: A Gene Set Enrichment Analysis. *J. Clin. Med.* **2020**, *9*, 1425. [CrossRef]
39. Muenst, S.; Schaerli, A.R.; Gao, F.; Däster, S.; Trella, E.; Droeser, R.A.; Muraro, M.G.; Zajac, P.; Zanetti, R.; Gillanders, W.E.; et al. Expression of programmed death ligand 1 (PD-L1) is associated with poor prognosis in human breast cancer. *Breast Cancer Res. Treat.* **2014**, *146*, 15–24. [CrossRef]
40. Lotfinejad, P.; Kazemi, T.; Safaei, S.; Amini, M.; Baghbani, E.; Shotorbani, S.S.; Niaragh, F.J.; Derakhshani, A.; Shadbad, M.A.; Silvestris, N. PD-L1 silencing inhibits triple-negative breast cancer development and upregulates T-cell-induced pro-inflammatory cytokines. *Biomed. Pharmacother.* **2021**, *138*, 111436. [CrossRef]
41. Setordzi, P.; Chang, X.; Liu, Z.; Wu, Y.; Zuo, D. The recent advances of PD-1 and PD-L1 checkpoint signaling inhibition for breast cancer immunotherapy. *Eur. J. Pharmacol.* **2021**, *895*, 173867. [CrossRef] [PubMed]
42. Schmid, P.; Adams, S.; Rugo, H.S.; Schneeweiss, A.; Barrios, C.H.; Iwata, H.; Diéras, V.; Hegg, R.; Im, S.-A.; Shaw Wright, G.; et al. Atezolizumab and Nab-Paclitaxel in Advanced Triple-Negative Breast Cancer. *N. Engl. J. Med.* **2018**, *379*, 2108–2121. [CrossRef] [PubMed]
43. Minn, A.J.; Wherry, E.J. Combination Cancer Therapies with Immune Checkpoint Blockade: Convergence on Interferon Signaling. *Cell* **2016**, *165*, 272–275. [CrossRef] [PubMed]
44. Abiko, K.; Matsumura, N.; Hamanishi, J.; Horikawa, N.; Murakami, R.; Yamaguchi, K.; Yoshioka, Y.; Baba, T.; Konishi, I.; Mandai, M. IFN-γ from lymphocytes induces PD-L1 expression and promotes progression of ovarian cancer. *Br. J. Cancer* **2015**, *112*, 1501–1509. [CrossRef] [PubMed]
45. Bouhet, S.; Lafont, V.; Billard, E.; Gross, A.; Dornand, J. The IFNgamma-induced STAT1-CBP/P300 association, required for a normal response to the cytokine, is disrupted in Brucella-infected macrophages. *Microb. Pathog.* **2009**, *46*, 88–97. [CrossRef] [PubMed]
46. Nakayama, Y.; Mimura, K.; Tamaki, T.; Shiraishi, K.; Kua, L.-F.; Koh, V.; Ohmori, M.; Kimura, A.; Inoue, S.; Okayama, H.; et al. Phospho-STAT1 expression as a potential biomarker for anti-PD-1/anti-PD-L1 immunotherapy for breast cancer. *Int. J. Oncol.* **2019**, *54*, 2030–2038. [CrossRef]
47. Calder, P.C. Foods to deliver immune-supporting nutrients. *Curr. Opin. Food Sci.* **2022**, *43*, 136–145. [CrossRef]
48. Calder, P.C.; Carr, A.G.; Gombart, A.F.; Eggersdorfer, M. Reply to Comment on: Optimal Nutritional Status for a Well-Functioning Immune System Is an Important Factor to Protect against Viral Infections. *Nutrients* **2020**, *12*, 1181. [CrossRef]
49. Chen, O.; Mah, E.; Dioum, E.; Marwaha, A.; Shanmugam, S.; Malleshi, N.; Sudha, V.; Gayathri, R.; Unnikrishnan, R.; Anjana, R.M.; et al. The Role of Oat Nutrients in the Immune System: A Narrative Review. *Nutrients* **2021**, *13*, 1048. [CrossRef]
50. Noor, S.; Piscopo, S.; Gasmi, A. Nutrients Interaction with the Immune System. *Arch. Razi. Inst.* **2021**, *76*, 1579–1588. [CrossRef]
51. Kichloo, A.; Albosta, M.; Dahiya, D.; Guidi, J.C.; Aljadah, M.; Singh, J.; Shaka, H.; Wani, F.; Kumar, A.; Lekkala, M. Systemic adverse effects and toxicities associated with immunotherapy: A review. *World J. Clin. Oncol.* **2021**, *12*, 150–163. [CrossRef]
52. Ticinesi, A.; Nouvenne, A.; Chiussi, G.; Castaldo, G.; Guerra, A.; Meschi, T. Calcium Oxalate Nephrolithiasis and Gut Microbiota: Not just a Gut-Kidney Axis. A Nutritional Perspective. *Nutrients* **2020**, *12*, 548. [CrossRef]
53. Taraszewska, A. Risk factors for gastroesophageal reflux disease symptoms related to lifestyle and diet. *Rocz Panstw Zakl Hig* **2021**, *72*, 21–28. [CrossRef] [PubMed]
54. Jadhav, A.; Bajaj, A.; Xiao, Y.; Markandey, M.; Ahuja, V.; Kashyap, P.C. Role of Diet–Microbiome Interaction in Gastrointestinal Disorders and Strategies to Modulate Them with Microbiome-Targeted Therapies. *Annu. Rev. Nutr.* **2023**, *43*, 355–383. [CrossRef]
55. Campmans-Kuijpers, M.J.E.; Dijkstra, G. Food and Food Groups in Inflammatory Bowel Disease (IBD): The Design of the Groningen Anti-Inflammatory Diet (GrAID). *Nutrients* **2021**, *13*, 1067. [CrossRef] [PubMed]
56. Tolkien, K.; Bradburn, S.; Murgatroyd, C. An anti-inflammatory diet as a potential intervention for depressive disorders: A systematic review and meta-analysis. *Clin. Nutr.* **2019**, *38*, 2045–2052. [CrossRef] [PubMed]
57. De Groot, S.; Lugtenberg, R.T.; Cohen, D.; Welters, M.J.P.; Ehsan, I.; Vreeswijk, M.P.G.; Smit, V.T.H.B.M.; de Graaf, H.; Heijns, J.B.; Portielje, J.E.A.; et al. Fasting mimicking diet as an adjunct to neoadjuvant chemotherapy for breast cancer in the multicentre randomized phase 2 DIRECT trial. *Nat. Commun.* **2020**, *11*, 3083. [CrossRef] [PubMed]
58. Arends, J.; Baracos, V.; Bertz, H.; Bozzetti, F.; Calder, P.C.; Deutz, N.E.P.; Erickson, N.; Laviano, A.; Lisanti, M.P.; Lobo, D.N.; et al. ESPEN expert group recommendations for action against cancer-related malnutrition. *Clin. Nutr.* **2017**, *36*, 1187–1196. [CrossRef]
59. Cheng, Y.; Zhang, J.; Zhang, L.; Wu, J.; Zhan, Z. Enteral immunonutrition versus enteral nutrition for gastric cancer patients undergoing a total gastrectomy: A systematic review and meta-analysis. *BMC Gastroenterol.* **2018**, *18*, 11. [CrossRef]
60. Greathouse, K.L.; Wyatt, M.; Johnson, A.J.; Toy, E.P.; Khan, J.M.; Dunn, K.; Clegg, D.J.; Reddy, S. Diet-microbiome interactions in cancer treatment: Opportunities and challenges for precision nutrition in cancer. *Neoplasia* **2022**, *29*, 100800. [CrossRef]
61. Owen, L.; Corfe, B. The role of diet and nutrition on mental health and wellbeing. *Proc. Nutr. Soc.* **2017**, *76*, 425–426. [CrossRef] [PubMed]
62. Berding, K.; Vlckova, K.; Marx, W.; Schellekens, H.; Stanton, C.; Clarke, G.; Jacka, F.; Dinan, T.G.; Cryan, J.F. Diet and the Microbiota–Gut–Brain Axis: Sowing the Seeds of Good Mental Health. *Adv. Nutr. Int. Rev. J.* **2021**, *12*, 1239–1285. [CrossRef] [PubMed]

63. Carreira, H.; Williams, R.; Müller, M.; Harewood, R.; Stanway, S.; Bhaskaran, K. Associations Between Breast Cancer Survivorship and Adverse Mental Health Outcomes: A Systematic Review. *J. Natl. Cancer Inst.* **2018**, *110*, 1311–1327. [CrossRef] [PubMed]
64. Fanakidou, I.; Zyga, S.; Alikari, V.; Tsironi, M.; Stathoulis, J.; Theofilou, P. Mental health, loneliness, and illness perception outcomes in quality of life among young breast cancer patients after mastectomy: The role of breast reconstruction. *Qual. Life Res.* **2018**, *27*, 539–543. [CrossRef] [PubMed]
65. Martínez-Garay, C.; Djouder, N. Dietary interventions and precision nutrition in cancer therapy. *Trends Mol. Med.* **2023**, *29*, 489–511. [CrossRef]
66. Vernieri, C.; Casola, S.; Foiani, M.; Pietrantonio, F.; De Braud, F.; Longo, V. Targeting Cancer Metabolism: Dietary and Pharmacologic Interventions. *Cancer Discov.* **2016**, *6*, 1315–1333. [CrossRef]
67. Bose, S.; Allen, A.E.; Locasale, J.W. The Molecular Link from Diet to Cancer Cell Metabolism. *Mol. Cell* **2020**, *78*, 1034–1044. [CrossRef]
68. Locasale, J.W. Diet and Exercise in Cancer Metabolism. *Cancer Discov.* **2022**, *12*, 2249–2257. [CrossRef]
69. Morita, M.; Kudo, K.; Shima, H.; Tanuma, N. Dietary intervention as a therapeutic for cancer. *Cancer Sci.* **2021**, *112*, 498–504. [CrossRef]
70. Patra, S.; Pradhan, B.; Nayak, R.; Behera, C.; Das, S.; Patra, S.K.; Efferth, T.; Jena, M.; Bhutia, S.K. Dietary polyphenols in chemoprevention and synergistic effect in cancer: Clinical evidences and molecular mechanisms of action. *Phytomedicine* **2021**, *90*, 153554. [CrossRef]
71. Zhou, Y.; Li, H. Neurological adverse events associated with PD-1/PD-L1 immune checkpoint inhibitors. *Front. Neurosci.* **2023**, *17*, 1227049. [CrossRef] [PubMed]
72. Alturki, N.A. Review of the Immune Checkpoint Inhibitors in the Context of Cancer Treatment. *J. Clin. Med.* **2023**, *12*, 4301. [CrossRef] [PubMed]
73. Zraik, I.M.; Heß-Busch, Y. Management of chemotherapy side effects and their long-term sequelae. *Urologe A* **2021**, *60*, 862–871. [CrossRef]
74. Buchholz, T.A. Radiation Therapy for Early-Stage Breast Cancer after Breast-Conserving Surgery. *New Engl. J. Med.* **2009**, *360*, 63–70. [CrossRef] [PubMed]
75. Zhang, C.; Xu, C.; Gao, X.; Yao, Q. Platinum-based drugs for cancer therapy and anti-tumor strategies. *Theranostics* **2022**, *12*, 2115–2132. [CrossRef] [PubMed]
76. Wu, Q.; Gao, Z.-J.; Yu, X.; Wang, P. Dietary regulation in health and disease. *Signal Transduct. Target. Ther.* **2022**, *7*, 252. [CrossRef]
77. Prado, C.M.; Antoun, S.; Sawyer, M.B.; Baracos, V.E. Two faces of drug therapy in cancer: Drug-related lean tissue loss and its adverse consequences to survival and toxicity. *Curr. Opin. Clin. Nutr. Metab. Care* **2011**, *14*, 250–254. [CrossRef]
78. Soldati, L.; Di Renzo, L.; Jirillo, E.; Ascierto, P.A.; Marincola, F.M.; De Lorenzo, A. The influence of diet on anti-cancer immune responsiveness. *J. Transl. Med.* **2018**, *16*, 75. [CrossRef]
79. Tao, J.; Li, S.; Gan, R.-Y.; Zhao, C.-N.; Meng, X.; Li, H.-B. Targeting gut microbiota with dietary components on cancer: Effects and potential mechanisms of action. *Crit. Rev. Food Sci. Nutr.* **2020**, *60*, 1025–1037. [CrossRef]
80. Dieli-Conwright, C.M.; Harrigan, M.; Cartmel, B.; Chagpar, A.; Bai, Y.; Li, F.-Y.; Rimm, D.L.; Pusztai, L.; Lu, L.; Sanft, T.; et al. Impact of a randomized weight loss trial on breast tissue markers in breast cancer survivors. *npj Breast Cancer* **2022**, *8*, 29. [CrossRef]
81. Puklin, L.; Cartmel, B.; Harrigan, M.; Lu, L.; Li, F.-Y.; Sanft, T.; Irwin, M.L. Randomized trial of weight loss on circulating ghrelin levels among breast cancer survivors. *npj Breast Cancer* **2021**, *7*, 49. [CrossRef] [PubMed]
82. Thomas, G.A.; Alvarez-Reeves, M.; Lu, L.; Yu, H.; Irwin, M.L. Effect of Exercise on Metabolic Syndrome Variables in Breast Cancer Survivors. *Int. J. Endocrinol.* **2013**, *2013*, 168797. [CrossRef] [PubMed]
83. Zeng, H.; Irwin, M.L.; Lu, L.; Risch, H.; Mayne, S.; Mu, L.; Deng, Q.; Scarampi, L.; Mitidieri, M.; Katsaros, D.; et al. Physical activity and breast cancer survival: An epigenetic link through reduced methylation of a tumor suppressor gene L3MBTL1. *Breast Cancer Res. Treat.* **2012**, *133*, 127–135. [CrossRef]
84. Garbiec, E.; Cielecka-Piontek, J.; Kowalówka, M.; Hołubiec, M.; Zalewski, P. Genistein—Opportunities Related to an Interesting Molecule of Natural Origin. *Molecules* **2022**, *27*, 815. [CrossRef] [PubMed]
85. Sharma, M.; Arora, I.; Chen, M.; Wu, H.; Crowley, M.R.; Tollefsbol, T.O.; Li, Y. Therapeutic Effects of Dietary Soybean Genistein on Triple-Negative Breast Cancer via Regulation of Epigenetic Mechanisms. *Nutrients* **2021**, *13*, 3944. [CrossRef]
86. Paul, B.; Li, Y.; Tollefsbol, T.O. The Effects of Combinatorial Genistein and Sulforaphane in Breast Tumor Inhibition: Role in Epigenetic Regulation. *Int. J. Mol. Sci.* **2018**, *19*, 1754. [CrossRef]
87. Chang, H.; Mi, M.; Ling, W.; Zhu, J.; Zhang, Q.; Wei, N.; Zhou, Y.; Tang, Y.; Yuan, J. Structurally related cytotoxic effects of flavonoids on human cancer cells in vitro. *Arch. Pharmacal Res.* **2008**, *31*, 1137–1144. [CrossRef]
88. Androutsopoulos, V.; Papakyriakou, A.; Vourloumis, D.; Spandidos, D.A. Comparative CYP1A1 and CYP1B1 substrate and inhibitor profile of dietary flavonoids. *Bioorg. Med. Chem.* **2011**, *19*, 2842–2849. [CrossRef]
89. Pal-Bhadra, M.; Ramaiah, M.J.; Reddy, T.L.; Krishnan, A.; Pushpavalli, S.; Babu, K.S.; Tiwari, A.K.; Rao, J.M.; Yadav, J.S.; Bhadra, U. Plant HDAC inhibitor chrysin arrest cell growth and induce p21 WAF1 by altering chromatin of STAT response element in A375 cells. *BMC Cancer* **2012**, *12*, 180. [CrossRef]

90. Sedlak, L.; Wojnar, W.; Zych, M.; Wyględowska-Promieńska, D.; Mrukwa-Kominek, E.; Kaczmarczyk-Sedlak, I. Effect of Resveratrol, a Dietary-Derived Polyphenol, on the Oxidative Stress and Polyol Pathway in the Lens of Rats with Streptozotocin-Induced Diabetes. *Nutrients* **2018**, *10*, 1423. [CrossRef]
91. Galiniak, S.; Aebisher, D.; Bartusik-Aebisher, D. Health benefits of resveratrol administration. *Acta Biochim. Pol.* **2019**, *66*, 13–21. [CrossRef]
92. Venturelli, S.; Berger, A.; Böcker, A.; Busch, C.; Weiland, T.; Noor, S.; Leischner, C.; Schleicher, S.; Mayer, M.; Weiss, T.S.; et al. Resveratrol as a pan-HDAC inhibitor alters the acetylation status of histone [corrected] proteins in human-derived hepatoblastoma cells. *PLoS ONE* **2013**, *8*, e73097. [CrossRef]
93. Izquierdo-Torres, E.; Hernández-Oliveras, A.; Meneses-Morales, I.; Rodríguez, G.; Fuentes-García, G.; Zarain-Herzberg, Á. Resveratrol up-regulates ATP2A3 gene expression in breast cancer cell lines through epigenetic mechanisms. *Int. J. Biochem. Cell Biol.* **2019**, *113*, 37–47. [CrossRef]
94. Zheng, Y.; Liu, Z.; Yang, X.; Liu, L.; Ahn, K.S. An updated review on the potential antineoplastic actions of oleuropein. *Phytother. Res.* **2022**, *36*, 365–379. [CrossRef] [PubMed]
95. Bayat, S.; Derakhshan, S.M.; Derakhshan, N.M.; Khaniani, M.S.; Alivand, M.R. Downregulation of *HDAC2* and *HDAC3* via oleuropein as a potent prevention and therapeutic agent in MCF-7 breast cancer cells. *J. Cell. Biochem.* **2019**, *120*, 9172–9180. [CrossRef] [PubMed]
96. Jabczyk, M.; Nowak, J.; Hudzik, B.; Zubelewicz-Szkodzińska, B. Curcumin in Metabolic Health and Disease. *Nutrients* **2021**, *13*, 4440. [CrossRef] [PubMed]
97. Chen, C.-Q.; Yu, K.; Yan, Q.-X.; Xing, C.-Y.; Chen, Y.; Yan, Z.; Shi, Y.-F.; Zhao, K.-W.; Gao, S.-M. Pure curcumin increases the expression of SOCS1 and SOCS3 in myeloproliferative neoplasms through suppressing class I histone deacetylases. *Carcinogenesis* **2013**, *34*, 1442–1449. [CrossRef]
98. Han, R.; Yang, H.; Li, Y.; Ling, C.; Lu, L. Valeric acid acts as a novel HDAC3 inhibitor against prostate cancer. *Med. Oncol.* **2022**, *39*, 213. [CrossRef]
99. Shi, F.; Li, Y.; Han, R.; Fu, A.; Wang, R.; Nusbaum, O.; Qin, Q.; Chen, X.; Hou, L.; Zhu, Y. Valerian and valeric acid inhibit growth of breast cancer cells possibly by mediating epigenetic modifications. *Sci. Rep.* **2021**, *11*, 2519. [CrossRef]
100. Wu, Y.; Duan, Z.; Qu, L.; Zhang, Y.; Zhu, C.; Fan, D. Gastroprotective effects of ginsenoside Rh4 against ethanol-induced gastric mucosal injury by inhibiting the MAPK/NF-κB signaling pathway. *Food Funct.* **2023**, *14*, 5167–5181. [CrossRef]
101. Dong, F.; Qu, L.; Duan, Z.; He, Y.; Ma, X.; Fan, D. Ginsenoside Rh4 inhibits breast cancer growth through targeting histone deacetylase 2 to regulate immune microenvironment and apoptosis. *Bioorganic Chem.* **2023**, *135*, 106537. [CrossRef]
102. Liu, H.; Wang, J.; He, T.; Becker, S.; Zhang, G.; Li, D.; Ma, X. Butyrate: A Double-Edged Sword for Health? *Adv. Nutr.* **2018**, *9*, 21–29. [CrossRef] [PubMed]
103. Fan, P.; Li, L.; Rezaei, A.; Eslamfam, S.; Che, D.; Ma, X. Metabolites of Dietary Protein and Peptides by Intestinal Microbes and their Impacts on Gut. *Curr. Protein Pept. Sci.* **2015**, *16*, 646–654. [CrossRef] [PubMed]
104. Canani, R.B.; Di Costanzo, M.; Leone, L.; Pedata, M.; Meli, R.; Calignano, A. Potential beneficial effects of butyrate in intestinal and extraintestinal diseases. *World J. Gastroenterol.* **2011**, *17*, 1519–1528. [CrossRef] [PubMed]
105. Andrade, F.; Nagamine, M.; De Conti, A.; Chaible, L.; Fontelles, C.; Junior, A.J.; Vannucchi, H.; Dagli, M.; Bassoli, B.; Moreno, F.; et al. Efficacy of the dietary histone deacetylase inhibitor butyrate alone or in combination with vitamin A against proliferation of MCF-7 human breast cancer cells. *Braz. J. Med. Biol. Res.* **2012**, *45*, 841–850. [CrossRef]
106. Chopin, V.; Slomianny, C.; Hondermarck, H.; Le Bourhis, X. Synergistic induction of apoptosis in breast cancer cells by cotreatment with butyrate and TNF-alpha, TRAIL, or anti-Fas agonist antibody involves enhancement of death receptors' signaling and requires P21(waf1). *Exp. Cell Res.* **2004**, *298*, 560–573. [CrossRef]
107. Thakur, V.S.; Gupta, K.; Gupta, S. Green tea polyphenols causes cell cycle arrest and apoptosis in prostate cancer cells by suppressing class I histone deacetylases. *Carcinogenesis* **2012**, *33*, 377–384. [CrossRef]
108. Wu, K.; Wei, Y.; Yu, Y.; Shan, M.; Tang, Y.; Sun, Y. Green tea polyphenols inhibit malignant melanoma progression via regulating circ_MITF/miR-30e-3p/HDAC2 axis. *Biotechnol. Appl. Biochem.* **2022**, *69*, 808–821. [CrossRef]
109. Jang, Y.-G.; Hwang, K.-A.; Choi, K.-C. Rosmarinic Acid, a Component of Rosemary Tea, Induced the Cell Cycle Arrest and Apoptosis through Modulation of HDAC2 Expression in Prostate Cancer Cell Lines. *Nutrients* **2018**, *10*, 1784. [CrossRef]
110. Kim, H.; Ramirez, C.N.; Su, Z.-Y.; Kong, A.-N.T. Epigenetic modifications of triterpenoid ursolic acid in activating Nrf2 and blocking cellular transformation of mouse epidermal cells. *J. Nutr. Biochem.* **2016**, *33*, 54–62. [CrossRef]
111. Çakır, I.; Pan, P.L.; Hadley, C.K.; El-Gamal, A.; Fadel, A.; Elsayegh, D.; Mohamed, O.; Rizk, N.M. Is a corresponding author Masoud Ghamari-Langroudi. Sulforaphane reduces obesity by reversing leptin resistance. *Elife* **2022**, *11*, e67368. [CrossRef] [PubMed]
112. Xie, Q.; Bai, Q.; Zou, L.-Y.; Zhang, Q.-Y.; Zhou, Y.; Chang, H.; Yi, L.; Zhu, J.-D.; Mi, M.-T. Genistein inhibits DNA methylation and increases expression of tumor suppressor genes in human breast cancer cells. *Genes Chromosom. Cancer* **2014**, *53*, 422–431. [CrossRef] [PubMed]
113. Tortorella, S.M.; Royce, S.G.; Licciardi, P.V.; Karagiannis, T.C. Dietary Sulforaphane in Cancer Chemoprevention: The Role of Epigenetic Regulation and HDAC Inhibition. *Antioxid. Redox Signal.* **2015**, *22*, 1382–1424. [CrossRef]
114. Middleton, E., Jr.; Kandaswami, C.; Theoharides, T.C. The effects of plant flavonoids on mammalian cells: Implications for inflammation, heart disease, and cancer. *Pharmacol. Rev.* **2000**, *52*, 673–751. [PubMed]

115. Davie, J.R. Inhibition of Histone Deacetylase Activity by Butyrate. *J. Nutr.* **2003**, *133* (Suppl. 7), 2485S–2493S. [CrossRef] [PubMed]
116. Wang, S.; Li, Z.; Ma, Y.; Liu, Y.; Lin, C.-C.; Li, S.; Zhan, J.; Ho, C.-T. Immunomodulatory Effects of Green Tea Polyphenols. *Molecules* **2021**, *26*, 3755. [CrossRef]
117. Han, R.; Yang, H.; Ling, C.; Lu, L. Neurospora crassa is a potential source of anti-cancer agents against breast cancer. *Breast Cancer* **2022**, *29*, 1032–1041. [CrossRef]
118. Sung, H.; Ferlay, J.; Siegel, R.L.; Laversanne, M.; Soerjomataram, I.; Jemal, A.; Bray, F. Global Cancer Statistics 2020: GLOBOCAN Estimates of Incidence and Mortality Worldwide for 36 Cancers in 185 Countries. *CA Cancer J. Clin.* **2021**, *71*, 209–249. [CrossRef]
119. Dima, C.; Assadpour, E.; Nechifor, A.; Dima, S.; Li, Y.; Jafari, S.M. Oral bioavailability of bioactive compounds; modulating factors, in vitro analysis methods, and enhancing strategies. *Crit. Rev. Food Sci. Nutr.* **2023**, 1–39. [CrossRef]
120. Rosenfeld, R.M.; Juszczak, H.M.; Wong, M.A. Scoping review of the association of plant-based diet quality with health out-comes. *Front. Nutr.* **2023**, *10*, 1211535. [CrossRef]
121. Weaver, C.M.; Alekel, D.L.; Ward, W.E.; Ronis, M.J. Flavonoid Intake and Bone Health. *J. Nutr. Gerontol. Geriatr.* **2012**, *31*, 239–253. [CrossRef] [PubMed]
122. Li, B.; Shao, H.; Gao, L.; Li, H.; Sheng, H.; Zhu, L. Nano-drug co-delivery system of natural active ingredients and chemotherapy drugs for cancer treatment: A review. *Drug Deliv.* **2022**, *29*, 2130–2161. [CrossRef] [PubMed]
123. Nakagawa, Y.; Mukai, S.; Yamada, S.; Matsuoka, M.; Tarumi, E.; Hashimoto, T.; Tamura, C.; Imaizumi, A.; Nishihira, J.; Nakamura, T. Short-term effects of highly-bioavailable curcumin for treating knee osteoarthritis: A randomized, double-blind, placebo-controlled prospective study. *J. Orthop. Sci.* **2014**, *19*, 933–939. [CrossRef] [PubMed]
124. Kanai, M.; Imaizumi, A.; Otsuka, Y.; Sasaki, H.; Hashiguchi, M.; Tsujiko, K.; Matsumoto, S.; Ishiguro, H.; Chiba, T. Dose-escalation and pharmacokinetic study of nanoparticle curcumin, a potential anticancer agent with improved bioavailability, in healthy human volunteers. *Cancer Chemother. Pharmacol.* **2012**, *69*, 65–70. [CrossRef]
125. Sasaki, H.; Sunagawa, Y.; Takahashi, K.; Imaizumi, A.; Fukuda, H.; Hashimoto, T.; Wada, H.; Katanasaka, Y.; Kakeya, H.; Fujita, M.; et al. Innovative Preparation of Curcumin for Improved Oral Bioavailability. *Biol. Pharm. Bull.* **2011**, *34*, 660–665. [CrossRef]
126. Gao, C.; Tang, F.; Gong, G.; Zhang, J.; Hoi, M.P.M.; Lee, S.M.Y.; Wang, R. pH-Responsive prodrug nanoparticles based on a sodium alginate derivative for selective co-release of doxorubicin and curcumin into tumor cells. *Nanoscale* **2017**, *9*, 12533–12542. [CrossRef]
127. Zhang, H.; Xue, Q.; Zhou, Z.; He, N.; Li, S.; Zhao, C. Co-delivery of doxorubicin and hydroxychloroquine via chitosan/alginate nanoparticles for blocking autophagy and enhancing chemotherapy in breast cancer therapy. *Front. Pharmacol.* **2023**, *14*, 1176232. [CrossRef]
128. Dong, X.; Sun, Y.; Li, Y.; Ma, X.; Zhang, S.; Yuan, Y.; Kohn, J.; Liu, C.; Qian, J. Synergistic Combination of Bioactive Hydroxyapatite Nanoparticles and the Chemotherapeutic Doxorubicin to Over-come Tumor Multidrug Resistance. *Small* **2021**, *17*, e2007672. [CrossRef]
129. Li, Z.; Wang, L.; Lin, X.; Shen, L.; Feng, Y. Drug delivery for bioactive polysaccharides to improve their drug-like properties and curative efficacy. *Drug Deliv.* **2017**, *24* (Suppl. 1), 70–80. [CrossRef]
130. Prasad, S.; Gupta, S.C.; Tyagi, A.K.; Aggarwal, B.B. Curcumin, a component of golden spice: From bedside to bench and back. *Biotechnol. Adv.* **2014**, *32*, 1053–1064. [CrossRef]
131. Passos, C.L.A.; Polinati, R.M.; Ferreira, C.; dos Santos, N.A.N.; Lima, D.G.V.; da Silva, J.L.; Fialho, E. Curcumin and melphalan cotreatment induces cell cycle arrest and apoptosis in MDA-MB-231 breast cancer cells. *Sci. Rep.* **2023**, *13*, 13446. [CrossRef]
132. Zhu, L.; Chen, L. Progress in research on paclitaxel and tumor immunotherapy. *Cell. Mol. Biol. Lett.* **2019**, *24*, 40. [CrossRef] [PubMed]
133. Nootim, P.; Kapol, N.; Bunchuailua, W.; Poompruek, P.; Tungsukruthai, P. Current state of cancer patient care incorporating Thai traditional medicine in Thailand: A qualitative study. *J. Integr. Med.* **2020**, *18*, 41–45. [CrossRef] [PubMed]
134. Yazdi, N.; Salehi, A.; Vojoud, M.; Sharifi, M.H.; Hoseinkhani, A. Use of complementary and alternative medicine in pregnant women: A cross-sectional survey in the south of Iran. *J. Integr. Med.* **2019**, *17*, 392–395. [CrossRef] [PubMed]
135. Ouyang, W.; Meng, Y.; Guo, G.; Zhao, C.; Zhou, X. Efficacy and safety of traditional Chinese medicine in the treatment of osteonecrosis of the femoral head. *J. Orthop. Surg. Res.* **2023**, *18*, 600. [CrossRef]
136. Bu, Z.-J.; Liu, Y.-N.; Shahjalal, M.; Zheng, Y.-Y.; Liu, C.-J.; Ye, M.-M.; Xu, J.-Y.; Peng, X.-Y.; Wang, X.-H.; Chen, X.; et al. Comparative effectiveness and safety of Chinese medicine belly button application for childhood diarrhea: A Bayesian network meta-analysis of randomized controlled trials. *Front. Pediatr.* **2023**, *11*, 1180694. [CrossRef]
137. Bushehri, R.H.; Navabi, P.; Saeedifar, A.M.; Keshavarzian, N.; Rouzbahani, N.H.; Mosayebi, G.; Ghazavi, A.; Ghorban, K.; Ganji, A. Integration of phytotherapy and chemotherapy: Recent advances in anticancer molecular pathways. *Iran J. Basic Med. Sci.* **2023**, *26*, 987–1000. [CrossRef]
138. Zhang, X.; Li, H.; Lv, X.; Hu, L.; Li, W.; Zi, M.; He, Y. Impact of Diets on Response to Immune Checkpoint Inhibitors (ICIs) Therapy against Tumors. *Life* **2022**, *12*, 409. [CrossRef]
139. Kromhout, D.; Yasuda, S.; Geleijnse, J.M.; Shimokawa, H. Fish oil and omega-3 fatty acids in cardiovascular disease: Do they really work? *Eur. Heart J.* **2012**, *33*, 436–443. [CrossRef]
140. Björkström, N.K.; Strunz, B.; Ljunggren, H.-G. Natural killer cells in antiviral immunity. *Nat. Rev. Immunol.* **2022**, *22*, 112–123. [CrossRef]

141. Thies, F.; Nebe-von-Caron, G.; Powell, J.R.; Yaqoob, P.; Newsholme, E.A.; Calder, P.C. Dietary supplementation with eicosapentaenoic acid, but not with other long-chain n-3 or n-6 polyunsaturated fatty acids, decreases natural killer cell activity in healthy subjects aged >55 y. *Am. J. Clin. Nutr.* **2001**, *73*, 539–548. [CrossRef] [PubMed]
142. Fortmann, S.P.; Burda, B.U.; Senger, C.A.; Lin, J.S.; Whitlock, E.P. Vitamin and Mineral Supplements in the Primary Prevention of Cardiovascular Disease and Cancer: An Updated Systematic Evidence Review for the U.S. Preventive Services Task Force. *Ann. Intern. Med.* **2013**, *159*, 824–834. [CrossRef]
143. Beck, K.L.; von Hurst, P.R.; O'Brien, W.J.; Badenhorst, C.E. Micronutrients and athletic performance: A review. *Food Chem. Toxicol.* **2021**, *158*, 112618. [CrossRef] [PubMed]
144. Daniel, C.; Sartory, N.A.; Zahn, N.; Radeke, H.H.; Stein, J.M. Immune modulatory treatment of trinitrobenzene sulfonic acid colitis with calcitriol is associated with a change of a T helper (Th) 1/Th17 to a Th2 and regulatory T cell profile. *J. Pharmacol. Exp. Ther.* **2008**, *324*, 23–33. [CrossRef] [PubMed]
145. Larkin, J.; Chiarion-Sileni, V.; Gonzalez, R.; Grob, J.-J.; Cowey, C.L.; Lao, C.D.; Schadendorf, D.; Dummer, R.; Smylie, M.; Rutkowski, P.; et al. Combined Nivolumab and Ipilimumab or Monotherapy in Untreated Melanoma. *N. Engl. J. Med.* **2015**, *373*, 23–34. [CrossRef] [PubMed]
146. Tobin, R.P.; Jordan, K.R.; Robinson, W.A.; Davis, D.; Borges, V.F.; Gonzalez, R.; Lewis, K.D.; McCarter, M.D. Targeting myeloid-derived suppressor cells using all-trans retinoic acid in melanoma patients treated with Ipili-mumab. *Int. Immunopharmacol.* **2018**, *63*, 282–291. [CrossRef]
147. Chen, L.; Diao, L.; Yang, Y.; Yi, X.; Rodriguez, B.L.; Li, Y.; Villalobos, P.A.; Cascone, T.; Liu, X.; Tan, L.; et al. CD38-Mediated Immunosuppression as a Mechanism of Tumor Cell Escape from PD-1/PD-L1 Blockade. *Cancer Discov.* **2018**, *8*, 1156–1175. [CrossRef]
148. Yuan, J.; Li, J.; Shang, M.; Fu, Y.; Wang, T. Identification of vitamin B6 as a PD-L1 suppressor and an adjuvant for cancer immunotherapy. *Biochem. Biophys. Res. Commun.* **2021**, *561*, 187–194. [CrossRef]
149. Kim, S.-K.; Guevarra, R.B.; Kim, Y.-T.; Kwon, J.; Kim, H.; Cho, J.H.; Kim, H.B.; Lee, J.-H. Role of Probiotics in Human Gut Microbiome-Associated Diseases. *J. Microbiol. Biotechnol.* **2019**, *29*, 1335–1340. [CrossRef]
150. Bedada, T.L.; Feto, T.K.; Awoke, K.S.; Garedew, A.D.; Yifat, F.T.; Birri, D.J. Probiotics for cancer alternative prevention and treatment. *BioMedicine* **2020**, *129*, 110409. [CrossRef]
151. Suez, J.; Zmora, N.; Zilberman-Schapira, G.; Mor, U.; Dori-Bachash, M.; Bashiardes, S.; Zur, M.; Regev-Lehavi, D.; Brik, R.B.-Z.; Federici, S.; et al. Post-Antibiotic Gut Mucosal Microbiome Reconstitution Is Impaired by Probiotics and Improved by Autologous FMT. *Cell* **2018**, *174*, 1406–1423.e16. [CrossRef] [PubMed]
152. Spencer, C.N.; Gopalakrishnan, V.; McQuade, J.; Andrews, M.C.; Helmink, B.; Khan, M.W.; Sirmans, E.; Haydu, L.; Cogdill, A.; Burton, E.; et al. Abstract 2838: The gut microbiome (GM) and immunotherapy response are influenced by host lifestyle factors. *Cancer Res* **2019**, *79* (Suppl. 13), 2838. [CrossRef]
153. Kuang, R.; Binion, D.G. Should high-fiber diets be recommended for patients with inflammatory bowel disease? *Curr. Opin. Gas-Troenterol.* **2022**, *38*, 168–172. [CrossRef] [PubMed]
154. Marques, F.Z.; Nelson, E.; Chu, P.-Y.; Horlock, D.; Fiedler, A.; Ziemann, M.; Tan, J.K.; Kuruppu, S.; Rajapakse, N.W.; El-Osta, A.; et al. High-Fiber Diet and Acetate Supplementation Change the Gut Microbiota and Prevent the Development of Hypertension and Heart Failure in Hypertensive Mice. *Circulation* **2017**, *135*, 964–977. [CrossRef] [PubMed]
155. Kocher, F.; Amann, A.; Zimmer, K.; Geisler, S.; Fuchs, D.; Pichler, R.; Wolf, D.; Kurz, K.; Seeber, A.; Pircher, A. High indoleamine-2,3-dioxygenase 1 (IDO) activity is linked to primary resistance to immunotherapy in non-small cell lung cancer (NSCLC). *Transl. Lung Cancer Res.* **2021**, *10*, 304–313. [CrossRef] [PubMed]
156. Weber, D.D.; Aminzadeh-Gohari, S.; Tulipan, J.; Catalano, L.; Feichtinger, R.G.; Kofler, B. Ketogenic diet in the treatment of cancer—Where do we stand? *Mol. Metab.* **2020**, *33*, 102–121. [CrossRef]
157. Lussier, D.M.; Woolf, E.C.; Johnson, J.L.; Brooks, K.S.; Blattman, J.N.; Scheck, A.C. Enhanced immunity in a mouse model of malignant glioma is mediated by a therapeutic ketogenic diet. *BMC Cancer* **2016**, *16*, 310. [CrossRef]
158. Rom-Jurek, E.-M.; Kirchhammer, N.; Ugocsai, P.; Ortmann, O.; Wege, A.K.; Brockhoff, G. Regulation of Programmed Death Ligand 1 (PD-L1) Expression in Breast Cancer Cell Lines In Vitro and in Immunodeficient and Humanized Tumor Mice. *Int. J. Mol. Sci.* **2018**, *19*, 563. [CrossRef]
159. Orillion, A.R.; Damayanti, N.P.; Shen, L.; Adelaiye-Ogala, R.; Affronti, H.C.; Elbanna, M.; Chintala, S.; Ciesielski, M.J.; Fontana, L.; Kao, C.; et al. Dietary Protein Restriction Reprograms Tumor-Associated Macrophages and Enhances Immunotherapy. *Clin. Cancer Res.* **2018**, *24*, 6383–6395. [CrossRef]
160. Nabe, S.; Yamada, T.; Suzuki, J.; Toriyama, K.; Yasuoka, T.; Kuwahara, M.; Shiraishi, A.; Takenaka, K.; Yasukawa, M.; Yamashita, M. Reinforce the antitumor activity of $CD8^+$ T cells via glutamine restriction. *Cancer Sci.* **2018**, *109*, 3737–3750. [CrossRef]

Disclaimer/Publisher's Note: The statements, opinions and data contained in all publications are solely those of the individual author(s) and contributor(s) and not of MDPI and/or the editor(s). MDPI and/or the editor(s) disclaim responsibility for any injury to people or property resulting from any ideas, methods, instructions or products referred to in the content.

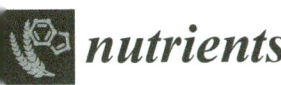

Review

Bergamot Byproducts: A Sustainable Source to Counteract Inflammation

Caterina Russo [1], Giovanni Enrico Lombardo [1], Giuseppe Bruschetta [2], Antonio Rapisarda [1], Alessandro Maugeri [2,*] and Michele Navarra [1]

1. Department of Chemical, Biological, Pharmaceutical and Environmental Sciences, University of Messina, Viale F. Stagno d'Alcontres 31, 98166 Messina, Italy; carusso@unime.it (C.R.); gelombardo@unime.it (G.E.L.); antonio.rapisarda@unime.it (A.R.); mnavarra@unime.it (M.N.)
2. Department of Veterinary Sciences, University of Messina, Viale G. Palatucci, 98168 Messina, Italy; giuseppe.bruschetta@unime.it
* Correspondence: amaugeri@unime.it

Abstract: Chronic inflammation is the result of an acute inflammatory response that fails to eliminate the pathogenic agent or heal the tissue injury. The consequence of this failure lays the foundations to the onset of several chronic ailments, including skin disorders, respiratory and neurodegenerative diseases, metabolic syndrome, and, eventually, cancer. In this context, the long-term use of synthetic anti-inflammatory drugs to treat chronic illnesses cannot be tolerated by patients owing to the severe side effects. Based on this, the need for novel agents endowed with anti-inflammatory effects prompted to search potential candidates also within the plant kingdom, being recognized as a source of molecules currently employed in several therapeutical areas. Indeed, the ever-growing evidence on the anti-inflammatory properties of dietary polyphenols traced the route towards the study of flavonoid-rich sources, such as *Citrus bergamia* (bergamot) and its derivatives. Interestingly, the recent paradigm of the circular economy has promoted the valorization of *Citrus* fruit waste and, in regard to bergamot, it brought to light new evidence corroborating the anti-inflammatory potential of bergamot byproducts, thus increasing the scientific knowledge in this field. Therefore, this review aims to gather the latest literature supporting the beneficial role of both bergamot derivatives and waste products in different models of inflammatory-based diseases, thus highlighting the great potentiality of a waste re-evaluation perspective.

Keywords: inflammation; *Citrus bergamia*; bergamot; polyphenols; byproducts; *Citrus* fruits; natural products; flavonoids; waste valorization

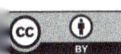

1. Introduction

The earliest records about plants having health benefits date back at least 5000 years ago, to the age of the Sumerians [1]. For thousands of years, plant kingdom represented the basis of traditional medicine and even today continues to be explored for the numerous remedies that it provides. The renewed interest of the scientific community towards natural products dramatically enhanced in the last two decades and resulted in the discovery of new plant sources and their byproducts for the prevention and treatment of several diseases, including inflammatory-based ones [2]. This is the case for *Citrus bergamia* Risso (bergamot), an endemic plant of the southern coast of the Calabria region (Italy), to which we have focused our studies for over a decade, thus documenting relevant pharmacological activities [3–5].

Chronic and age-related diseases, including metabolic, autoimmune, cardiovascular and neurodegenerative ones, are primarily associated with a status of systemic and low-grade chronic inflammation, as well as oxidative stress. In particular, a dysregulation of the cytokine network along with a redox imbalance and DNA damage leads to the activation of a cytosolic protein complex called inflammasome. This complex is known to stimulate nuclear factor kappa B (NF-κB), mitogen-activated protein kinases (MAPKs), Janus kinase (JAK) signal transducer and the activator of transcription (STAT) signaling pathways, thus triggering the interleukin (IL)–1β-mediated inflammatory cascade [6]. Therefore, the resolution of this process constitutes a strategy to improve the symptoms and quality of life of patients with chronic inflammatory diseases. However, the severe side effects and/or high costs of conventional therapies, consisting of the use of corticosteroids, nonsteroidal anti-inflammatory drugs (NSAIDs) or biologic drugs, impair their tolerability and the compliance of patients. Thereby, the route towards natural products has led to the evaluation of the potential anti-inflammatory effects of bioactive molecules and phytocomplexes, also obtained from the waste of food processing [7].

In the last years, significant advancements have been reached on the study of the anti-inflammatory properties of bergamot derivatives and byproducts, observing its beneficial effects in different models of disease [8]. On this basis, we aimed at gathering the recent literature on the anti-inflammatory potential of bergamot, with the purpose to shed light on its role for each inflammatory disease.

2. Inflammatory Process

Inflammation is an immune response to injurious stimuli, including pathogens, damaged cells and toxins, which can cause tissue or organ damage. It is a defense mechanism triggered with the aim of removing the harmful agent and thus initiating a healing process leading to restoration of tissue or organ homeostasis. At the local level, inflammation is characterized by redness, heat, swelling, pain and loss of tissue function, occurring as result of an increase in vascular permeability, leukocyte recruitment and the accumulation and release of inflammatory mediators (such as cytokines, chemokines and complement proteins). Although the etiology of inflammation may be infectious (caused by bacteria, viruses or other microorganisms) or non-infectious (caused by physical, chemical and biological stimuli), the processing of the inflammatory response involves common events [9].

The first event consists of the recognition by pattern receptors, located on the surface of immune cells and named pattern-recognition receptors (PRRs), of specific signals, which are released during tissue cell damage. These signals, known as pathogen-associated molecular patterns (PAMPs), include microbial structures, which account for the activation of an infectious inflammatory response; on the contrary, other signals, known as danger-associated molecular patterns (DAMPs), including endogenous biomolecules, are responsible for the triggering of non-infectious inflammatory responses. Among PRRs, the most known class is that of Toll-like receptors (TLRs) [10]. Of note, signal transmission between PAMPs/DAMPs and TLRs, such as TLR4, is mediated by myeloid differentiation factor-88 (MyD88) and culminates in the nuclear translocation of downstream transcription factors, such as NF-κB, the activator protein 1 (AP-1) or the interferon regulatory factor 3 (IRF3) [11,12].

The second event of the inflammatory response reflects the activation of specific pathways of inflammation, mainly NF-κB, MAPKs and JAK-STAT pathways. In the presence of an inflammatory stimulus, the PRRs activate the IκB-kinase (IKK), which in turn promotes the activation of NF-κB via phosphorylation and degradation of the inhibitor of nuclear factor kappa B (IκB). The activation of NF-κB implies the release of pro-inflammatory cytokines (such as IL-1β, IL-6, IL-8, IL-12 or tumor necrosis factor-TNF-α), chemokines (monocyte chemoattractant protein-MCP-1 or macrophage-inflammatory protein-MIP-2) and immune cells in the focus of inflammation [13]. A phlogosis state also involves the activation of extracellular signal-regulated kinase (ERK), c-Jun N-terminal kinase (JNK) and p38 MAP kinases [14]. The JAK-STAT signaling pathway converts the inflammatory signal into a transcriptional response, thus regulating the expression of a variety of inflammatory genes such as cytokines, chemokines, interferons, colony stimulating factors (CSFs) or transforming growth factors (TGFs) [15].

The third event characterizing the inflammatory process is the release of specific markers of inflammation. They mainly include chemokines and inflammatory cytokines, subdivided into interleukins (such as IL-1β, IL-6 and IL-10), tumor necrosis factors (TNFs, such as TNF-α), interferons (IFNs, such as IFN-γ), colony stimulating factors (CSFs, such as granulocyte macrophage (GM)-CSF), and transforming growth factors (TGFs, such as TGF-β). The release of these molecules by immune cells is functional at recruiting leukocytes to the site of inflammation, via establishing a complex network of interactions [16]. In addition, high production of oxidative biomarkers, such as reactive oxygen species (ROS), 8-oxo-2′-deoxyguanosine (8-oxo-dG) as well as high levels of malondialdehyde (MDA) may represent the prelude to an inflammatory response or oxidative disorders [17]. The inflammatory process also implies the alteration of C-reactive protein (CRP) levels, the impaired activity of nuclear factor erythroid-2-related factor 2 (Nrf2) and several enzymes, such as inducible nitric oxide synthase (iNOS), prostaglandin-endoperoxide synthase (PTGS)-2, known as cyclooxygenase (COX)-2, NADPH oxidase (NOX), superoxide dismutase (SOD), catalase (CAT), glutathione peroxidase (GPx) and high mobility group box 1 (HMGB1) [18–20].

The fourth event determining phlogosis is the recruitment of specific cells at the site of inflammation. Based on the stage of the ongoing inflammatory process, neutrophils, monocytes/macrophages, lymphocytes, mast cells and platelets are involved [21]. All these cells, in turn, amplify the acute inflammatory response by releasing inflammatory mediators at local levels.

However, it is essential that inflammation resolves in a timely and controlled way [22]. This is because uncontrolled acute inflammation can evolve into chronic inflammation, becoming the cause of several chronic inflammatory diseases.

3. Main Pathological Conditions Linked to Inflammation

Inflammation represents the pathogenesis of many chronic diseases by involving common mediators and pathways. Indeed, specific markers can be predictive of some pathologies and functional to define their diagnosis, prognosis and treatment. A high production of inflammatory cytokines, an abnormal activation of inflammatory enzymes and/or proteins along with immune alterations and severe conditions of oxidative stress can cause tissue damage and organ failure [9].

Various types of skin disorders can exhibit an inflammatory etiology. This is the case of acne vulgaris, a dermatological disease caused by altered keratinization, androgen-induced sebum, inflammation and *Propionibacterium acne* colonization [23]. Patients with atopic dermatitis, driven by the JAK pathway, are highly exposed to *Staphylococcus aureus* that contributes to the generation of an inflammatory state, where pro-inflammatory cytokines (IL-13, 31 and 33) are massively released [24]. Clinically, psoriasis can exhibit highly inflammatory, pustular or erythrodermic forms. In this case timely treatment is necessary because of the possible increase in inflammation, mediated by TNF-α, IL-17, IL-23 cytokines, throughout the organism with consequent systemic impairment of other organs [25]. Like psoriasis, rheumatoid arthritis represents an immune-based inflammatory disease with high levels for TNF-α and IL-6 cytokines [6].

Chronic respiratory diseases can be caused from unresolved acute inflammation, which in turn provokes pulmonary fibrosis and impaired gas exchange through the airways. This occurs in pathologies such as cystic fibrosis, acute respiratory distress syndrome, asthma and chronic obstructive pulmonary disease (COPD) [26]. In asthma, the activation of the MAPKs pathway stimulates immune cells to release pro-inflammatory factors as well as induces goblet cells to produce mucus, causing hyperresponsiveness and obstruction of airways [27]. The JAK-STAT pathway is also responsible for the activation of inflammatory processes leading to the impairment of airways [28]. The COX-2 enzyme is implied in spasms of airways via the production of prostaglandin E2 (PGE2) [29]. In the same context, the peroxisome proliferator-activated receptors (PPARs) have been shown to influence the gene expression of lipid mediators of inflammation, such as leukotrienes [30,31].

Inflammation and oxidative stress are pillars of diseases like obesity [32]. In particular, overnutrition causes saturation of fat deposits and malfunction of tissue adipose, which becomes hypertrophied. Here, the fat accumulation triggers a pro-inflammatory state, promoting the recruitment of inflammatory cells, with release of TNF-α and IL-6 cytokines and MCP-1 chemokines. Both cytokines and chemokines impair the responsiveness of adipose tissue to insulin, meaning adipocytes are unable to capture fatty acids in excess in circulation. As a result, circulating fatty acids are accumulated in the liver, thus triggering the process of steatosis [33]. Then, the excessive inflammation which affects hepatic parenchyma increases the risk of development of non-alcoholic fatty liver disease (NAFLD) [34]. Moreover, the liver also represents a target for infectious inflammatory diseases like viral hepatitis [35].

Inevitably, the onset of metabolic syndrome, a cluster of obesity, insulin resistance and cardiovascular disorders, underlies an inflammatory pathogenesis. In particular, the adipocytes secrete MCP-1, TNF-α and IL-6, which promote the infiltration of macrophages into adipose tissue [36]. In turn, TNF-α activates the JNK and IKK kinases, which phosphorylate the insulin receptor substrate (IRS)-1 and then impair the insulin-induced uptake of glucose, resulting in insulin resistance [37]. At the same time, high levels of TNF-α as well as IL-6 amplify the inflammatory response, through the activation of NF-κB [38]. Consequently, NF-κB increases the release of chemokines and cytokines, the recruitment of inflammatory cells and the expression of adhesion molecules on endothelial cells (such as vascular cell adhesion molecule-VCAM-1, intracellular adhesion molecule-ICAM-1 and E-selectin), leading to formation of foam cells and then to atherosclerosis [39].

Several inflammatory mediators come into play during the atherosclerotic process, where the activation of nucleotide-binding domain leucine-rich repeat protein 3 (NLRP3) inflammasome by oxidized low-density lipoproteins (LDLs) stimulates the IL-1β signaling pathway [40]. Moreover, inflammatory biomarkers such as CRP and TNF-α seem to be predictors for type 2 diabetes and some cardiovascular events [41,42].

Again, the complex of inflammatory bowel diseases, known as IBD, including ulcerative colitis (UC) and Crohn disease (CD), is caused by chronic inflammation of the gastrointestinal tract [43]. The etiology of these conditions is still elusive, though it is thought that a compromised immune system, due to a hereditary component, can possibly react improperly to environmental stimuli such as viruses or bacteria, resulting in gastrointestinal inflammation [44]. Their development is cytokine-mediated, in particular by IL-17, IL-12 and IL-23 cytokines [45]. Other cytokines also involved are TNF-α, IL-1β and IL-6, along with NF-κB factor, which plays a key role in the pathogenesis of these diseases by stimulating the production of the COX-2 enzyme [46].

Kidneys are organs frequently exposed to damage by toxicants since their function consists of maintaining cell homeostasis and reaching a balance between the extracellular and intracellular environment by removing toxic substances from the organism. This also reflects on the adrenal glands, which respond to stress via altering neuroendocrine equilibrium [47,48]. In the kidneys, interstitial and tubular inflammation is recurrent in cases of acute and chronic renal disease, or glomerulonephritis may also occur. Following an inflammatory stimulus (DAMPS, PAMPS, high levels of glucose, etc.), epithelial renal cells promote the release of cytokines (TNF-α and IL-1β) and leukocyte infiltration, resulting in the activation of the NF-κB and MAPKs pathways [49].

Inflammation and oxidative stress have also been established as the major causes of neurodegeneration in the brain [50]. In Parkinson's and Alzheimer's diseases, specific central events occur, including the activation of the NLRP3 inflammasome and NF-κB pathway as well as of astrocytes and microglia, the main effectors of neuroinflammation. These cells release IL-1β, IL-6, TNF-α and IL-18 pro-inflammatory cytokines, accounting for the neuronal dysfunction and death [51].

Finally, prolonged inflammation can be pathological and lead to a malignant progression. In particular, bacterial and viral infections evolving chronic inflammation can represent a contributory factor for oncogenesis [52].

Given the key role of inflammation in several diseases, the unceasing research for valuable anti-inflammatory agents appears to still be an open challenge.

4. Bergamot Derivatives and Byproducts

Several studies have shed light on the value of *Citrus* fruits, encouraging their cultivation and widespread nutraceutical interest [53,54]. This is the case of bergamot, for which 90% of the global production occurs along the Ionian coast of the province of Reggio Calabria (Italy), finding a favorable microclimate for cultivation. Here, bergamot fruit is called "green gold" due to its economic value and its greenish color, which changes to straw yellow when it ripens. The remaining 5% of bergamot production come from Greece, Morocco, Turkey, Iran, Ivory Coast, Argentina and Brazil.

Citrus bergamia Risso, bergamot, is considered a cross between *Citrus aurantium* L. (sour orange) and *Citrus aurantiifolia* (Christm.) Swingle (lime) or *Citrus limon* L. (limon), although its botanical and geographical origins still remain uncertain [55]. Bergamot fruit, from the Turkish "beg armūdi" meaning "prince's pear", is a pyriform hesperidium with a weight of between 80 and 200 g. It is characterized by a thin epicarp (flavedo), covered with waxes, rich in schizolysigenous oil glands, accounting for the distinctive aromatic oil, colored from light yellow to orange or green, with various shades depending on the degree of ripeness of the fruit, and consists of small, dense collenchyma cells, which contain chromoplasts. Internally, it has a white, spongy and dry mesocarp (albedo), consisting of loosely connected, colorless cells and numerous air spaces in it, hence conferring a white color to this part of the hesperidium. Below the albedo is the endocarp, divided into septa resulting from the modification of the carpel leaves arranged with radial symmetry around the axis. The endocarp is relatively thin and is made up of very elongated, thick-walled epidermal cells, from which spindle-shaped pedunculated vesicles rich in juice develop; citric acid, together with a complex mix of other acids and sugars, is present in the juice vesicles, which gives the characteristic flavor to fruit [56]. The fruit contains white ovoid seeds. However, the molecular composition of each fruit can be influenced by harvesting time (from October to March), type of cultivar (Femminello, Castagnaro or Fantastico) and its degree of ripeness [57].

The fame of bergamot is linked first and foremost to its essential oil (namely BEO), which is isolated from the peel by cold-pressing or steam distillation procedures. BEO consists of a volatile fraction (93–96%), constituted by monoterpenes such as limonene, linalool, linalyl acetate, and a non-volatile fraction (4–7%), including coumarins and psoralens, such as bergamottin, bergapten and citropten [58]. Its use is well-established in the cosmetic industry as the base of many perfumes and fragrances and in the food industry where it is employed as a flavoring ingredient in the preparations of teas, liqueurs and confectionery products. Noteworthy is the role of BEO as an antiseptic due its antimicrobial activity [59]. Moreover, in vitro experiments documented the potential anticancerogenic effect of BEO [60,61].

Approximately 50–65% of the waste generated during the BEO extraction process (peel, albedo and juice) must be properly handled by the manufacturing industry. If this does not occur, the large quantity of waste created yearly might be a serious environmental hazard. As a result, recovering phytochemicals endowed with high biological value from bergamot waste may provide a viable sustainable option [62] (Figure 1).

In this frame, bergamot juice (BJ), obtained by pressing of the remaining fruit pulp, has long been considered a waste product for the essence industry. Nevertheless, in the last ten years, BJ has attracted the attention of the scientific community, being recognized as a source of countless bioactive compounds. The chemical composition of BJ mainly consists of a high content of flavonoids, including naringin, neohesperidin, neoeriocitrin, melitidin, brutieridin and in diosmin, and traces of poncirin and rhoifolin [63], whose biological activity is widely acknowledged [64]. In addition, it is rich in vitamins, minerals, organic acids, sugars, proteins, dietary fiber, pectin and phosphates.

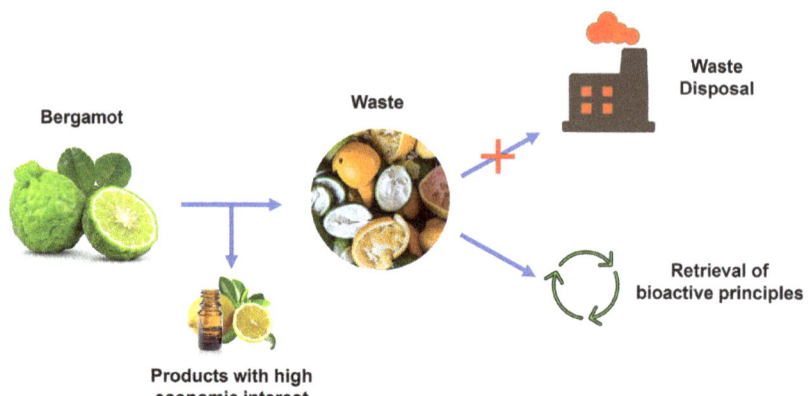

Figure 1. Path of bergamot processing from obtaining products with high economic interest to waste disposal. The waste valorization represents a great strategy both for recovery of compounds endowed with pharmacological properties and reduction of environmental disposal costs.

Finally, the seeds and leaves of bergamot have been recently revaluated. An extract obtained from bergamot seeds, including nomilin and limonin as major components, was shown to possess antiretroviral activity against human T-lymphotropic virus type 1 (HTLV-1) infection [65]. Potentially bioactive compounds such as linalyl acetate, linalool, and α-terpineol were also identified in bergamot leaf oil [66]. Figure 2 depicts chemical structures of the main bioactive components characterizing bergamot derivatives and byproducts.

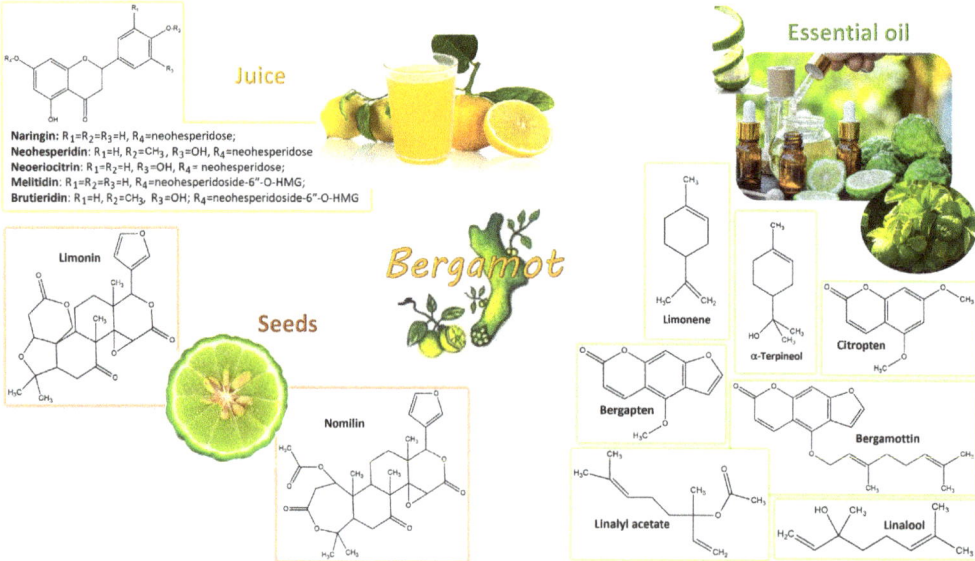

Figure 2. Main chemical composition of bergamot derivatives and byproducts. Bergamot juice is mostly characterized by flavonoids (i.e., naringin, neohesperidin, neoeriocitrin, melitidin and brutieridin), whereas bergamot seeds are characterized by limonoids (i.e., limonin and nomilin). Bergamot leaf oil is rich in monoterpenes (i.e., linalool, linalyl acetate and α-terpineol) and bergamot essential oil obtained from fruit peel is mainly composed of monoterpenes (i.e., limonene, linalool and linalyl acetate), coumarins (i.e., citropten) and psoralens (i.e., bergamottin and bergapten).

5. Anti-Inflammatory Activity of Bergamot Derivatives and Byproducts

5.1. Bergamot Derivatives and Byproducts against Acute Inflammation

Bergamot was shown to be able to exert anti-inflammatory effects on experimental models of acute inflammation. In an in vitro model, a flavonoid-rich extract of bergamot juice (BJe) attenuated the inflammatory response in the leukemic monocyte THP-1 exposed to lipopolysaccharide (LPS) via the activation of the adenosine monophosphate-activated protein kinase (AMPK)/sirtuin (SIRT)1 axis [67]. Consistently, the same extract also unveiled its anti-inflammatory potential in an in vivo model by improving LPS-induced gingival inflammation in rats. Here, BJe reduced the nuclear translocation of NF-κB, the expression of TNF-α and IL-1β cytokines and ICAM and P-selectin adhesion molecules, as well as the myeloperoxidase activity at the gingival tissue level [68]. Similar to BJe, a BEO fraction deprived of furocoumarins (BEO-FF) produced anti-inflammatory effects on an animal model of acute inflammation. In this latter case, BEO-FF significantly reduced the carrageenan-induced paw edema in rats, decreasing levels of IL-1β, IL-6 and TNF-α in the paw homogenates, and those of nitrite/nitrate and PGE2 in exudates [69]. In Table 1, evidence on the effects of bergamot derivatives and byproducts against acute inflammation is reported.

Table 1. Effects of bergamot derivatives and byproducts in acute inflammation models.

Derivatives/Byproducts	Inflammation-Related Disease	Experimental Model		Inflammatory Biomarkers	References
A flavonoid-rich extract of bergamot juice	Acute inflammation	In vitro	Leukemic monocytes THP-1 exposed to LPS	AMPK/SIRT1 axis	[67]
A flavonoid-rich extract of bergamot juice	Periodontitis	In vivo	LPS-induced gingival inflammation in rats	NF-κB, TNF-α, IL-1β, ICAM, P-selectin and myeloperoxidase	[68]
Bergamot essential oil fraction deprived of furocoumarins	Acute inflammation		Carrageenan-induced paw edema in rats	IL-1β, IL-6, TNF-α, nitrite/nitrate and PGE2	[69]

5.2. Bergamot Derivatives and Byproducts in Inflammatory-Based Respiratory Ailments

Regarding chronic respiratory diseases, BEO exhibited relevant anti-asthmatic effects both in vitro and in vivo models. In the first case, BEO was able to suppress the release of inflammatory cytokines (IL-6, IL-1β and TNF-α) and inhibited their gene expression (*Il6*, *Il1b* and *Tnf-alpha*) in MH-S cells exposed to LPS. Here, it also hampered the activation of MAPKs and JAK-STAT signaling pathways and lowered the levels for key genes PTGS2 (*Ptgs2*) and PPARα (*Ppara*) [70]. Again, recent insights into anti-inflammatory potential have emerged for bergapten, a psoralen present in BEO. This component exerted a negative modulation of iNOS, COX-2 and levels of PGE2 and nitric oxide (NO) and increased the release of IL-10 in RAW264.7 cells exposed to LPS [71]. Of note, both BEO and bergapten were also shown to be effective on more complex models of respiratory inflammation such as the animal ones. In this line, the inhaling of BEO by ovalbumin-induced mice improved lung inflammation and airway narrowing, via the reduction in IL-4, IL-5, IL-13 (both at gene and protein levels), IL-6, IL-1β and TNF-α levels, and inhibited collagen deposition [70]. On the other hand, bergapten was able to ameliorate the inflammatory symptoms associated with combined allergic rhinitis and asthma syndrome (CARAS) in a mouse model. Indeed, the administration of bergapten limited the release of pro-inflammatory cytokines, the activation of STAT3 and MAPKs signaling pathways, the infiltration of inflammatory cells and collagen deposition at the level of nasal mucosa and lung tissue [72]. Table 2 shows the effects of BEO on inflammatory-based respiratory ailments.

Table 2. Anti-inflammatory effects of bergamot essential oil on asthma experimental models.

Derivatives/Byproducts	Inflammation-Related Disease	Experimental Model		Inflammatory Biomarkers	References
Bergamot essential oil	Asthma	In vitro	MH-S cells exposed to LPS	IL-6 (*Il6*), IL-1β (*Il1b*), TNF-α (*Tnf-alpha*), MAPKs1,3,8,14, Jak2, Stat3, Ptgs2 and Ppara	[70]
		In vivo	Ovalbumin-induced mice	IL-4 (*Il4*), IL-5 (*Il5*), IL-13 (*Il13*), IL-6, IL-1β, TNF-α and collagen deposition	

5.3. Bergamot Derivatives and Byproducts against Metabolic Syndrome

Inflammation precedes and aggravates the cluster of metabolic and cardiovascular disorders known as "metabolic syndrome" [73]. In this context, several studies documented the protective role of bergamot derivatives and byproducts associated with their numerous biological effects, including relevant anti-inflammatory activity. In detail, two polyphenol fractions isolated from the bergamot leaf (BLPF) and fruit (BFPF) were able to inhibit the translocation and activation of NF-κB in a cellular model of IL-1α-induced inflammation, although to a different extent. Here, by comparing the analytical profile and anti-inflammatory activity of both fractions, bergamot leaves were found to be a richer source of polyphenols with respect to the fruit [74]. The same anti-inflammatory mechanism was observed for a byproduct of the BEO industry obtained by squeezing the solid residue that remains after fruit pressing, called PBJ, which reduced nuclear translocation of NF-κB in a cellular model of TNF-α-induced inflammation. PBJ proved to also be effective in an in vivo model of metabolic syndrome induced by a high-sugar and high-fat diet (HSF) [75]. Also noteworthy were the protective effects of a bergamot leaf extract (BLE) against the comorbidities associated with metabolic syndrome, such as the impaired function of skeletal muscles. In this context, BLE reduced oxidative stress and levels of TNF-α, IL-6 and IL-10 in the muscles of rats with metabolic syndrome [76]. Again, BJ was shown to alleviate hepatic steatosis in an animal model of diet-induced metabolic syndrome and cardiovascular risk via the reduction in IL-6 and TNF-α plasma levels and ROS generation [77].

It is known that the Mediterranean diet represents the gold standard among dietary patterns for its ability to counteract inflammation and related pathologies [78]. In this regard, it has been shown that the supplementation of an extract of bergamot polyphenols (BPF) in diet-induced hyperlipemic Wistar rats ameliorated several serum parameters. This has also occurred clinically in patients suffering from hyperlipemia and/or hyperglycemia, thus suggesting the BPF potential in counteracting metabolic syndrome [79].

A pilot study investigated the effects of a phytocomplex, including BJ, on untreated subjects with metabolic syndrome who followed the Mediterranean diet. It was shown that this nutraceutical complex was able to boost the beneficial effects of this type of diet through controlling metabolic syndrome parameters (total cholesterol, LDLs, high-density lipoproteins (HDLs), triglycerides (TGs) and glucose) and inflammation markers, like CRP [80]. Other causes thought to unleash metabolic syndrome are suggested to be gastric infections; indeed, it was shown that *Helicobacter pylori* is positively linked to such a condition [81]. In this field, bergamot juice effectively inhibited the viability of clinical isolates of *H. pylori*, while also synergistically boosting the effect of common antibiotics [82]. On this basis, Carresi and co-workers [83] defined the protective role of bergamot derivatives and their flavonoids in metabolic syndrome, indicating pleiotropic antioxidant, anti-inflammatory and lipid-lowering effects. Among these, the anti-inflammatory properties of bergamot derivatives and by-products have been highlighted in Table 3.

Table 3. Anti-inflammatory effects of bergamot derivatives and byproducts on metabolic syndrome.

Derivatives/Byproducts	Inflammation-Related Disease	Experimental Model		Inflammatory Biomarkers	References
Enriched polyphenol fraction from bergamot fruit and leaves	Metabolic syndrome	In vitro	IL-1α-induced inflammation in R3/1 NF-κB cell line	NF-κB	[74]
Powder from bergamot juice	Metabolic syndrome		TNF-α-induced inflammation in R3/1 NF-κB cell line	NF-κB	[75]
Bergamot leaf extract	Metabolic syndrome and impaired function of skeletal muscle	In vivo	Rats fed with high-sugar diet	TNF-α, IL-6 and IL-10	[76]
Bergamot juice	Metabolic syndrome		High-fat-diet-induced steatosis in rats	IL-6 and TNF-α	[77]
Nutraceutical multicompound including bergamot juice	Metabolic syndrome	Clinical trial	Untreated subjects with metabolic syndrome	CRP	[80]

5.4. Bergamot Derivatives and Byproducts in Obesity and Overweight

Obesity and being overweight, which also occur in more complex conditions such as that of metabolic syndrome, are triggers for the inflammatory process. Thereby, anti-inflammatory approaches are suggested in the management of these pathologies [84]. Regarding the role of bergamot derivatives and byproducts on metabolic disorders, it was seen that a bergamot leaf extract (BLE) is able to decrease inflammation (TNF-α and IL-6 levels) and oxidative stress, acting on the adipose tissue–liver axis of obese rats, with an effect which might improve both insulin resistance and dyslipidemia conditions [85]. In the same experimental model, BLE was also studied at the hypothalamic level, where it reduced the inflammation (decreasing the production of cytokine signaling (SOCS) 3, IL-6 and TNF-α and activating the JAK2/STAT3 pathway) and oxidative stress, thus counteracting the resistance to leptin (known as the "satiety hormone") of obese rats [86]. Clinically, a nutraceutical containing bergamot extract was shown to improve systemic inflammation, significantly reducing high-sensitivity C-reactive protein (hs-CRP) and TNF-α levels in dyslipidemic overweight subjects [87]. The beneficial role of bergamot derivatives and byproducts in counteracting obesity/overweight is collected in Table 4.

Table 4. Anti-inflammatory effects of bergamot derivatives and byproducts against obesity and overweight.

Derivatives/Byproducts	Inflammation-Related Disease	Experimental Model		Inflammatory Biomarkers	References
Bergamot leaf extract	Obesity	In vivo	Diet-induced obese rats	TNF-α, IL-6	[85]
Bergamot leaf extract	Obesity		Obese rats fed with high-sugar and high-fat diet	TNF-α, IL-6, JAK2/STAT3 pathway and SOCS3	[86]
Nutraceutical containing a bergamot standardized flavonoid extract	Overweight	Clinical trial	Dyslipidemic overweight patients	hs-CRP and TNF-α	[87]

5.5. Bergamot Derivatives and Byproducts in Liver Diseases

It is known that the accumulation of triglycerides in hepatocytes accompanied by inflammation or cell injury is the leading cause of non-alcoholic fatty liver disease (NAFLD), which may progress into the more aggressive form of non-alcoholic steatohepatitis (NASH).

In this context, BPF has been shown to decrease hepatic inflammation in rats with cafeteria diet-induced NAFLD. In detail, BPF lowered *Il-6* gene expression and increased *Il-10* mRNA levels, which were related to a reduced number of Kupffer cells and inflammatory foci in the liver [88]. Again, bergamot polyphenolic formulation (BPF99) reduced inflammation in a mouse model of NAFLD by inhibiting the activation of the JNK and p38 MAPKs pathways responsible for an overproduction of pro-inflammatory cytokines and collagen deposition, which may precede liver fibrosis [89]. Interestingly, a synergistic combination between BPF and *Cynara cardunculus* extract (CyC), namely Bergacyn, counteracted NAFLD-related symptoms in a clinical setting, inducing anti-inflammatory effects. In particular, oral administration of Bergacyn® reduced oxidative stress (GPx, SOD and MDA) and inflammatory biomarkers (TNF-α), contributing to a significant improvement of vascular inflammation and NO-mediated vasodilation in patients with NAFLD and type 2 diabetes [90]. The anti-inflammatory effects described for bergamot derivatives and byproducts in the context of liver diseases are gathered in Table 5.

Table 5. Anti-inflammatory effects of bergamot derivatives and byproducts in liver diseases.

Derivatives/Byproducts	Inflammation-Related Disease	Experimental Model		Inflammatory Biomarkers	References
Bergamot polyphenol fraction	Non-alcoholic steatohepatitis (NASH)	In vivo	Rats exposed to a cafeteria diet	*Il-6* and *Il-10*	[88]
Bergamot polyphenolic formulation	Non-alcoholic fatty liver disease (NAFLD)		Mice fed with a Western diet	JNK, p38, procollagen I and III	[89]
Bergacyn (combination between bergamot polyphenolic fraction and *Cynara cardunculus* extract)	NAFLD	Clinical trial	Patients with NAFLD and type 2 diabetes	TNF-α	[90]

5.6. Bergamot Derivatives and Byproducts in Dyslipidemic Disorders

Of note, systemic inflammation and elevated serum cholesterol concentrations are predisposing factors for the development and progression of cardiovascular diseases, such as atherosclerosis. Interestingly, bergamot juice flavanones were shown to play a key role in restoring the endothelial functionality impaired by lipotoxic effects, a common cause of atherosclerosis. In detail, Spigoni and co-workers [91] indicated that some flavanone metabolites (i.e., hesperetin-7-O-glucuronide, hesperetin-3′-O-glucuronide, naringenin-7-O-glucuronide and naringenin-4′-O-glucuronide) were able to mitigate the stearate-induced inflammation (reducing the *Il-1b*, *Il-6*, *Il-8* and *Tnf-alpha* mRNA levels) in human pro-angiogenic cells. From a clinical point of view, a polyphenolic fraction of bergamot juice was previously shown to reduce plasma lipids and improve the lipoprotein profile in patients with moderate hyperlipidemia [4]. In this frame, Fogacci and collaborators [92] recently proved significant improvements in subjects with moderate hypercholesterolemia after dietary supplementation with a nutraceutical containing a standardized bergamot polyphenolic fraction (Eufortyn® Colesterolo Plus, Scharper, Milano, Italia). This mixture reduced the levels of hs-CRP as well as the indexes of endothelial reactivity (ER) and NAFLD. Inflammation-lowering effects were also observed for another dietary supplement (BruMeChol™, Mivell, Jesi, Italia), composed of a mixture of flavonoids extracted from bergamot, olive polyphenols, plant sterols and vitamin K2, in patients with mild hypercholesterolemia. In this case, the nutraceutical combination significantly lowered circulating levels of inflammatory mediators, such as IL-6, IL-32, IL-37 and IL-38, hs-CRP, and inflamma-microRNA miR-21 and miR-146a [93]. The effects of bergamot derivatives and byproducts on dyslipidemias are described in Table 6.

Table 6. Effects of bergamot derivatives and byproducts against dyslipidemias.

Derivatives/Byproducts	Inflammation-Related Disease	Experimental Model	Experimental Model	Inflammatory Biomarkers	References
Bergamot juice flavanones (i.e., hesperetin-7-O-glucuronide, hesperetin-3′-O-glucuronide, naringenin-7-O-glucuronide and naringenin-4′-O-glucuronide)	Endothelial dysfunction	In vitro	Stearate-induced inflammation in myeloid angiogenic cells.	*Il-1b, Il-6, Il-8* and *Tnf-alpha*	[91]
Eufortyn® Colesterolo Plus (a nutraceutical containing a standardized bergamot polyphenolic fraction)	Hypercholesterolemia	Clinical trial	Patients with moderate hypercholesterolemia	hs-CRP and ER	[92]
BruMeChol™ (supplement composed by a mixture of flavonoids extracted from bergamot, olive polyphenols, plant sterols and vitamin K2)	Hypercholesterolemia		Patients with mild hypercholesterolemia	IL-6, IL-32, IL-37, IL-38, hs-CRP, miR-21 and miR-146a	[93]

5.7. Bergamot Derivatives and Byproducts in Renal, Gynecological and Rectal Dysfunctions

The frequent exposure of kidneys to drugs and toxic agents is the major cause of renal injury. In this regard, a bergamot extract exerted preventive effects against amikacin-induced nephrotoxicity in rats, restoring the kidney function and IL-6 serum levels that were raised by the drug [94]. Similarly, a flavonoid-rich extract of bergamot juice (BJe), alone or in association with curcumin (Cur) and resveratrol (Re), counteracted the cadmium-induced kidney damage in a murine model, restoring the antioxidant defense systems and reducing the expression of *Nos2, Il1b, Nrf2* and heme oxygenase (*Hmox*)1 pro-inflammatory genes [95]. In addition, BEO, and to a minor extent BJ and an ethanol bergamot extract, was shown to be effective in gynecological disorders such as primary dysmenorrhea induced by estradiol benzoate and oxytocin in rats. These bergamot derivatives alleviated dysmenorrhea, regulating the levels of $PGF_{2\alpha}$ and PGE_2 prostaglandins and the release of inflammatory mediators such as iNOS as well as activating the antioxidant defense mechanisms in the uterine tissue of rats [96]. Clinically, innovative results came from the treatment of patients affected by anitis/proctitis after treatment with a bergamot oil (known as Benebeo® gel, Wellvit, Cosenza, Italia). The local administration of bergamot gel, containing hesperidin, naringenin, apigenin and eriocitrin as major components, produced anti-inflammatory effects (improvement in local bleeding and hyperemia), promoting a fast-healing process in situ [97]. The evidence of bergamot derivatives and byproducts against the abovementioned disorders is reported in Table 7.

5.8. Bergamot Derivatives and Byproducts in Neurological Disorders

Neuronal disorders in most cases recognize an inflammatory component at the basis of their etiology. In this regard, neuroprotective effects of *Citrus bergamia* juice extract were documented in an in vitro model of Alzheimer's disease (AD), where BJe decreased the pro-inflammatory stimulus induced by β-amyloid on THP-1 cells [98].

In vivo, BEO attenuated anxiety in rats, counteracting the oxidative stress, the neuroinflammation and GABA changes induced after exposure to aluminum. As an anti-inflammatory agent, BEO significantly reduced the content of IL-6, IL-1β and TNF-α both at the hippocampal and frontal cortex levels of rats [99]. In a clinical trial, the oral administration of a bergamot polyphenolic fraction (BPF) was associated with a significant improvement in cognitive functioning, which had been impaired by ongoing inflammatory processes in schizophrenic patients [100]. The effects on neurological disorders of bergamot derivatives and byproducts are reported in Table 8.

Table 7. Anti-inflammatory effects of bergamot derivatives on inflammation-related diseases affecting renal, gynecological and rectal districts.

Derivatives/Byproducts	Inflammation-Related Disease	Experimental Model	Experimental Model	Inflammatory Biomarkers	References
Bergamot extract	Nephrotoxicity		Amikacin-induced nephrotoxicity in rats	IL-6	[94]
A flavonoid-rich extract of bergamot juice, alone or in association with curcumin and resveratrol	Nephrotoxicity	In vivo	Cadmium-induced kidney damage in a murine model	Nos2, Il1b, Nrf2 and Nqo1	[95]
Bergamot essential oil, bergamot juice and ethanol extract of bergamot	Primary dysmenorrhea		Dysmenorrhea induced by estradiol benzoate and oxytocin in rats	PGF2α, PGE2 and iNOS	[96]
Benebeo® gel (Bergamot oil)	Anitis/proctitis	Clinical trial	Patients with anitis/proctitis	Local bleeding and hyperemia	[97]

Table 8. Effects of bergamot derivatives and byproducts on inflammatory-based neurological disorders.

Derivatives/Byproducts	Inflammation-Related Disease	Experimental Model	Experimental Model	Inflammatory Biomarkers	References
Bergamot juice extract	Alzheimer's disease	In vitro	THP-1 cells exposed to β-amyloid	IL-6 (Il-6), IL-1β (Il1b), NF-κB, AP-1 and MAPKs pathway	[98]
Bergamot essential oil	Anxiety	In vivo	Rats exposed to aluminum	IL-6, IL-1β and TNF-α	[99]

5.9. Bergamot Derivatives and Byproducts in Cancer

The weak balance between the inflammatory status and unsuccessful anti-inflammatory response is at the basis of cellular degeneration, an event that may lead to serious outcomes such as cancer [53]. Within this frame, bergamot byproducts were shown to play a relevant role against several types of cancer. In vitro, BJ was able to counteract the malignant proliferation of neuroblastoma SH-SY5Y cells [101] as well as that one of human hepatocellular carcinoma HepG2 cells via targeting NF-κB, a central factor in both inflammation and cancer [102]. This is in line with the evidence of the anti-proliferative effects observed for a flavonoid-rich extract of BJ in human colon cancer HT-29 cells [103]. However, in a complex context like the tumor microenvironment, other factors come into play including the family of sirtuins. Interestingly, the antileukemic effects observed for BJe and some flavanones it contains on leukemic THP-1 cells were mediated by the inhibition of the SIRT2 enzyme [104,105]. Anticancer effects induced by bergamot derivatives were also observed in murine models [106]. In particular, anti-inflammatory mechanisms were related to the potentiality of BJe to prevent colorectal carcinogenesis in Pirc rats (F344/NTac-Apc^{am1137}). Here, a significant reduction in colon tumors and mucin-depleted foci was recorded in BJe-treated groups. This effect was ascribed to the extract's capacity to inhibit apoptosis and decrease the expression of Ptgs2, iNos, Il-1b, Il-6, Il-10 and Arginase (Arg)1 pro-inflammatory biomarkers [107]. The beneficial role of bergamot derivatives and byproducts against cancerous pathways are presented in Table 9.

Table 9. Anti-inflammatory effects of bergamot derivatives on inflammation markers related to cancer.

Derivatives/Byproducts	Inflammation-Related Disease	Experimental Model		Inflammatory Biomarkers	References
Bergamot juice	Hepatocellular carcinoma	In vitro	HepG2 cells	NF-κB	[102]
Bergamot juice extract	Colorectal cancer	In vivo	Pirc rat (F344/NTac-Apc^{am1137})	*Ptgs2, iNos, Il-1b, Il-6, Il-10* and *Arg1*	[107]

5.10. Bergamot Derivatives and Byproducts in Skin Disorders

In the field of skin diseases, BEO with its major components, namely limonene, linalyl acetate and linalool, showed significant antiproliferative activity on a pre-inflamed human dermal system, consisting of primary fibroblasts stimulated with a mixture of IL-1β, TNF-α, IFN-γ, basic fibroblast growth factor (bFGF), epidermal growth factor (EGF) and platelet-derived growth factor (PDGF) to simulate chronic inflammation. In the same model, BEO significantly inhibited the expression of proteins related to inflammation (MCP-1, VCAM-1, ICAM-1, interferon gamma-induced protein (IP-10), interferon-inducible T cell alpha chemoattractant (I-TAC) and monokine induced by gamma interferon (MIG)) and tissue remodeling processes (collagen I, collagen III, plasminogen activator inhibitor (PAI) 1, tissue inhibitor of metalloproteinase (TIMP) 1 and 2), thus exhibiting anti-inflammatory and wound healing properties [108]. The anti-inflammatory role of bergamot derivatives was also documented in vivo, considering that BJ improved the acne vulgaris lesions caused by an excessive secretion of androgen via reducing the release of inflammatory IL-1α, IL-6, TNF-α cytokines and the levels of matrix metalloprotease (MMP)-2 and -9 in the sebaceous gland of golden hamsters, though to a lesser extent than BEO [109]. This study is resulted in line with a previous clinical application in which a nano-phytosome (NP) formulation was developed to optimize the BEO topical delivery, experiencing synergic effects between BEO-NPs and spironolactone in acne patients [110]. Interestingly, ultradeformable nanocarriers were designed for a transdermal delivery of naturally derived compounds such as BEO and ammonium glycyrrhizinate (AG) since the proper deformability of these nanosystems facilitates movement through the skin barrier, ensuring a topical application. In particular, the co-encapsulation of BEO into AG-loaded nanoparticles preserved their degree of deformability, thus efficiently counteracting the skin inflammatory states on human volunteers [111]. In Table 10, the effects of bergamot derivatives and byproducts against skin disorders are listed.

Table 10. Anti-inflammatory effects of bergamot derivatives and byproducts on skin disorders.

Derivatives/Byproducts	Inflammation-Related Disease	Experimental Model	Experimental Model	Inflammatory Biomarkers	References
Bergamot essential oil	Chronic skin inflammation	In vitro	Primary fibroblasts stimulated with a mixture of IL-1β, TNF-α, IFNγ, bFGF, EGF and PDGF	MCP-1, VCAM-1, ICAM-1, IP-10, I-TAC, MIG, collagen I and III, PAI-1 and TIMP-1 and -2	[108]
Bergamot essential oil and juice	Acne vulgaris	In vivo	Administration of compound pearl acne capsules on golden hamsters	IL-1α, IL-6, TNF-α, MMP-2 and MMP-9	[109]
Encapsulation of bergamot essential oil into ammonium glycyrrhizinate-loaded nanoparticles	Skin inflammation	Clinical trial	Human volunteers subjected to methylnicotinate solution on specific skin sites	Erythema index	[111]

6. Conclusions

Inflammation is a complex process, which affects organs and tissue with high costs for human health. Many disorders arise from an unresolved inflammatory response, evolving into chronic inflammatory pathologies. Thereby, the resolution of the phlogistic process represents the goal strategy to prevent or limit the progression of inflammatory illnesses by exerting control on the production of mediators such as the release of pro-inflammatory cytokines, the activation of specific pathways or the recruitment of infiltrating cells at the site of inflammation.

The waste from bergamot processing has long been considered byproducts, leading not solely to a loss of valuable molecules but also increasing the environmental cost of its appropriate disposal. For over a decade, bergamot derivatives and byproducts have been demonstrated to be a relevant source of bioactive molecules, which can play a significant role in several diseases thanks to their considerable pharmacological properties, including anti-inflammatory ones (Figure 3).

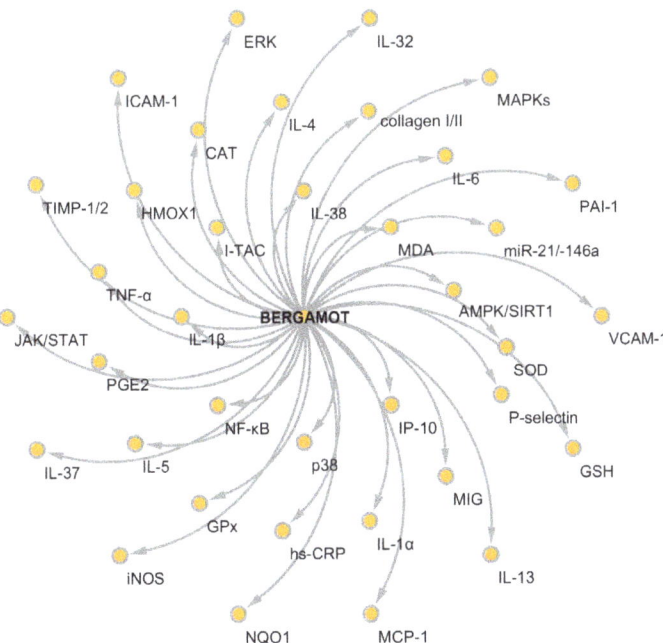

Figure 3. Radial map of the chemokines, enzymes and nuclear factors influenced by bergamot derivatives and byproducts.

Recently, new outcomes in both preclinical studies and human trials have been reached on the beneficial properties of bergamot that we summarized here, thus deciding to update our previous review on this topic. The reinforced data on the effectiveness of bergamot derivatives and byproducts on modulating the expression and release of chemokines, as well as the activity of nuclear factors and enzymes linked to the onset and progression of inflammation, contribute to the amelioration of current therapeutical strategies. Therefore, bergamot can represent a sustainable and powerful resource in the management of several inflammatory-based ailments given the robust and deep evidence in this regard.

Author Contributions: C.R. performed the literature review and drafted this paper; G.E.L. assisted in preparing this review; G.B. assisted in the literature search; A.M. and A.R. critically revised this paper; M.N. conceived and designed this study and critically revised this paper. All authors have read and agreed to the published version of the manuscript.

Funding: This research received no external funding.

Institutional Review Board Statement: Not applicable.

Informed Consent Statement: Not applicable.

Data Availability Statement: Not applicable.

Acknowledgments: The A PON Industrial PhD fellowship from the Italian Minister of Instruction, University and Research (MIUR) to Caterina Russo (CUP: J11B21008430007) is gratefully acknowledged.

Conflicts of Interest: The authors declare no conflicts of interest.

References

1. Langgut, D. The citrus route revealed: From Southeast Asia into the Mediterranean. *HortScience* **2017**, *52*, 814–822. [CrossRef]
2. Wang, R.X.; Zhou, M.; Ma, H.L.; Qiao, Y.B.; Li, Q.S. The Role of Chronic Inflammation in Various Diseases and Anti-inflammatory Therapies Containing Natural Products. *ChemMedChem* **2021**, *16*, 1576–1592. [CrossRef] [PubMed]

3. Cirmi, S.; Navarra, M.; Woodside, J.V.; Cantwell, M.M. Citrus fruits intake and oral cancer risk: A systematic review and meta-analysis. *Pharmacol. Res.* **2018**, *133*, 187–194. [CrossRef] [PubMed]
4. Mannucci, C.; Navarra, M.; Calapai, F.; Squeri, R.; Gangemi, S.; Calapai, G. Clinical Pharmacology of *Citrus bergamia*: A Systematic Review. *Phytother. Res.* **2017**, *31*, 27–39. [CrossRef]
5. Marino, A.; Paterniti, I.; Cordaro, M.; Morabito, R.; Campolo, M.; Navarra, M.; Esposito, E.; Cuzzocrea, S. Role of natural antioxidants and potential use of bergamot in treating rheumatoid arthritis. *PharmaNutrition* **2015**, *3*, 53–59. [CrossRef]
6. Rea, I.M.; Gibson, D.S.; McGilligan, V.; McNerlan, S.E.; Alexander, H.D.; Ross, O.A. Age and Age-Related Diseases: Role of Inflammation Triggers and Cytokines. *Front. Immunol.* **2018**, *9*, 586. [CrossRef]
7. Russo, C.; Maugeri, A.; Lombardo, G.E.; Musumeci, L.; Barreca, D.; Rapisarda, A.; Cirmi, S.; Navarra, M. The Second Life of Citrus Fruit Waste: A Valuable Source of Bioactive Compounds. *Molecules* **2021**, *26*, 5991. [CrossRef]
8. Ferlazzo, N.; Cirmi, S.; Calapai, G.; Ventura-Spagnolo, E.; Gangemi, S.; Navarra, M. Anti-Inflammatory Activity of *Citrus bergamia* Derivatives: Where Do We Stand? *Molecules* **2016**, *21*, 1273. [CrossRef]
9. Chen, L.; Deng, H.; Cui, H.; Fang, J.; Zuo, Z.; Deng, J.; Li, Y.; Wang, X.; Zhao, L. Inflammatory responses and inflammation-associated diseases in organs. *Oncotarget* **2018**, *9*, 7204–7218. [CrossRef]
10. Li, D.; Wu, M. Pattern recognition receptors in health and diseases. *Signal Transduct. Target. Ther.* **2021**, *6*, 291. [CrossRef]
11. Kawasaki, T.; Kawai, T. Toll-like receptor signaling pathways. *Front. Immunol.* **2014**, *5*, 461. [CrossRef] [PubMed]
12. Cirmi, S.; Maugeri, A.; Russo, C.; Musumeci, L.; Navarra, M.; Lombardo, G.E. Oleacein Attenuates Lipopolysaccharide-Induced Inflammation in THP-1-Derived Macrophages by the Inhibition of TLR4/MyD88/NF-kappaB Pathway. *Int. J. Mol. Sci.* **2022**, *23*, 1206. [CrossRef] [PubMed]
13. Liu, T.; Zhang, L.; Joo, D.; Sun, S.C. NF-kappaB signaling in inflammation. *Signal Transduct. Target. Ther.* **2017**, *2*, 17023. [CrossRef] [PubMed]
14. Kaminska, B. MAPK signalling pathways as molecular targets for anti-inflammatory therapy—From molecular mechanisms to therapeutic benefits. *Biochim. Biophys. Acta* **2005**, *1754*, 253–262. [CrossRef] [PubMed]
15. Morris, R.; Kershaw, N.J.; Babon, J.J. The molecular details of cytokine signaling via the JAK/STAT pathway. *Protein Sci.* **2018**, *27*, 1984–2009. [CrossRef] [PubMed]
16. Turner, M.D.; Nedjai, B.; Hurst, T.; Pennington, D.J. Cytokines and chemokines: At the crossroads of cell signalling and inflammatory disease. *Biochim. Biophys. Acta* **2014**, *1843*, 2563–2582. [CrossRef] [PubMed]
17. Abbate, F.; Maugeri, A.; Laura, R.; Levanti, M.; Navarra, M.; Cirmi, S.; Germana, A. Zebrafish as a Useful Model to Study Oxidative Stress-Linked Disorders: Focus on Flavonoids. *Antioxidants* **2021**, *10*, 668. [CrossRef] [PubMed]
18. Cheng, Y.; Wang, D.; Wang, B.; Li, H.; Xiong, J.; Xu, S.; Chen, Q.; Tao, K.; Yang, X.; Zhu, Y.; et al. HMGB1 translocation and release mediate cigarette smoke-induced pulmonary inflammation in mice through a TLR4/MyD88-dependent signaling pathway. *Mol. Biol. Cell* **2017**, *28*, 201–209. [CrossRef]
19. Murakami, A.; Ohigashi, H. Targeting NOX, INOS and COX-2 in inflammatory cells: Chemoprevention using food phytochemicals. *Int. J. Cancer* **2007**, *121*, 2357–2363. [CrossRef]
20. Sproston, N.R.; Ashworth, J.J. Role of C-Reactive Protein at Sites of Inflammation and Infection. *Front. Immunol.* **2018**, *9*, 754. [CrossRef]
21. Rossaint, J.; Margraf, A.; Zarbock, A. Role of Platelets in Leukocyte Recruitment and Resolution of Inflammation. *Front. Immunol.* **2018**, *9*, 2712. [CrossRef] [PubMed]
22. Sugimoto, M.A.; Sousa, L.P.; Pinho, V.; Perretti, M.; Teixeira, M.M. Resolution of Inflammation: What Controls Its Onset? *Front. Immunol.* **2016**, *7*, 160. [CrossRef]
23. Williams, H.C.; Dellavalle, R.P.; Garner, S. Acne vulgaris. *Lancet* **2012**, *379*, 361–372. [CrossRef] [PubMed]
24. Misery, L.; Pierre, O.; Le Gall-Ianotto, C.; Lebonvallet, N.; Chernyshov, P.V.; Le Garrec, R.; Talagas, M. Basic mechanisms of itch. *J. Allergy Clin. Immunol.* **2023**, *152*, 11–23. [CrossRef] [PubMed]
25. Ujiie, H.; Rosmarin, D.; Schon, M.P.; Stander, S.; Boch, K.; Metz, M.; Maurer, M.; Thaci, D.; Schmidt, E.; Cole, C.; et al. Unmet Medical Needs in Chronic, Non-communicable Inflammatory Skin Diseases. *Front. Med.* **2022**, *9*, 875492. [CrossRef]
26. Barnes, P.J. Cellular and molecular mechanisms of asthma and COPD. *Clin. Sci.* **2017**, *131*, 1541–1558. [CrossRef]
27. Chung, K.F. p38 mitogen-activated protein kinase pathways in asthma and COPD. *Chest* **2011**, *139*, 1470–1479. [CrossRef]
28. Calbet, M.; Ramis, I.; Calama, E.; Carreno, C.; Paris, S.; Maldonado, M.; Orellana, A.; Calaf, E.; Pauta, M.; De Alba, J.; et al. Novel Inhaled Pan-JAK Inhibitor, LAS194046, Reduces Allergen-Induced Airway Inflammation, Late Asthmatic Response, and pSTAT Activation in Brown Norway Rats. *J. Pharmacol. Exp. Ther.* **2019**, *370*, 137–147. [CrossRef]
29. Gao, Y.; Zhao, C.; Wang, W.; Jin, R.; Li, Q.; Ge, Q.; Guan, Y.; Zhang, Y. Prostaglandins E2 signal mediated by receptor subtype EP2 promotes IgE production in vivo and contributes to asthma development. *Sci. Rep.* **2016**, *6*, 20505. [CrossRef]
30. Luczak, E.; Wieczfinska, J.; Sokolowska, M.; Pniewska, E.; Luczynska, D.; Pawliczak, R. Troglitazone, a PPAR-gamma agonist, decreases LTC(4) concentration in mononuclear cells in patients with asthma. *Pharmacol. Rep.* **2017**, *69*, 1315–1321. [CrossRef]
31. Devchand, P.R.; Keller, H.; Peters, J.M.; Vazquez, M.; Gonzalez, F.J.; Wahli, W. The PPARalpha-leukotriene B4 pathway to inflammation control. *Nature* **1996**, *384*, 39–43. [CrossRef]
32. Russo, C.; Maugeri, A.; Musumeci, L.; De Sarro, G.; Cirmi, S.; Navarra, M. Inflammation and Obesity: The Pharmacological Role of Flavonoids in the Zebrafish Model. *Int. J. Mol. Sci.* **2023**, *24*, 2899. [CrossRef]

33. Kanda, H.; Tateya, S.; Tamori, Y.; Kotani, K.; Hiasa, K.; Kitazawa, R.; Kitazawa, S.; Miyachi, H.; Maeda, S.; Egashira, K.; et al. MCP-1 contributes to macrophage infiltration into adipose tissue, insulin resistance, and hepatic steatosis in obesity. *J. Clin. Investig.* **2006**, *116*, 1494–1505. [CrossRef]
34. Jorge, A.S.B.; Andrade, J.M.O.; Paraiso, A.F.; Jorge, G.C.B.; Silveira, C.M.; de Souza, L.R.; Santos, E.P.; Guimaraes, A.L.S.; Santos, S.H.S.; De-Paula, A.M.B. Body mass index and the visceral adipose tissue expression of IL-6 and TNF-alpha are associated with the morphological severity of non-alcoholic fatty liver disease in individuals with class III obesity. *Obes. Res. Clin. Pract.* **2018**, *12*, 1–8. [CrossRef] [PubMed]
35. Montanari, N.R.; Ramirez, R.; Aggarwal, A.; van Buuren, N.; Doukas, M.; Moon, C.; Turner, S.; Diehl, L.; Li, L.; Debes, J.D.; et al. Multi-parametric analysis of human livers reveals variation in intrahepatic inflammation across phases of chronic hepatitis B infection. *J. Hepatol.* **2022**, *77*, 332–343. [CrossRef] [PubMed]
36. Panahi, Y.; Hosseini, M.S.; Khalili, N.; Naimi, E.; Simental-Mendia, L.E.; Majeed, M.; Sahebkar, A. Effects of curcumin on serum cytokine concentrations in subjects with metabolic syndrome: A post-hoc analysis of a randomized controlled trial. *Biomed. Pharmacother.* **2016**, *82*, 578–582. [CrossRef] [PubMed]
37. Park, J.E.; Kang, E.; Han, J.S. HM-chromanone attenuates TNF-alpha-mediated inflammation and insulin resistance by controlling JNK activation and NF-kappaB pathway in 3T3-L1 adipocytes. *Eur. J. Pharmacol.* **2022**, *921*, 174884. [CrossRef] [PubMed]
38. Fusco, R.; Cirmi, S.; Gugliandolo, E.; Di Paola, R.; Cuzzocrea, S.; Navarra, M. A flavonoid-rich extract of orange juice reduced oxidative stress in an experimental model of inflammatory bowel disease. *J. Funct. Foods* **2017**, *30*, 168–178. [CrossRef]
39. Plotkin, J.D.; Elias, M.G.; Dellinger, A.L.; Kepley, C.L. NF-kappaB inhibitors that prevent foam cell formation and atherosclerotic plaque accumulation. *Nanomedicine* **2017**, *13*, 2037–2048. [CrossRef]
40. Lu, N.; Cheng, W.; Liu, D.; Liu, G.; Cui, C.; Feng, C.; Wang, X. NLRP3-Mediated Inflammation in Atherosclerosis and Associated Therapeutics. *Front. Cell Dev. Biol.* **2022**, *10*, 823387. [CrossRef]
41. Lainampetch, J.; Panprathip, P.; Phosat, C.; Chumpathat, N.; Prangthip, P.; Soonthornworasiri, N.; Puduang, S.; Wechjakwen, N.; Kwanbunjan, K. Association of Tumor Necrosis Factor Alpha, Interleukin 6, and C-Reactive Protein with the Risk of Developing Type 2 Diabetes: A Retrospective Cohort Study of Rural Thais. *J. Diabetes Res.* **2019**, *2019*, 9051929. [CrossRef] [PubMed]
42. Singh, T.P.; Morris, D.R.; Smith, S.; Moxon, J.V.; Golledge, J. Systematic Review and Meta-Analysis of the Association Between C-Reactive Protein and Major Cardiovascular Events in Patients with Peripheral Artery Disease. *Eur. J. Vasc. Endovasc. Surg.* **2017**, *54*, 220–233. [CrossRef]
43. Adolph, T.E.; Meyer, M.; Schwarzler, J.; Mayr, L.; Grabherr, F.; Tilg, H. The metabolic nature of inflammatory bowel diseases. *Nat. Rev. Gastroenterol. Hepatol.* **2022**, *19*, 753–767. [CrossRef] [PubMed]
44. Cirmi, S.; Randazzo, B.; Russo, C.; Musumeci, L.; Maugeri, A.; Montalbano, G.; Guerrera, M.C.; Lombardo, G.E.; Levanti, M. Anti-inflammatory effect of a flavonoid-rich extract of orange juice in adult zebrafish subjected to Vibrio anguillarum-induced enteritis. *Nat. Prod. Res.* **2021**, *35*, 5350–5353. [CrossRef]
45. Moschen, A.R.; Tilg, H.; Raine, T. IL-12, IL-23 and IL-17 in IBD: Immunobiology and therapeutic targeting. *Nat. Rev. Gastroenterol. Hepatol.* **2019**, *16*, 185–196. [CrossRef] [PubMed]
46. Cianciulli, A.; Calvello, R.; Cavallo, P.; Dragone, T.; Carofiglio, V.; Panaro, M.A. Modulation of NF-kappaB activation by resveratrol in LPS treated human intestinal cells results in downregulation of PGE2 production and COX-2 expression. *Toxicol. Vitro* **2012**, *26*, 1122–1128. [CrossRef]
47. Bruschetta, G.; Fazio, E.; Cravana, C.; Ferlazzo, A.M. Effects of partial versus complete separation after weaning on plasma serotonin, tryptophan and pituitary-adrenal pattern of Anglo-Arabian foals. *Livest. Sci.* **2017**, *198*, 157–161. [CrossRef]
48. Bruschetta, G.; Medica, P.; Fazio, E.; Cravana, C.; Ferlazzo, A.M. The effect of training sessions and feeding regimes on neuromodulator role of serotonin, tryptophan, and β-endorphin of horses. *J. Vet. Behav.* **2018**, *23*, 82–86. [CrossRef]
49. Wang, M.; Xu, H.; Chong Lee Shin, O.L.; Li, L.; Gao, H.; Zhao, Z.; Zhu, F.; Zhu, H.; Liang, W.; Qian, K.; et al. Compound alpha-keto acid tablet supplementation alleviates chronic kidney disease progression via inhibition of the NF-kB and MAPK pathways. *J. Transl. Med.* **2019**, *17*, 122. [CrossRef]
50. Milo, R.; Korczyn, A.D.; Manouchehri, N.; Stuve, O. The temporal and causal relationship between inflammation and neurodegeneration in multiple sclerosis. *Mult. Scler.* **2020**, *26*, 876–886. [CrossRef]
51. Song, L.; Pei, L.; Yao, S.; Wu, Y.; Shang, Y. NLRP3 Inflammasome in Neurological Diseases, from Functions to Therapies. *Front. Cell Neurosci.* **2017**, *11*, 63. [CrossRef] [PubMed]
52. Filaly, H.E.; Outlioua, A.; Medyouf, H.; Guessous, F.; Akarid, K. Targeting IL-1beta in patients with advanced Helicobacter pylori infection: A potential therapy for gastric cancer. *Future Microbiol.* **2022**, *17*, 633–641. [CrossRef] [PubMed]
53. Maugeri, A.; Cirmi, S.; Minciullo, P.L.; Gangemi, S.; Calapai, G.; Mollace, V.; Navarra, M. Citrus fruits and inflammaging: A systematic review. *Phytochem. Rev.* **2019**, *18*, 1025–1049. [CrossRef]
54. Mannucci, C.; Calapai, F.; Cardia, L.; Inferrera, G.; D'Arena, G.; Di Pietro, M.; Navarra, M.; Gangemi, S.; Ventura Spagnolo, E.; Calapai, G. Clinical Pharmacology of Citrus aurantium and Citrus sinensis for the Treatment of Anxiety. *Evid. Based Complement. Altern. Med.* **2018**, *2018*, 3624094. [CrossRef] [PubMed]
55. Rapisarda, A.; Germanò, M.P. Citrus × bergamia Risso & Poiteau Botanical classification, Morphology and Anatomy. In *Citrus bergamia: Bergamot and Its Derivatives*; CRC Press: Boca Raton, FL, USA, 2014; pp. 9–11.
56. Liu, Y.; Heying, E.; Tanumihardjo, S.A. History, global distribution, and nutritional importance of citrus fruits. *Compr. Rev. Food Sci. Food Saf.* **2012**, *11*, 530–545. [CrossRef]

57. Giuffre, A.M. Bergamot (*Citrus bergamia*, Risso): The Effects of Cultivar and Harvest Date on Functional Properties of Juice and Cloudy Juice. *Antioxidants* **2019**, *8*, 221. [CrossRef]
58. Gonzalez-Mas, M.C.; Rambla, J.L.; Lopez-Gresa, M.P.; Blazquez, M.A.; Granell, A. Volatile Compounds in Citrus Essential Oils: A Comprehensive Review. *Front. Plant Sci.* **2019**, *10*, 12. [CrossRef]
59. Cirmi, S.; Bisignano, C.; Mandalari, G.; Navarra, M. Anti-infective potential of *Citrus bergamia* Risso et Poiteau (bergamot) derivatives: A systematic review. *Phytother. Res.* **2016**, *30*, 1404–1411. [CrossRef]
60. Navarra, M.; Ferlazzo, N.; Cirmi, S.; Trapasso, E.; Bramanti, P.; Lombardo, G.E.; Minciullo, P.L.; Calapai, G.; Gangemi, S. Effects of bergamot essential oil and its extractive fractions on SH-SY5Y human neuroblastoma cell growth. *J. Pharm. Pharmacol.* **2015**, *67*, 1042–1053. [CrossRef]
61. Maugeri, A.; Lombardo, G.E.; Musumeci, L.; Russo, C.; Gangemi, S.; Calapai, G.; Cirmi, S.; Navarra, M. Bergamottin and 5-Geranyloxy-7-methoxycoumarin Cooperate in the Cytotoxic Effect of *Citrus bergamia* (Bergamot) Essential Oil in Human Neuroblastoma SH-SY5Y Cell Line. *Toxins* **2021**, *13*, 275. [CrossRef]
62. Gattuso, A.; Piscopo, A.; Romeo, R.; De Bruno, A.; Poiana, M. Recovery of Bioactive Compounds from Calabrian Bergamot Citrus Waste: Selection of Best Green Extraction. *Agriculture* **2023**, *13*, 1095. [CrossRef]
63. Salerno, R.; Casale, F.; Calandruccio, C.; Procopio, A. Characterization of flavonoids in *Citrus bergamia* (Bergamot) polyphenolic fraction by liquid chromatography–high resolution mass spectrometry (LC/HRMS). *PharmaNutrition* **2016**, *4*, S1–S7.
64. Musumeci, L.; Maugeri, A.; Russo, C.; Lombardo, G.E.; Cirmi, S.; Navarra, M. Citrus Flavonoids and Autoimmune Diseases: A Systematic Review of Clinical Studies. *Curr. Med. Chem.* **2023**, *30*, 2191–2204. [CrossRef] [PubMed]
65. Balestrieri, E.; Pizzimenti, F.; Ferlazzo, A.; Giofre, S.V.; Iannazzo, D.; Piperno, A.; Romeo, R.; Chiacchio, M.A.; Mastino, A.; Macchi, B. Antiviral activity of seed extract from *Citrus bergamia* towards human retroviruses. *Bioorg Med. Chem.* **2011**, *19*, 2084–2089. [CrossRef]
66. Kirbaslar, Ş.İ.; Kirbaslar, F.G. Composition of Turkish mandarin and bergamot leaf oils. *J. Essent. Oil Res.* **2006**, *18*, 318–327. [CrossRef]
67. Maugeri, A.; Ferlazzo, N.; De Luca, L.; Gitto, R.; Navarra, M. The link between the AMPK/SIRT1 axis and a flavonoid-rich extract of *Citrus bergamia* juice: A cell-free, in silico, and in vitro study. *Phytother. Res.* **2019**, *33*, 1805–1814. [CrossRef]
68. Gugliandolo, E.; Fusco, R.; D'Amico, R.; Peditto, M.; Oteri, G.; Di Paola, R.; Cuzzocrea, S.; Navarra, M. Treatment with a Flavonoid-Rich Fraction of Bergamot Juice Improved Lipopolysaccharide-Induced Periodontitis in Rats. *Front. Pharmacol.* **2018**, *9*, 1563. [CrossRef]
69. Lombardo, G.E.; Cirmi, S.; Musumeci, L.; Pergolizzi, S.; Maugeri, A.; Russo, C.; Mannucci, C.; Calapai, G.; Navarra, M. Mechanisms Underlying the Anti-Inflammatory Activity of Bergamot Essential Oil and Its Antinociceptive Effects. *Plants* **2020**, *9*, 704. [CrossRef]
70. Feng, S.; Xu, G.; Fu, Y.; Ding, Q.; Shi, Y. Exploring the Mechanism of Bergamot Essential Oil against Asthma Based on Network Pharmacology and Experimental Verification. *ACS Omega* **2023**, *8*, 10202–10213. [CrossRef]
71. Zhou, Y.; Wang, J.; Yang, W.; Qi, X.; Lan, L.; Luo, L.; Yin, Z. Bergapten prevents lipopolysaccharide-induced inflammation in RAW264.7 cells through suppressing JAK/STAT activation and ROS production and increases the survival rate of mice after LPS challenge. *Int. Immunopharmacol.* **2017**, *48*, 159–168. [CrossRef]
72. Jiang, Y.; Nguyen, T.V.; Jin, J.; Yu, Z.N.; Song, C.H.; Chai, O.H. Bergapten ameliorates combined allergic rhinitis and asthma syndrome after PM2.5 exposure by balancing Treg/Th17 expression and suppressing STAT3 and MAPK activation in a mouse model. *Biomed. Pharmacother.* **2023**, *164*, 114959. [CrossRef] [PubMed]
73. Reddy, P.; Lent-Schochet, D.; Ramakrishnan, N.; McLaughlin, M.; Jialal, I. Metabolic syndrome is an inflammatory disorder: A conspiracy between adipose tissue and phagocytes. *Clin. Chim. Acta* **2019**, *496*, 35–44. [CrossRef]
74. Baron, G.; Altomare, A.; Mol, M.; Garcia, J.L.; Correa, C.; Raucci, A.; Mancinelli, L.; Mazzotta, S.; Fumagalli, L.; Trunfio, G.; et al. Analytical Profile and Antioxidant and Anti-Inflammatory Activities of the Enriched Polyphenol Fractions Isolated from Bergamot Fruit and Leave. *Antioxidants* **2021**, *10*, 141. [CrossRef] [PubMed]
75. Della Vedova, L.; Gado, F.; Vieira, T.A.; Grandini, N.A.; Palacio, T.L.N.; Siqueira, J.S.; Carini, M.; Bombardelli, E.; Correa, C.R.; Aldini, G.; et al. Chemical, Nutritional and Biological Evaluation of a Sustainable and Scalable Complex of Phytochemicals from Bergamot By-Products. *Molecules* **2023**, *28*, 2964. [CrossRef] [PubMed]
76. Palacio, T.L.N.; Siqueira, J.S.; de Paula, B.H.; Rego, R.M.P.; Vieira, T.A.; Baron, G.; Altomare, A.; Ferron, A.J.T.; Aldini, G.; Kano, H.T.; et al. Bergamot (*Citrus bergamia*) leaf extract improves metabolic, antioxidant and anti-inflammatory activity in skeletal muscles in a metabolic syndrome experimental model. *Int. J. Food Sci. Nutr.* **2023**, *74*, 64–71. [CrossRef]
77. De Leo, M.; Piragine, E.; Pirone, A.; Braca, A.; Pistelli, L.; Calderone, V.; Miragliotta, V.; Testai, L. Protective Effects of Bergamot (*Citrus bergamia* Risso & Poiteau) Juice in Rats Fed with High-Fat Diet. *Planta Med.* **2020**, *86*, 180–189. [CrossRef]
78. Montano, L.; Maugeri, A.; Volpe, M.G.; Micali, S.; Mirone, V.; Mantovani, A.; Navarra, M.; Piscopo, M. Mediterranean Diet as a Shield against Male Infertility and Cancer Risk Induced by Environmental Pollutants: A Focus on Flavonoids. *Int. J. Mol. Sci.* **2022**, *23*, 1568. [CrossRef]
79. Mollace, V.; Sacco, I.; Janda, E.; Malara, C.; Ventrice, D.; Colica, C.; Visalli, V.; Muscoli, S.; Ragusa, S.; Muscoli, C.; et al. Hypolipemic and hypoglycaemic activity of bergamot polyphenols: From animal models to human studies. *Fitoterapia* **2011**, *82*, 309–316. [CrossRef]

80. Di Folco, U.; Pollakova, D.; De Falco, D.; Nardone, M.R.; Tubili, F.; Tubili, C. Effects of a nutraceutical multicompound including bergamot (*Citrus bergamia* Risso) juice on metabolic syndrome: A pilot study. *Mediterr. J. Nutr. Metab.* **2018**, *11*, 119–126. [CrossRef]
81. Upala, S.; Jaruvongvanich, V.; Riangwiwat, T.; Jaruvongvanich, S.; Sanguankeo, A. Association between Helicobacter pylori infection and metabolic syndrome: A systematic review and meta-analysis. *J. Dig. Dis.* **2016**, *17*, 433–440. [CrossRef]
82. Filocamo, A.; Bisignano, C.; Ferlazzo, N.; Cirmi, S.; Mandalari, G.; Navarra, M. In vitro effect of bergamot (*Citrus bergamia*) juice against cagA-positive and-negative clinical isolates of Helicobacter pylori. *BMC Complement. Altern. Med.* **2015**, *15*, 256. [CrossRef] [PubMed]
83. Carresi, C.; Gliozzi, M.; Musolino, V.; Scicchitano, M.; Scarano, F.; Bosco, F.; Nucera, S.; Maiuolo, J.; Macri, R.; Ruga, S.; et al. The Effect of Natural Antioxidants in the Development of Metabolic Syndrome: Focus on Bergamot Polyphenolic Fraction. *Nutrients* **2020**, *12*, 1504. [CrossRef] [PubMed]
84. Ellulu, M.S.; Patimah, I.; Khaza'ai, H.; Rahmat, A.; Abed, Y. Obesity and inflammation: The linking mechanism and the complications. *Arch. Med. Sci.* **2017**, *13*, 851–863. [CrossRef] [PubMed]
85. Siqueira, J.S.; Nakandakare-Maia, E.T.; Vieira, T.A.; Palacio, T.L.N.; Grandini, N.A.; Belin, M.A.F.; Nai, G.A.; Moreto, F.; Altomare, A.; Baron, G. Effect of Bergamot Leaves (*Citrus bergamia*) in the Crosstalk between Adipose Tissue and Liver of Diet-Induced Obese Rats. *Livers* **2023**, *3*, 258–270. [CrossRef]
86. Nakandakare-Maia, E.T.; Siqueira, J.S.; Ferron, A.J.T.; Vieira, T.A.; Palacio, T.L.N.; Grandini, N.A.; Garcia, J.L.; Belin, M.A.; Altomare, A.; Baron, G.; et al. Treatment with bergamot (*Citrus bergamia*) leaves extract attenuates leptin resistance in obese rats. *Mol. Cell Endocrinol.* **2023**, *566–567*, 111908. [CrossRef]
87. Cicero, A.F.G.; Fogacci, F.; Bove, M.; Giovannini, M.; Borghi, C. Three-arm, placebo-controlled, randomized clinical trial evaluating the metabolic effect of a combined nutraceutical containing a bergamot standardized flavonoid extract in dyslipidemic overweight subjects. *Phytotherapy Res.* **2019**, *33*, 2094–2101. [CrossRef]
88. Parafati, M.; Lascala, A.; La Russa, D.; Mignogna, C.; Trimboli, F.; Morittu, V.M.; Riillo, C.; Macirella, R.; Mollace, V.; Brunelli, E.; et al. Bergamot Polyphenols Boost Therapeutic Effects of the Diet on Non-Alcoholic Steatohepatitis (NASH) Induced by "Junk Food": Evidence for Anti-Inflammatory Activity. *Nutrients* **2018**, *10*, 1604. [CrossRef]
89. Musolino, V.; Gliozzi, M.; Scarano, F.; Bosco, F.; Scicchitano, M.; Nucera, S.; Carresi, C.; Ruga, S.; Zito, M.C.; Maiuolo, J.; et al. Bergamot Polyphenols Improve Dyslipidemia and Pathophysiological Features in a Mouse Model of Non-Alcoholic Fatty Liver Disease. *Sci. Rep.* **2020**, *10*, 2565. [CrossRef]
90. Musolino, V.; Gliozzi, M.; Bombardelli, E.; Nucera, S.; Carresi, C.; Maiuolo, J.; Mollace, R.; Paone, S.; Bosco, F.; Scarano, F.; et al. The synergistic effect of *Citrus bergamia* and Cynara cardunculus extracts on vascular inflammation and oxidative stress in non-alcoholic fatty liver disease. *J. Tradit. Complement. Med.* **2020**, *10*, 268–274. [CrossRef]
91. Spigoni, V.; Mena, P.; Fantuzzi, F.; Tassotti, M.; Brighenti, F.; Bonadonna, R.C.; Del Rio, D.; Dei Cas, A. Bioavailability of Bergamot (*Citrus bergamia*) Flavanones and Biological Activity of Their Circulating Metabolites in Human Pro-Angiogenic Cells. *Nutrients* **2017**, *9*, 1328. [CrossRef]
92. Fogacci, F.; Rizzoli, E.; Giovannini, M.; Bove, M.; D'Addato, S.; Borghi, C.; Cicero, A.F.G. Effect of Dietary Supplementation with Eufortyn((R)) Colesterolo Plus on Serum Lipids, Endothelial Reactivity, Indexes of Non-Alcoholic Fatty Liver Disease and Systemic Inflammation in Healthy Subjects with Polygenic Hypercholesterolemia: The ANEMONE Study. *Nutrients* **2022**, *14*, 2099. [CrossRef] [PubMed]
93. Bonfigli, A.R.; Protic, O.; Olivieri, F.; Montesanto, A.; Malatesta, G.; Di Pillo, R.; Antonicelli, R. Effects of a novel nutraceutical combination (BruMeChol) in subjects with mild hypercholesterolemia: Study protocol of a randomized, double-blind, controlled trial. *Trials* **2020**, *21*, 616. [CrossRef] [PubMed]
94. Dari, F.F.; Jaccob, A.A.; AL-Moziel, M.S. The potential protective effects of citrus bergamot extract against amikacin-induced nephrotoxicity in male albino rats. *Toxicol. Environ. Health Sci.* **2023**, *15*, 9–17. [CrossRef]
95. Cirmi, S.; Maugeri, A.; Micali, A.; Marini, H.R.; Puzzolo, D.; Santoro, G.; Freni, J.; Squadrito, F.; Irrera, N.; Pallio, G.; et al. Cadmium-Induced Kidney Injury in Mice Is Counteracted by a Flavonoid-Rich Extract of Bergamot Juice, Alone or in Association with Curcumin and Resveratrol, via the Enhancement of Different Defense Mechanisms. *Biomedicines* **2021**, *9*, 1797. [CrossRef] [PubMed]
96. Zhang, N.; Kong, F.; Zhao, L.; Yang, X.; Wu, W.; Zhang, L.; Ji, B.; Zhou, F. Essential oil, juice, and ethanol extract from bergamot confer improving effects against primary dysmenorrhea in rats. *J. Food Biochem.* **2021**, *45*, e13614. [CrossRef]
97. Cafaro, D.; Celedon, F.; Sturiale, A.; Sinicropi, M.S. Innovative results in the treatment of inespecific anusitis-proctitis with the use of bergamot gel (Benebeo gel)®. *Insights Clin. Cell. Immunol.* **2019**, *3*, 020–024.
98. Curro, M.; Risitano, R.; Ferlazzo, N.; Cirmi, S.; Gangemi, C.; Caccamo, D.; Ientile, R.; Navarra, M. *Citrus bergamia* Juice Extract Attenuates beta-Amyloid-Induced Pro-Inflammatory Activation of THP-1 Cells Through MAPK and AP-1 Pathways. *Sci. Rep.* **2016**, *6*, 20809. [CrossRef]
99. Cui, Y.; Che, Y.; Wang, H. Bergamot essential oil attenuate aluminum-induced anxiety-like behavior through antioxidation, anti-inflammatory and GABA regulation in rats. *Food Chem. Toxicol.* **2020**, *145*, 111766. [CrossRef]
100. Bruno, A.; Pandolfo, G.; Crucitti, M.; Cedro, C.; Zoccali, R.A.; Muscatello, M.R.A. Bergamot Polyphenolic Fraction Supplementation Improves Cognitive Functioning in Schizophrenia: Data From an 8-Week, Open-Label Pilot Study. *J. Clin. Psychopharmacol.* **2017**, *37*, 468–471. [CrossRef]

101. Delle Monache, S.; Sanità, P.; Trapasso, E.; Ursino, M.R.; Dugo, P.; Russo, M.; Ferlazzo, N.; Calapai, G.; Angelucci, A.; Navarra, M. Mechanisms underlying the anti-tumoral effects of *Citrus bergamia* juice. *PLoS ONE* **2013**, *8*, e61484. [CrossRef]
102. Ferlazzo, N.; Cirmi, S.; Russo, M.; Trapasso, E.; Ursino, M.R.; Lombardo, G.E.; Gangemi, S.; Calapai, G.; Navarra, M. NF-kappaB mediates the antiproliferative and proapoptotic effects of bergamot juice in HepG2 cells. *Life Sci.* **2016**, *146*, 81–91. [CrossRef] [PubMed]
103. Visalli, G.; Ferlazzo, N.; Cirmi, S.; Campiglia, P.; Gangemi, S.; Di Pietro, A.; Calapai, G.; Navarra, M. Bergamot juice extract inhibits proliferation by inducing apoptosis in human colon cancer cells. *Anticancer Agents Med. Chem.* **2014**, *14*, 1402–1413. [CrossRef]
104. Maugeri, A.; Russo, C.; Musumeci, L.; Lombardo, G.E.; De Sarro, G.; Barreca, D.; Cirmi, S.; Navarra, M. The Anticancer Effect of a Flavonoid-Rich Extract of Bergamot Juice in THP-1 Cells Engages the SIRT2/AKT/p53 Pathway. *Pharmaceutics* **2022**, *14*, 2168. [CrossRef] [PubMed]
105. Russo, C.; Maugeri, A.; De Luca, L.; Gitto, R.; Lombardo, G.E.; Musumeci, L.; De Sarro, G.; Cirmi, S.; Navarra, M. The SIRT2 Pathway Is Involved in the Antiproliferative Effect of Flavanones in Human Leukemia Monocytic THP-1 Cells. *Biomedicines* **2022**, *10*, 2383. [CrossRef] [PubMed]
106. Navarra, M.; Ursino, M.R.; Ferlazzo, N.; Russo, M.; Schumacher, U.; Valentiner, U. Effect of *Citrus bergamia* juice on human neuroblastoma cells in vitro and in metastatic xenograft models. *Fitoterapia* **2014**, *95*, 83–92. [CrossRef] [PubMed]
107. Navarra, M.; Femia, A.P.; Romagnoli, A.; Tortora, K.; Luceri, C.; Cirmi, S.; Ferlazzo, N.; Caderni, G. A flavonoid-rich extract from bergamot juice prevents carcinogenesis in a genetic model of colorectal cancer, the Pirc rat (F344/NTac-Apc(am1137)). *Eur. J. Nutr.* **2020**, *59*, 885–894. [CrossRef]
108. Han, X.; Beaumont, C.; Stevens, N. Chemical composition analysis and in vitro biological activities of ten essential oils in human skin cells. *Biochim. Open* **2017**, *5*, 1–7. [CrossRef]
109. Sun, P.; Zhao, L.; Zhang, N.; Wang, C.; Wu, W.; Mehmood, A.; Zhang, L.; Ji, B.; Zhou, F. Essential Oil and Juice from Bergamot and Sweet Orange Improve Acne Vulgaris Caused by Excessive Androgen Secretion. *Mediat. Inflamm.* **2020**, *2020*, 8868107. [CrossRef]
110. Albash, R.; Badawi, N.M.; Hamed, M.I.A.; Ragaie, M.H.; Mohammed, S.S.; Elbesh, R.M.; Darwish, K.M.; Lashkar, M.O.; Elhady, S.S.; Mosallam, S. Exploring the Synergistic Effect of Bergamot Essential Oil with Spironolactone Loaded Nano-Phytosomes for Treatment of Acne Vulgaris: In Vitro Optimization, In Silico Studies, and Clinical Evaluation. *Pharmaceuticals* **2023**, *16*, 128. [CrossRef]
111. Cristiano, M.C.; d'Avanzo, N.; Mancuso, A.; Tarsitano, M.; Barone, A.; Torella, D.; Paolino, D.; Fresta, M. Ammonium Glycyrrhizinate and Bergamot Essential Oil Co-Loaded Ultradeformable Nanocarriers: An Effective Natural Nanomedicine for In Vivo Anti-Inflammatory Topical Therapies. *Biomedicines* **2022**, *10*, 1039. [CrossRef]

Disclaimer/Publisher's Note: The statements, opinions and data contained in all publications are solely those of the individual author(s) and contributor(s) and not of MDPI and/or the editor(s). MDPI and/or the editor(s) disclaim responsibility for any injury to people or property resulting from any ideas, methods, instructions or products referred to in the content.

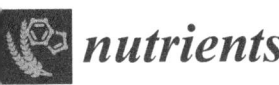

Article

Inulin Prebiotic Protects against Lethal *Pseudomonas aeruginosa* Acute Infection via γδ T Cell Activation

Emilie Boucher [1,†], Caroline Plazy [2,†], Audrey Le Gouellec [2], Bertrand Toussaint [2] and Dalil Hannani [1,*]

1. Univ. Grenoble Alpes, CNRS, UMR 5525, VetAgro Sup, Grenoble INP, TIMC, 38000 Grenoble, France; emilie.boucher@univ-grenoble-alpes.fr
2. Univ. Grenoble Alpes, CNRS, UMR 5525, VetAgro Sup, Grenoble INP, CHU Grenoble Alpes, TIMC, 38000 Grenoble, France; cplazy@chu-grenoble.fr (C.P.); alegouellec@chu-grenoble.fr (A.L.G.); btoussaint@chu-grenoble.fr (B.T.)
* Correspondence: dalil.hannani@univ-grenoble-alpes.fr
† These authors contributed equally to this work.

Abstract: *Pseudomonas aeruginosa* (*P. aeruginosa*) causes harmful lung infections, especially in immunocompromised patients. The immune system and Interleukin (IL)-17-producing γδ T cells (γδ T) are critical in controlling these infections in mice. The gut microbiota modulates host immunity in both cancer and infection contexts. Nutritional intervention is a powerful means of modulating both microbiota composition and functions, and subsequently the host's immune status. We have recently shown that inulin prebiotic supplementation triggers systemic γδ T activation in a cancer context. We hypothesized that prophylactic supplementation with inulin might protect mice from lethal *P. aeruginosa* acute lung infection in a γδ T-dependent manner. C57Bl/6 mice were supplemented with inulin for 15 days before the lethal *P. aeruginosa* lung infection, administered intranasally. We demonstrate that prophylactic inulin supplementation triggers a higher proportion of γδ T in the blood, accompanied by a higher infiltration of IL-17-producing γδ T within the lungs, and protects 33% of infected mice from death. This observation relies on γδ T, as in vivo γδ TcR blocking using a monoclonal antibody completely abrogates inulin-mediated protection. Overall, our data indicate that inulin supplementation triggers systemic γδ T activation, and could help resolve lung *P. aeruginosa* infections. Moreover, our data suggest that nutritional intervention might be a powerful way to prevent/reduce infection-related mortality, by reinforcing the microbiota-dependent immune system.

Keywords: prebiotic; inulin; γδ T cells; *Pseudomonas aeruginosa*; immunity; gut–lung axis

1. Introduction

Pseudomonas aeruginosa (*P. aeruginosa*) is a common gram-negative environmental bacterium. This opportunistic bacterium causes nosocomial infections and is highly virulent in immunodeficient patients. Indeed, pulmonary infection with *P. aeruginosa* is one of the leading causes of death in ventilator-associated pneumonia (VAP), cystic fibrosis, and chronic obstructive pulmonary disease (COPD) patients [1–3]. Due to its adaptability, *P. aeruginosa* strains have become increasingly more resistant to antibiotics [4,5]. As a result, in 2017, the World Health Organization classified *P. aeruginosa* as an antibiotic-resistant "critical priority pathogen" among the bacteria species causing the greatest menace to the global population [6].

In an acute *P. aeruginosa* infection mouse model, several studies support the idea that the immune system, especially pulmonary γδ T lymphocytes, plays a key role in fighting such infection [7–9]. γδ T cells are unconventional innate T cells, primarily activated during *P. aeruginosa* infection [10]. This early activation makes them the first pulmonary producers of interleukin 17 (IL-17), and highly protective cells, during *P. aeruginosa* infection. In addition, lung γδ T cell infiltration is a good prognostic marker in the lethal *P. aeruginosa* acute infection mouse model and might, therefore, be an attractive therapeutic target [7–10].

Indeed, an active immune system is crucial for eliminating this opportunistic pathogen that has many virulence factors and easily acquires many antibiotic resistance determinants [5]. In immunodeficient patients, therapies and interventions reinforcing host immunity are therefore urgently required.

The modulation of the immune system can be achieved in several ways, including the use of recombinant cytokines or monoclonal antibodies. Monoclonal antibodies can either act as agonists, activating receptors, or antagonists, inhibiting receptors or cytokines. These therapeutic strategies are currently being investigated in bacterial lung infections caused by *Mycobacterium tuberculosis* or *P. aeruginosa*, for example [11–13]. While vaccine approaches for *P. aeruginosa* infections have been ineffective so far, some immunotherapies, particularly monoclonal antibodies, are currently under investigation [14]. For over a decade, the gut microbiota has been shown to play a fundamental role in the induction, education, and function of the mammalian immune system [15]. The gut microbiota is composed of bacteria, fungi, archaea, and viruses that are in constant interaction with their host. Among these, bacteria have been the most extensively studied and have been shown to interact with host gut immunity [16,17]. Immune system modulation is balanced between pro- and anti-inflammatory signals produced by bacteria [17]. These signals include microorganisms-associated molecular patterns (MAMPs) and metabolites. Some metabolites derived from the gut microbiota can act as potent immune modulators [18]. These metabolites not only act on local (gut) immunity but also have an impact on distal, systemic immunity [15]. For instance, gut microbiota-derived aryl hydrocarbon receptor (AhR) ligands can influence the function of dendritic epidermal T cells, a type of T cell residing in the skin epidermis [19]. Additionally, short-chain fatty acids (SCFAs), which are metabolites produced through fiber fermentation by commensal bacteria, can directly modulate the function of various immune cells [20]. SCFAs can also enhance host hematopoiesis, promoting the generation of macrophage and dendritic cell (DC) precursors in the blood [21]. Consequently, they facilitate the migration of DCs with high phagocytic capacity to the lung [21]. These findings illustrate the gut–lung axis, where the gut microbiota and its derived metabolites potently regulate lung immunity under homeostatic conditions [22]. Since some studies have implicated the gut microbiome in certain bacterial pulmonary infection-associated diseases, targeting it could represent a promising therapeutic approach, particularly through nutritional interventions [23]. For example, COPD patients have an altered gut microbiome that correlates with disease features [24]. In the nontuberculous mycobacterial pulmonary disease (NTM-PDs) mouse model, modulation of the gut microbiome through L-arginine administration has shown a protective effect, even against multi-drug resistant *Mycobacterium abscessus* [25].

Based on these studies, the development of optimal strategies for modulating the composition and function of the gut microbiota for therapeutic purposes is highly appealing. As diet is one of the most potent modulators of the microbiota, nutritional intervention could significantly improve host anti-bacterial immunity [26]. A promising nutritional intervention approach involves diet supplementation with dietary fibers that exhibit prebiotic activity. Prebiotics are indigestible compounds found in vegetables, fermented by commensal bacteria of the gut microbiota [27]. A diet rich in prebiotics promotes the growth and metabolic activity of beneficial bacteria in the colon, thus favoring gut-associated benefits [28,29]. Among prebiotics, inulin is a fructooligosaccharide (FOS) primarily found in chicory roots, composed of a fructosyl chain ending with a glucosyl moiety. Dietary supplementation with inulin has shown beneficial effect in several pathologies. In Type 2 diabetes patients, inulin consumption helps to regulate the glycemia [30]. In addition, dietary supplementation with inulin showed anti-tumor effect in several tumor-bearing mouse models [31]. Inulin is known to enhance the colonization of the gut by profitable bacteria, including *Bifidobacterium*, which has been described as an immuno-stimulatory species [32,33]. However, its biological mode of action still remains unknown.

We previously demonstrated that a 15-day diet supplementation with inulin efficiently modulates the gut microbiota and promotes the growth of *Bifidobacterium* in mice [34].

This modulation of the microbiota led to the activation of colonic γδ T intraepithelial lymphocytes (IELs), notably enhancing their capacity to produce pro-inflammatory cytokines. Local γδ T cell activation was accompanied by systemic γδ T cell activation, as evidenced by enhanced cancer immunosurveillance. In contrast to mice on a control diet, mice supplemented with inulin exhibited a significant reduction in the size of subcutaneously transplanted melanoma tumors. This effect was dependent on the microbiota and γδ T cells, as simultaneous treatment with broad-spectrum antibiotics or administration of an anti-γδ TcR blocking antibody completely abolished the efficacy of inulin-mediated protection. Collectively, our findings demonstrate that this prebiotic strategy holds great potential for activating systemic host immunity, particularly γδ T cells, in a cancer context [34]. Considering the protective role of γδ T cells in *P. aeruginosa* infections [7–9], we hypothesized that prophylactic nutritional intervention with inulin supplementation could trigger a protective systemic activation of γδ T cell, potentially safeguarding against lethal *P. aeruginosa* infection. To evaluate this scenario, we conducted the present study.

2. Materials and Methods

2.1. Animals

Female C57Bl/6 mice (aged 5 weeks) were provided by Janvier SA Laboratory (Le Genest-Saint-Isle, France) and housed at "Plateforme de Haute Technologie Animale (PHTA)" UGA core facility (Grenoble, France), EU0197, Agreement C38-51610006, under specific pathogen-free conditions, in a temperature-controlled environment with a 12 h light/dark cycle and ad libitum access to water and diet. Animal housing and procedures were conducted in accordance with the recommendations from the Direction des Services Vétérinaires, Ministry of Agriculture of France, according to European Communities Council Directive 2010/63/EU, and according to recommendations for health monitoring from the Federation of European Laboratory Animal Science Associations. Protocols involving animals were reviewed by the local ethics committee, "Comité d'Ethique pour l'Expérimentation Animale no.#12, Cometh-Grenoble", and approved by the Ministry of Research (APAFIS#21249-2019062715154462.v4, on 19 July 2019). Only female mice were used in this project, to avoid housing issues after group randomization. After a 1-week adaptation, the mice were randomly assigned to 2 groups, according to their diet.

(1) Healthy control group (Control), $n = 16$

$n = 10$: *P. aeruginosa* infected ($n = 6$ were used for survival assessment, and $n = 4$ were used for lung and blood-immunity analysis).

$n = 6$: Non-infected mice, used for lung and blood-immunity analysis.

(2) Inulin-supplemented group (Inulin) $n = 24$

$n = 12$: *P. aeruginosa* infected ($n = 6$ were used for survival assessment, and $n = 6$ were used for lung and blood-immunity analysis).

$n = 6$: *P. aeruginosa* infected + anti-γδ TcR, used for survival assessment.

$n = 6$: Non-infected mice, used for lung and blood-immunity analysis.

For inulin treatment, mice received a standard diet and drinking water supplemented with 7.2% inulin, starting 15 days before *P. aeruginosa* intranasal infection. Drinking bottles supplemented with inulin were renewed 3 times a week. All experiments were conducted with 6 mice per group, except when indicated in the figure legend.

2.2. Bacterial Culture

A clinical strain of *P. aeruginosa*, named CHA, was used for intrapulmonary infections [35]. Bacteria were cultured in Lysogeny Broth (LB) medium, under agitation at 37 °C. Bacterial growth, followed by optical density (OD) at 600 nm, was stopped at the exponential phase, corresponding to OD = 1. After centrifugation, bacteria were resuspended at a concentration of 1.25×10^8 CFU/mL in Phosphate Buffer Saline 1X (PBS) (Gibco). The number of bacteria administered was confirmed by colony-forming unit (CFU) count after 24 h of culture at 37 °C on LB agar.

2.3. Intranasal Inoculation of P. aeruginosa

Mice were anesthetized with 4% isoflurane and infected intranasally with 3×10^6 CFU *P. aeruginosa*, in 40 µL PBS. After 14 h, half of the mice were euthanized for pulmonary immunity analysis. The other half were under acute surveillance for 96 h. The severity of the symptoms was evaluated regularly by calculating a clinical score, as follows:

Score 1: normal clinical condition, may have slight piloerection, normal activity and no weight loss.
Score 2: slight piloerection, slight prostration, weight loss < 20%.
Score 3: piloerection, moderate prostration, weight loss < 20%, slightly closed eyes, irregular breathing, slightly reduced mobility, slightly reduced activity.
Score 4: piloerection, prostration, weight loss > 20%, closed eyes, reduced breathing rate, increased breathing depth, reduced activity: animal has reached moderate endpoint and should be euthanized.

When a score reached 3, animals were monitored every hour. Animals reaching a score of 4 were euthanized, to avoid any unnecessary suffering, and reported as dead from the infection.

2.4. In Vivo Blocking of γδ-TcR

Mice received 100 µg of the anti-γδTcR monoclonal antibody (clone UC7-13D5, Euromedex, Souffekweyersheim, France) intraperitoneally, in 100 µL PBS 1X. Anti-γδTcR antibodies were injected the day before and after the bacterial challenge.

2.5. Lung Harvest

Lung lobes were collected in Roswell Park Memorial Institute (RPMI) complete medium (supplemented with 1% non-essential amino acids, 1 mM sodium pyruvate, 50 U/mL penicillin and 50 µg/mL streptomycin (all from Life technologies, Courtaboeuf, France)). Each lobe was lacerated into small pieces using scalpels, and digested with Liberase^{TM} (25 µg/mL, Roche, Meylan, France) for 30 min at 37 °C. Finally, the digested lungs were passed through a 70 µm cell strainer, washed, and cells were resuspended in 10% Fetal Bovine Serum (FBS) (Life technologies, Courtaboeuf, France) RPMI complete medium.

2.6. Blood Sample Preparation

Blood was collected via retro-orbital sampling in K2E tubes (BD Medical, Le Pont-de-Claix, France). After centrifugation, blood pellets were resuspended in 1 mL Red Blood Cell Lysis buffer 1X (Sigma, Saint-Quentin Fallavier, France) and washed with 10% FBS complete RPMI.

2.7. Flow Cytometry

To allow intracellular cytokine detection, cell suspensions were stimulated for 4 h at 37 °C with 50 ng/mL phorbol 12-myristate 13-acetate (PMA) (Sigma, Saint-Quentin Fallavier, France), 1 µg/mL ionomycin (Sigma, Saint-Quentin Fallavier, France), in the presence of Golgi Stop^{TM} (BD Biosciences, Le Pont-de-Claix, France). Following activation, cells were stained for extracellular markers and incubated with 200 ng of each antibody for 15 min in the dark at RT. The antibodies targeting extracellular proteins were CD45 (30-F11), CD3 (17A2), CD4 (GK1.5) (Biolegend, Amsterdam, The Netherlands), γδ-TcR (eBioGL3 (GL-3, GL3)) (BD Biosciences, Le Pont-de-Claix, France). To allow intracellular labeling, cells were first permeabilized using a FoxP3 staining buffer kit (Life technologies, Courtaboeuf, France) before being incubated with intracellular antibodies for 1 h in the dark at RT. Antibodies targeting intracellular cytokines were IFNγ (XMG1.2) (Biolegend, Amsterdam, The Netherlands), IL-10 (JES5-16E3) (Life technologies, Courtaboeuf, France), and IL-17A (TC11-18H10) (BD Biosciences, Le Pont-de-Claix, France). After intracellular labeling, cells were fixed with FACS (fluorescence-activated cell sorting) Lysing Solution 1X (BD Biosciences, Le Pont-de-Claix, France) and stored at +4 °C until acquisition. All data were acquired on a BD Biosciences FACS Canto II and analyzed using FlowJo Software V10.4.2. The gating strategy is shown in Figure S1.

2.8. Statistical Analysis

Statistical analyses were performed on GraphPad PRISM software. Mann–Whitney tests were used to compare 2 groups; ns corresponds to non-significant and * corresponds to p-value < 0.05.

3. Results

3.1. An Inulin-Enriched Diet Protects Mice against Lethal P. aeruginosa Infection and Enhances Pulmonary IL-17-Producing γδ T Cells

We have recently described how an inulin-enriched diet promotes systemic γδ T cell activation through microbiota modulation [19]. Since γδ T cells are critical players in controlling acute *P. aeruginosa* infections, we assessed the potential anti-bacterial effect of such an inulin-mediated immune boost. To do so, mice were fed either a standard diet or an inulin-enriched diet for 2 weeks before being intranasally challenged with a lethal dose of *P. aeruginosa* (Figure 1A). Only the two-week inulin-enriched diet efficiently protected 33% of infected mice from death (two out of six mice) (Figure 1B).

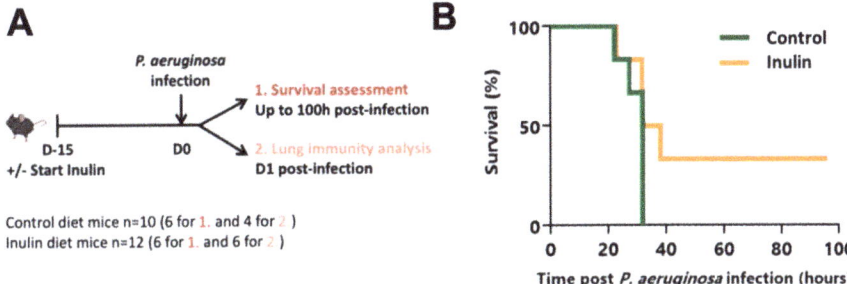

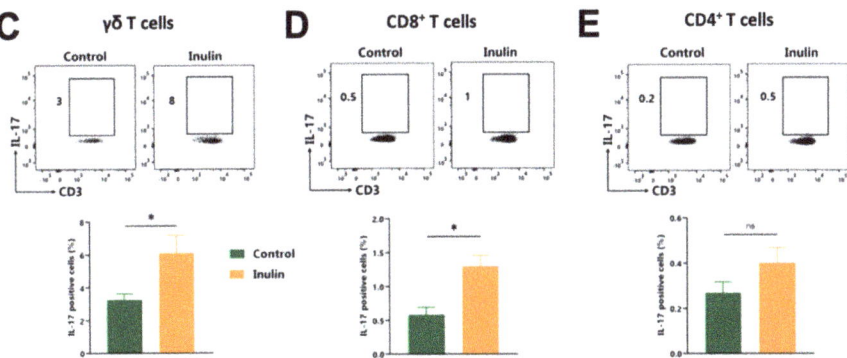

Figure 1. The inulin-enriched diet protects against lethal *P. aeruginosa* infection by reinforcing γδ T cells. (**A**) Experimental schedule. C57BL/6 mice were fed a control or an inulin-enriched diet (7.2% in drinking water) (n = 4–6 mice per group) starting 15 days before intranasal infection with 3×10^6 CFU of *P. aeruginosa*. (**B**) Survival curves of mice treated and infected as described in (**A**). (**C–E**) Frequency of pulmonary IL-17-producing cells gated on CD45$^+$ CD3$^+$ γδ TcR $^+$, defined as γδ T cells (**C**), CD45$^+$ CD3$^+$ γδ TcR$^-$ CD4$^-$, defined as CD8$^+$ T cells (**D**) or CD45$^+$ CD3$^+$ γδ TcR$^-$, CD4$^+$, defined as CD4$^+$ T cells (**E**) from mice treated as in (**A**) 12 h post-infection. Graphs show the mean ± SEM. Statistically significant results are indicated by: ns = non-significant, * p < 0.05, by Mann–Whitney tests.

To better understand the mechanisms behind this observation, we analyzed lung immunity by flow cytometry 12 h post-infection. While the inulin-enriched diet did not affect the infiltration of CD45$^+$ and CD3$^+$ in the lung (Figure S2), it significantly increased the proportion of pulmonary IL-17-producing γδ T lymphocytes (Figure 1C) and CD8$^+$ T lymphocytes (Figure 1D), from 3% to 8%, and 0.5% to 1%, respectively. The frequency of IL-17-producing CD4$^+$ T cells also tended to increase, although non significantly (Figure 1E). The proportions of Interferon γ (IFNγ)-producing T lymphocytes in the lungs were not affected by the inulin-enriched diet (Figure S3A), but the proportion of IL-10-producing CD8$^+$ T cells was increased in the lungs of infected mice (Figure S3B).

IL-17-producing γδ T lymphocytes have already been described as potent protective immune cells against *P. aeruginosa* infection. To confirm that the inulin-mediated protection was immune-dependent, and particularly dependent on γδ T cell-dependent, the same experiment was repeated, with one group receiving a blocking γδ TcR antibody the day before and the day after intranasal infection (Figure 2A). While 33% of inulin-treated mice were protected against *P. aeruginosa* infection (two out of six mice), the administration of the γδ TcR-blocking antibody completely abrogated this protective effect (Figure 2B), and none of the mice from either the control or the inulin + blocking γδ TcR group survived. These results collectively indicate that inulin triggered a Th17-polarized antibacterial lung immunity strongly supported by γδ T lymphocytes. Indeed, γδ T lymphocytes, and more likely their γδ TcR engagement, are mandatory for inulin's protection against *P. aeruginosa*.

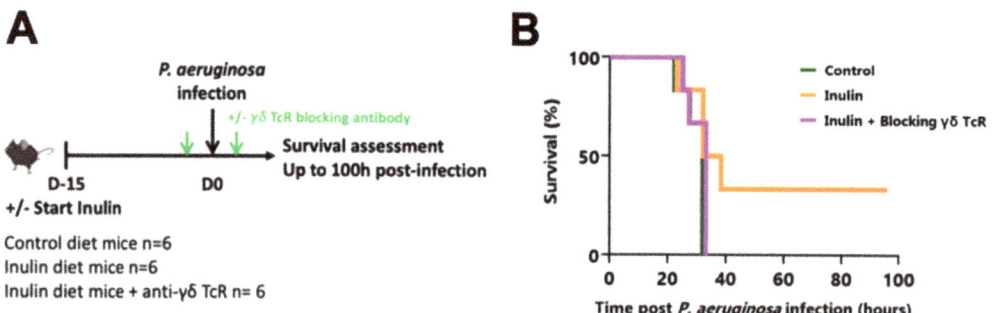

Figure 2. The inulin-mediated protective effect against *P. aeruginosa* depends on γδ T cells. (**A**) Experimental schedule. C57BL/6 mice were fed a control or an inulin-enriched diet (7.2% in drinking water) (*n* = 6 mice per group) starting 15 days before intranasal infection with 3 × 10^6 CFU *P. aeruginosa*. Anti-γδ TcR antibodies were injected intraperitoneally (i.p.) into 6 mice from the inulin group the days before and after bacterial infection. (**B**) Survival curves of mice treated and infected as described in (**A**).

3.2. The Inulin Diet Reinforces Blood Circulating Immunity

We have previously shown that a 15-day inulin-enriched diet triggers γδ T cell activation in the gut [34], specifically within colon IntraEpithelial Lymphocytes (IELs) γδ T cells. The gut microbiota can induce immune modulation in distal sites, including the lungs (known as gut-lung axis) [22]. Therfore, we investigated whether an inulin-enriched diet modulates lung γδ T cell infiltration under steady-state conditions or if these cells are only recruited from the periphery upon infection. To adress this, we analyzed both the immune cells infiltrating the lungs and the immune cells circulating in the blood following a 15-day inulin-enriched diet (Figure 3A), corresponding to the day of infection (Figure 1A).

The inulin-enriched diet did not trigger higher lung leukocyte (CD45$^+$) or T cell infiltration compared to mice on the control diet (Figure S4). Among the T cells, we did not observe any differences in the proportions of γδ, CD4$^+$, and CD8$^+$ T cells (Figure 3B–D). The cytokine patterns of lung-infiltrating T cells, particularly IFNγ, IL-17, and IL-10, were comparable in both groups (Figure S5A,B), except for the proportion of the IL-10-producing CD8$^+$ T cells, which was found to be higher under the inulin diet (Figure S5C). While the inulin diet did not affect the proportions of pulmonary T lymphocytes, it significantly increased the proportion of γδ T and CD4$^+$ T cells in the blood, from 0.08% to 0.14%, and from 3.9% to 8.3%, respectively (Figure 3E,G). The proportion of CD8$^+$ T cells also showed a tendency to increase, but did not reach statistical significance (Figure 3F). Regarding the cytokine patterns of circulating T cells in the blood, the proportion of IL-17- and IL-10-producing T lymphocytes were comparable between both groups (Figure S5D,F), while the proportions of IFNγ-producing γδ and CD8$^+$ T cells were reduced (Figure S5E).

Altogether, these observations suggest that the inulin diet promotes the circulation of γδ T cells and conventional T cells within the blood, but does not enhance their infiltration into the lung under steady-state conditions. However, upon acute infection, these cells are recruited to the lungs.

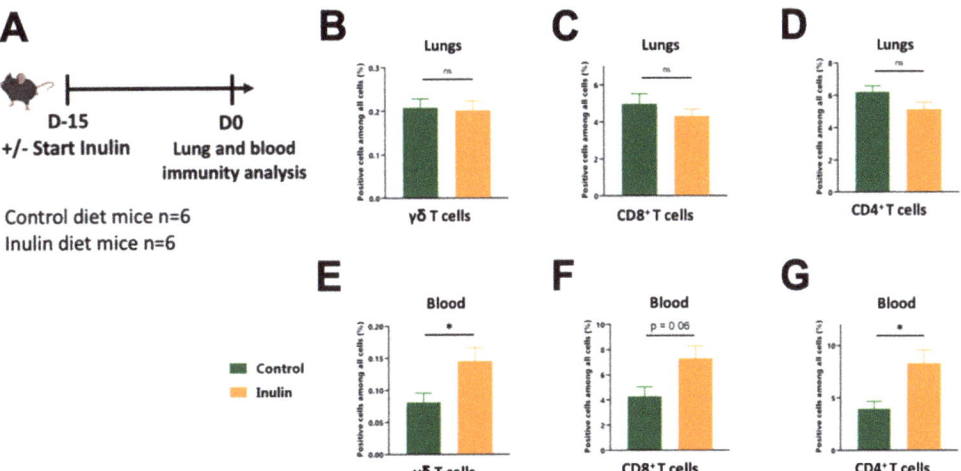

Figure 3. Pulmonary-activated T cells probably originate from the blood. (**A**) Experimental schedule. C57BL/6 mice were fed a control or an inulin-enriched diet (7.2% in drinking water) (*n* = 6 mice per group) starting 15 days before the analysis of the lung-infiltrated and blood-circulating immune cells. (**B–D**) Frequency of lung-infiltrated immune cells gated on CD45$^+$ CD3$^+$ γδ TcR$^+$, defined as γδ T cells (**B**), CD45$^+$ CD3$^+$ γδ TcR$^-$ CD4$^-$, defined as CD8$^+$ T cells (**C**) or CD45$^+$ CD3$^+$ γδ TcR$^-$, CD4$^+$, defined as CD4$^+$ T cells (**D**) from mice treated as in (**A**). (**E–G**) Frequency of blood-circulating cells gated on CD45$^+$ CD3$^+$ γδ TcR$^+$, defined as γδ T cells (**E**), CD45$^+$ CD3$^+$ γδ TcR$^-$ CD4$^-$, defined as CD8$^+$ T cells (**F**) or CD45$^+$ CD3$^+$ γδ TcR$^-$, CD4$^+$, defined as CD4$^+$ T cells (**G**) from mice treated as in (**A**). Graphs show the mean ± SEM. Statistically significant results are indicated by: ns = non-significant, * $p < 0.05$, by Mann–Whitney tests.

4. Discussion

P. aeruginosa is widely recognized as a priority pathogen with respect to its high pathogenicity and the development of antibiotic resistance. There is an urgent need for emerging strategies that target the immune system, particularly those focusing on γδ T cells, which have been shown to play a critical role in combatting such infections [7–9]. In this study, we propose to harness the prebiotic and immune-stimulatory properties of inulin. It has been demonstrated, by ourselves and others, that this dietary fiber promotes the growth of immune-stimulatory bacteria such as *Bifidobacterium* [34,36], consequently leading to γδ T cell activation. Additionally, inulin promotes gut health by facilitating the production of SCFAs by the gut microbiota, which possess anti-inflammatory properties and support gut barrier integrity [37–39]. Strategies that reinforce the immune system through modulations of the gut microbiota are being increasingly investigated. Among the various gut microbiota modulators, inulin holds the advantage of being a widely consumed prebiotic, available either through diet source or as a supplement.

In the present study, we report that an inulin-enriched diet has the capacity to protect 33% of mice against lethal infection with *P. aeruginosa*. This protective effect was accompanied by an increased proportion of IL-17-producing γδ T lymphocytes infiltrating the lungs, which play a critical role in this process, as blocking the γδ TcR in vivo abolished the protective effect mediated by inulin. Previous studies have also highlighted the importance of these cells in immune defense against *P. aeruginosa* infections [7–9], which our results confirm. Prior to infection, at a steady state, the proportion of immune cells in the lungs did not appear to be affected by inulin consumption. However, there was an increase in the proportion of patrolling T lymphocytes in the bloodstream. It is possible that the production of SCFAs or other metabolites induced by the inulin modulate γδ T cell proportion through the stimulation of lymphoid hematopoiesis, as has been described for the myeloid compartment [20,21]. As a result, an inulin-enriched diet enhances systemic immunosurveillance, making it more responsive to lung infiltration upon infection and thereby protecting the host from death.

The molecular mechanisms underlying the activation of systemic γδ T lymphocyte are still unclear. In addition to establishing the essential role of γδ T lymphocytes as mediators, our data indicate that their activation is TcR-mediated rather than mediated through NKR (natural killer receptor) or TLR molecules. Since γδ T cells detect metabolites such as (E)-4-Hydroxy-3-methyl-but-2-enyl pyrophosphate (HMB-PP) derived from bacteria or isopentenyl-pyrophosphate (IPP) derived from tumors via their TcR [40], our findings strongly suggest that their activation may be mediated by microbiota-derived metabolites. Further research is needed to unravel the exact mechanisms and identify the specific metabolites that activate γδ T cells. The identification of these metabolites would be highly valuable for developing future post-biotic therapeutic strategies based on metabolites, particularly for immunocompromised or dysbiotic patients who are already infected, as nutritional interventions would require significant time to achieve the optimal modulation of the microbiota.

In addition to immune-stimulatory metabolites, we also hypothesized that anti-inflammatory and tissue repair signals (metabolites/mediators) could play a role. These signals would have a protective effect by preventing a harmful immune response from the host, which could lead to the destruction of lung tissue and, ultimately, death. Among the metabolites derived from inulin that have been described, SCFAs are known to promote the integrity of the gut epithelial barrier through IL-22 production, and possess anti-inflammatory properties [41]. In the protective effect observed in the acute *P. aeruginosa* infection mouse model due to inulin consumption, SCFAs could also regulate immunity, preventing mice from succumbing to excessive inflammation. Consistent with this, we observed a slight increase in the proportion of IL-10-producing $CD8^+$ T cells in the lungs when the mice were on an inulin diet, supporting this hypothesis. We previously demonstrated that an inulin diet promotes IL-22, a cytokine involved in tissue repair, in the lamina propria of the gut [34]. It is conceivable that such modulation occurs at distant sites such as the lungs.

Beyond *P. aeruginosa* infection-related issues, the immune state of patients prior to any infection is a determining factor in clinical outcome. This has been exemplified by the severe acute respiratory syndrome coronavirus 2 (SARS-CoV-2) pandemic, where individuals with microbiota-related disorders (such as obesity and diabetes) were more prone to developing severe disease [42]. This can be attributed to pre-existing immune dysregulation (chronic systemic inflammatory state) and a compromised gut barrier, which facilitates the spread of the virus and subsequent multi-organ failure [43]. Both of these factors are associated with a dysbiotic state of the gut microbiota [44]. In a state of eubiosis, beneficial bacteria that are part of the microbiota produce key metabolites, notably SCFAs, which are crucial for gut health. SCFAs promote mucus production by goblet cells, preventing excessive inflammation [45]. The mucus acts as a barrier, shielding epithelial cells from bacteria and thus preventing tissue inflammation through Toll-like receptors (TLRs) and/or tissue damage caused by bacterial toxins [46]. SCFAs also possess anti-inflammatory properties [41], which help prevent autoimmunity and subsequent tissue damage. Additionally, SCFAs promote the expression of the tight junction protein by epithelial cells, maintaining the integrity of the intestinal barrier and preventing the translocation of bacteria or bacterial products from the gut lumen into the bloodstream [45]. On the other hand, dysbiosis, characterized by a loss or reduction of beneficial bacteria and decreased or absent SFCA production, leads to a thinner mucus layer, a decrease in anti-inflammatory signals, and compromised barrier integrity, due to the downregulation of tight junctions. Dysbiosis promotes local and systemic inflammation, particularly through bacterial product translocation. This systemic inflammation can trigger metabolic syndromes such as insulin resistance, diabetes, and obesity. It has been demonstrated that the initial response to SARS-CoV-2 infection is crucial in rapidly reducing viral load and preventing a later exacerbated immune response that could be detrimental and even fatal for patients [43]. However, individuals with metabolic syndromes may already have a pre-existing chronic inflammation that impairs the initial anti-SARS-CoV-2 response. Importantly, since the virus has a tropism for the gut due to the expression of the angiotensin-converting enzyme 2 (ACE2) in gut cells [47], a compromised gut epithelial barrier due to dysbiosis can facilitate viral propagation in the body. The virus can then reach vital organs, multiply, and cause death through immune exacerbation and multiple organ failure [43]. Similar scenarios could arise in future pandemics, especially if caused by an enterotropic pathogen (virus or bacteria) capable of eliciting exacerbated and harmful immune responses. Based on this knowledge and lessons learned, one can envision strategies to attenuate the severity and clinical outcome of viral and bacterial infections, as well as future pandemics, by promoting the optimization of the gut microbiota, particularly through nutritional intervention, within the general population. We believe that this should be given priority as a preventive strategy for various health issues, including infections. Inulin is a very interesting prebiotic for prevention, because it has been shown that this fiber could ameliorate mucus production, decrease gut permeability and reduce inflammation in obese patients [48]. Additionally, in line with our preclinical data, inulin profoundly modifies the composition of the gut microbiota in humans, in a bifidogenic manner [49]. Since inulin is a natural fiber, it is possible to enrich people's daily diet in a simple way by increasing the intake of inulin-rich vegetables and fruits, and/or through supplementation.

To conclude, our study has identified inulin as a promising fiber capable of triggering host immune reinforcement, which can protect certain individuals from lethal infections, in a microbiota- and $\gamma\delta$ T cell-dependent manner. This research provides the groundwork for promoting a fiber-rich diet among the general population as a significant preventive strategy against current and future infection-related issues. In order to exploit these findings for severe acute infections, it is imperative that we urgently identify the microbiota-derived metabolites involved to develop post-biotic metabolite-based immunotherapy.

Supplementary Materials: The following supporting information can be downloaded at: https://www.mdpi.com/article/10.3390/nu15133037/s1, Figure S1: Flow cytometry gating strategy; Figure S2: CD45+ and CD3+ cell lung infiltration, upon *P. aeruginosa* infection. Figure S3: IFNγ- and IL-10-producing T cell lung infiltration, upon *P. aeruginosa* infection. Figure S4: CD45+ and CD3+ cell lung infiltration at steady state. Figure S5: Cytokine production by pulmonary and blood T Lymphocytes at steady state.

Author Contributions: Conceptualization, D.H., B.T. and E.B.; methodology, D.H.; validation, D.H., E.B. and C.P.; formal analysis, E.B., C.P. and D.H.; investigation, E.B., C.P., A.L.G. and D.H.; data curation, E.B., C.P. and D.H.; writing—original draft preparation, E.B., C.P. and D.H.; writing—review and editing, B.T.; supervision, D.H.; project administration, D.H.; funding acquisition, D.H. All authors have read and agreed to the published version of the manuscript.

Funding: D.H is supported by la Fondation du Souffle et de la Santé Respiratoire, GEFLUC Dauphiné-Savoie, Ligue contre le Cancer Comité Isère, Ligue contre le Cancer Comité Savoie, Université Grenoble Alpes IDEX Initiatives de Recherche Stratégiques, Université Grenoble Alpes IRGA grant program, and TIMC lab grant «Emergence 2023». E.B. is supported by a grant salary from the French Ministry of Higher Education, Research and Innovation. The funders had no role in study design, data collection, or analysis.

Institutional Review Board Statement: The animal study was reviewed and approved by "Comité d'Ethique pour l'Expérimentation Animale no.#12, Cometh-Grenoble" and approved by the Ministry of Research (APAFIS#21249-2019062715154462.v4).

Informed Consent Statement: Not applicable.

Acknowledgments: We would like to thank Sylvie Berthier (Cytometry Platform, CHUGA), Hervé Lerat, Kevin Escot, and Laurie Arnaud (PHTA Animal Facility), for their technical assistance.

Conflicts of Interest: The authors declare no conflict of interest.

References

1. Zaragoza, R.; Vidal-cortés, P.; Aguilar, G.; Borges, M.; Diaz, E.; Ferrer, R.; Maseda, E.; Nieto, M.; Nuvials, F.X.; Ramirez, P.; et al. Update of the Treatment of Nosocomial Pneumonia in the ICU. *Crit. Care* **2020**, *24*, 383. [CrossRef]
2. Malhotra, S.; Hayes, D.; Wozniak, D.J. Cystic Fibrosis and Pseudomonas Aeruginosa: The Host-Microbe Interface. *Clin. Microbiol. Rev.* **2019**, *32*, e00138-18. [CrossRef]
3. Tiew, P.Y.; Jaggi, T.K.; Chan, L.L.Y.; Chotirmall, S.H. The Airway Microbiome in COPD, Bronchiectasis and Bronchiectasis-COPD Overlap. *Clin. Respir. J.* **2021**, *15*, 123–133. [CrossRef] [PubMed]
4. Gellatly, S.L.; Hancock, R.E.W. Pseudomonas Aeruginosa: New Insights into Pathogenesis and Host Defenses. *Pathog. Dis.* **2013**, *67*, 159–173. [CrossRef] [PubMed]
5. López-Causapé, C.; Cabot, G.; del Barrio-Tofiño, E.; Oliver, A. The Versatile Mutational Resistome of Pseudomonas Aeruginosa. *Front. Microbiol.* **2018**, *9*, 685. [CrossRef]
6. World Health Organization. WHO Publishes List of Bacteria for Which New Antibiotics Are Urgently Needed. *Saudi Med. J.* **2017**, *38*, 444–445.
7. Liu, J.; Qu, H.; Li, Q.; Ye, L.; Ma, G.; Wan, H. The Responses of Γδ T-Cells against Acute Pseudomonas Aeruginosa Pulmonary Infection in Mice via Interleukin-17. *Pathog. Dis.* **2013**, *68*, 44–51. [CrossRef] [PubMed]
8. Omar, T.; Ziltener, P.; Chamberlain, E. Mice Lacking Γδ T Cells Exhibit Impaired Clearance of Pseudomonas Aeruginosa Lung Infection and Excessive Production of Inflammatory Cytokines. *Infect. Immun.* **2020**, *88*, e00171-20. [CrossRef] [PubMed]
9. Pan, T.; Tan, R.; Li, M.; Liu, Z.; Wang, X.; Tian, L.; Liu, J.; Qu, H. IL17-Producing Γδ T Cells May Enhance Humoral Immunity during Pulmonary Pseudomonas Aeruginosa Infection in Mice. *Front. Cell. Infect. Microbiol.* **2016**, *6*, 170. [CrossRef]
10. Liu, J.; Feng, Y.; Yang, K.; Li, Q.; Ye, L.; Han, L.; Wan, H. Early Production of IL-17 Protects against Acute Pulmonary Pseudomonas Aeruginosa Infection in Mice. *FEMS Immunol. Med. Microbiol.* **2011**, *61*, 179–188. [CrossRef]
11. Giver, C.R.; Shaw, P.A.; Fletcher, H.; Kaushal, D.; Pamela, G.; Omoyege, D.; Bisson, G.; Gumbo, T.; Wallis, R.; Waller, E.K.; et al. IMPACT-TB*: A Phase II Trial Assessing the Capacity of Low Dose Imatinib to Induce Myelopoiesis and Enhance Host Anti-Microbial Immunity Against Tuberculosis. *Imatinib Mesylate per Oral As a Clinical Therapeutic for TB. *Blood* **2019**, *134*, 1050. [CrossRef]
12. Wallis, R.S.; O'Garra, A.; Sher, A.; Wack, A. Host-Directed Immunotherapy of Viral and Bacterial Infections: Past, Present and Future. *Nat. Rev. Immunol.* **2023**, *23*, 121–133. [CrossRef] [PubMed]
13. Hurley, M.N.; Cámara, M.; Smyth, A.R. Novel Approaches to the Treatment of Pseudomonas Aeruginosa Infections in Cystic Fibrosis. *Eur. Respir. J.* **2012**, *40*, 1014–1023. [CrossRef] [PubMed]
14. Reig, S.; Le Gouellec, A.; Bleves, S. What Is New in the Anti–Pseudomonas Aeruginosa Clinical Development Pipeline Since the 2017 WHO Alert? *Front. Cell. Infect. Microbiol.* **2022**, *12*, 862. [CrossRef]
15. Belkaid, Y.; Harrison, O.J. Homeostatic Immunity and the Microbiota. *Immunity* **2017**, *46*, 562–576. [CrossRef]
16. Parigi, S.M.; Eldh, M.; Larssen, P.; Gabrielsson, S.; Villablanca, E.J. Breast Milk and Solid Food Shaping Intestinal Immunity. *Front. Immunol.* **2015**, *6*, 415. [CrossRef]
17. Kamada, N.; Seo, S.U.; Chen, G.Y.; Núñez, G. Role of the Gut Microbiota in Immunity and Inflammatory Disease. *Nat. Rev. Immunol.* **2013**, *13*, 321–335. [CrossRef]
18. Caffaratti, C.; Plazy, C.; Mery, G.; Tidjani, A.R.; Fiorini, F.; Thiroux, S.; Toussaint, B.; Hannani, D.; Le Gouellec, A. What We Know so Far about the Metabolite-Mediated Microbiota-Intestinal Immunity Dialogue and How to Hear the Sound of This Crosstalk. *Metabolites* **2021**, *11*, 406. [CrossRef]
19. Li, Y.; Innocentin, S.; Withers, D.R.; Roberts, N.A.; Gallagher, A.R.; Grigorieva, E.F.; Wilhelm, C.; Veldhoen, M. Exogenous Stimuli Maintain Intraepithelial Lymphocytes via Aryl Hydrocarbon Receptor Activation. *Cell* **2011**, *147*, 629–640. [CrossRef]
20. Rooks, M.G.; Garrett, W.S. Gut Microbiota, Metabolites and Host Immunity. *Nat. Rev. Immunol.* **2016**, *16*, 341–352. [CrossRef]
21. Trompette, A.; Gollwitzer, E.S.; Yadava, K.; Sichelstiel, A.K.; Sprenger, N.; Ngom-Bru, C.; Blanchard, C.; Junt, T.; Nicod, L.P.; Harris, N.L.; et al. Gut Microbiota Metabolism of Dietary Fiber Influences Allergic Airway Disease and Hematopoiesis. *Nat. Med.* **2014**, *20*, 159–166. [CrossRef]
22. Dang, A.T.; Marsland, B.J. Microbes, Metabolites, and the Gut–Lung Axis. *Mucosal Immunol.* **2019**, *12*, 843–850. [CrossRef]
23. Collins, N.; Belkaid, Y. Control of Immunity via Nutritional Interventions. *Immunity* **2022**, *55*, 210–223. [CrossRef] [PubMed]
24. Bowerman, K.L.; Rehman, S.F.; Vaughan, A.; Lachner, N.; Budden, K.F.; Kim, R.Y.; Wood, D.L.A.; Gellatly, S.L.; Shukla, S.D.; Wood, L.G.; et al. Disease-Associated Gut Microbiome and Metabolome Changes in Patients with Chronic Obstructive Pulmonary Disease. *Nat. Commun.* **2020**, *11*, 5886. [CrossRef]
25. Kim, Y.J.; Lee, J.Y.; Lee, J.J.; Jeon, S.M.; Silwal, P.; Kim, I.S.; Kim, H.J.; Park, C.R.; Chung, C.; Han, J.E.; et al. Arginine-Mediated Gut Microbiome Remodeling Promotes Host Pulmonary Immune Defense against Nontuberculous Mycobacterial Infection. *Gut Microbes* **2022**, *14*, 2073132. [CrossRef] [PubMed]

26. Kim, J.H.; Kim, D.H.; Jo, S.; Cho, M.J.; Cho, Y.R.; Lee, Y.J.; Byun, S. Immunomodulatory Functional Foods and Their Molecular Mechanisms. *Exp. Mol. Med.* **2022**, *54*, 1–11. [CrossRef]
27. Holmes, E.; Li, J.V.; Marchesi, J.R.; Nicholson, J.K. Gut Microbiota Composition and Activity in Relation to Host Metabolic Phenotype and Disease Risk. *Cell Metab.* **2012**, *16*, 559–564. [CrossRef] [PubMed]
28. Fehlbaum, S.; Prudence, K.; Kieboom, J.; Heerikhuisen, M.; van den Broek, T.; Schuren, F.H.J.; Steinert, R.E.; Raederstorff, D. In Vitro Fermentation of Selected Prebiotics and Their Effects on the Composition and Activity of the Adult Gut Microbiota. *Int. J. Mol. Sci.* **2018**, *19*, 3097. [CrossRef]
29. Gibson, G.R.; Hutkins, R.; Sanders, M.E.; Prescott, S.L.; Reimer, R.A.; Salminen, S.J.; Scott, K.; Stanton, C.; Swanson, K.S.; Cani, P.D.; et al. Expert Consensus Document: The International Scientific Association for Probiotics and Prebiotics (ISAPP) Consensus Statement on the Definition and Scope of Prebiotics. *Nat. Rev. Gastroenterol. Hepatol.* **2017**, *14*, 491–502. [CrossRef] [PubMed]
30. Dehghan, P.; Pourghassem Gargari, B.; Asgharijafarabadi, M. Effects of High Performance Inulin Supplementation on Glycemic Status and Lipid Profile in Women with Type 2 Diabetes: A Randomized, Placebo-Controlled Clinical Trial. *Health Promot. Perspect.* **2013**, *3*, 55–63. [CrossRef]
31. Li, Y.; Elmén, L.; Segota, I.; Xian, Y.; Tinoco, R.; Feng, Y.; Fujita, Y.; Segura Muñoz, R.R.; Schmaltz, R.; Bradley, L.M.; et al. Prebiotic-Induced Anti-Tumor Immunity Attenuates Tumor Growth. *Cell Rep.* **2020**, *30*, 1753–1766.e6. [CrossRef]
32. Cherbut, C. Inulin and Oligofructose in the Dietary Fibre Concept. *Br. J. Nutr.* **2002**, *87*, S159–S162. [CrossRef] [PubMed]
33. Ruiz, L.; Delgado, S.; Ruas-Madiedo, P.; Sánchez, B.; Margolles, A. Bifidobacteria and Their Molecular Communication with the Immune System. *Front. Microbiol.* **2017**, *8*, 2345. [CrossRef] [PubMed]
34. Boucher, E.; Plazy, C.; Richard, M.L.; Suau, A.; Mangin, I.; Cornet, M.; Aldebert, D.; Toussaint, B.; Hannani, D. Inulin Prebiotic Reinforces Host Cancer Immunosurveillance via γδ T Cell Activation. *Front. Immunol.* **2023**, *14*, 1104224. [CrossRef]
35. Toussaint, B.; Delic-Attree, I.; Vignais, P.M. Pseudomonas Aeruginosa Contains an IHF-like Protein That Binds to the AlgD Promoter. *Biochem. Biophys. Res. Commun.* **1993**, *196*, 416–421. [CrossRef]
36. Sivan, A.; Corrales, L.; Hubert, N.; Williams, J.B.; Aquino-Michaels, K.; Earley, Z.M.; Benyamin, F.W.; Lei, Y.M.; Jabri, B.; Alegre, M.L.; et al. Commensal Bifidobacterium Promotes Antitumor Immunity and Facilitates Anti-PD-L1 Efficacy. *Science* **2015**, *350*, 1084–1089. [CrossRef] [PubMed]
37. Yao, Y.; Cai, X.; Fei, W.; Ye, Y.; Zhao, M.; Zheng, C. The Role of Short-Chain Fatty Acids in Immunity, Inflammation and Metabolism. *Crit. Rev. Food Sci. Nutr.* **2022**, *62*, 1–12. [CrossRef]
38. Kim, C.H. Control of Lymphocyte Functions by Gut Microbiota-Derived Short-Chain Fatty Acids. *Cell. Mol. Immunol.* **2021**, *18*, 1161–1171. [CrossRef]
39. Kelly, C.J.; Zheng, L.; Campbell, E.L.; Saeedi, B.; Scholz, C.C.; Bayless, A.J.; Wilson, K.E.; Glover, L.E.; Kominsky, D.J.; Magnuson, A.; et al. Crosstalk between Microbiota-Derived Short-Chain Fatty Acids and Intestinal Epithelial HIF Augments Tissue Barrier Function. *Cell Host Microbe* **2015**, *17*, 662–671. [CrossRef]
40. Herrmann, T.; Fichtner, A.S.; Karunakaran, M.M. An Update on the Molecular Basis of Phosphoantigen Recognition by Vγ9vδ2 t Cells. *Cells* **2020**, *9*, 1433. [CrossRef]
41. Yang, W.; Yu, T.; Huang, X.; Bilotta, A.J.; Xu, L.; Lu, Y.; Sun, J.; Pan, F.; Zhou, J.; Zhang, W.; et al. Intestinal Microbiota-Derived Short-Chain Fatty Acids Regulation of Immune Cell IL-22 Production and Gut Immunity. *Nat. Commun.* **2020**, *11*, 4457. [CrossRef]
42. Jabczyk, M.; Nowak, J.; Hudzik, B.; Zubelewicz-Szkodzińska, B. Microbiota and Its Impact on the Immune System in COVID-19—A Narrative Review. *J. Clin. Med.* **2021**, *10*, 4537. [CrossRef]
43. Kim, H.S. Do an Altered Gut Microbiota and an Associated Leaky Gut Affect COVID-19 Severity? *MBio* **2021**, *12*, 1–9. [CrossRef] [PubMed]
44. Rivera-Piza, A.; Lee, S.J. Effects of Dietary Fibers and Prebiotics in Adiposity Regulation via Modulation of Gut Microbiota. *Appl. Biol. Chem.* **2020**, *63*, 2. [CrossRef]
45. Ma, J.; Piao, X.; Mahfuz, S.; Long, S.; Wang, J. The Interaction among Gut Microbes, the Intestinal Barrier and Short Chain Fatty Acids. *Anim. Nutr.* **2022**, *9*, 159–174. [CrossRef] [PubMed]
46. Herath, M.; Hosie, S.; Bornstein, J.C.; Franks, A.E.; Hill-Yardin, E.L. The Role of the Gastrointestinal Mucus System in Intestinal Homeostasis: Implications for Neurological Disorders. *Front. Cell. Infect. Microbiol.* **2020**, *10*, 248. [CrossRef]
47. Penninger, J.M.; Grant, M.B.; Sung, J.J.Y. The Role of Angiotensin Converting Enzyme 2 in Modulating Gut Microbiota, Intestinal Inflammation, and Coronavirus Infection. *Gastroenterology* **2021**, *160*, 39–46. [CrossRef]
48. Fernandes, R.; do Rosario, V.A.; Mocellin, M.C.; Kuntz, M.G.F.; Trindade, E.B.S.M. Effects of Inulin-Type Fructans, Galacto-Oligosaccharides and Related Synbiotics on Inflammatory Markers in Adult Patients with Overweight or Obesity: A Systematic Review. *Clin. Nutr.* **2017**, *36*, 1197–1206. [CrossRef]
49. Ramirez-Farias, C.; Slezak, K.; Fuller, Z.; Duncan, A.; Holtrop, G.; Louis, P. Effect of Inulin on the Human Gut Microbiota: Stimulation of Bifidobacterium Adolescentis and Faecalibacterium Prausnitzii. *Br. J. Nutr.* **2009**, *101*, 541–550. [CrossRef]

Disclaimer/Publisher's Note: The statements, opinions and data contained in all publications are solely those of the individual author(s) and contributor(s) and not of MDPI and/or the editor(s). MDPI and/or the editor(s) disclaim responsibility for any injury to people or property resulting from any ideas, methods, instructions or products referred to in the content.

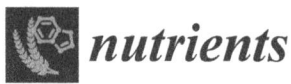

Article

No Associations between Dairy Intake and Markers of Gastrointestinal Inflammation in Healthy Adult Cohort

Yasmine Y. Bouzid [1,2], Elizabeth L. Chin [1,2], Sarah S. Spearman [2], Zeynep Alkan [1], Charles B. Stephensen [1,2] and Danielle G. Lemay [1,2,*]

1 USDA ARS Western Human Nutrition Research Center, Davis, CA 95616, USA
2 Department of Nutrition, University of California, Davis, CA 95616, USA
* Correspondence: danielle.lemay@usda.gov; Tel.: +1-(530)-752-4748

Abstract: Dairy products are a good source of essential nutrients and past reviews have shown associations of dairy consumption with decreased systemic inflammation. Links between dairy intake and gastrointestinal (GI) inflammation are under-investigated. Therefore, we examined associations between reported dairy intake and markers of GI inflammation in healthy adults in a cross-sectional observational study, hypothesizing a negative association with yogurt intake, suggesting a protective effect, and no associations with total dairy, fluid milk, and cheese intake. Participants completed 24-h dietary recalls and a food frequency questionnaire (FFQ) to assess recent and habitual intake, respectively. Those who also provided a stool sample ($n = 295$), and plasma sample ($n = 348$) were included in analysis. Inflammation markers from stool, including calprotectin, neopterin, and myeloperoxidase, were measured along with LPS-binding protein (LBP) from plasma. Regression models tested associations between dairy intake variables and inflammation markers with covariates: age, sex, and body mass index (BMI). As yogurt is episodically consumed, we examined differences in inflammation levels between consumers (>0 cup equivalents/day reported in recalls) and non-consumers. We found no significant associations between dairy intake and markers of GI inflammation. In this cohort of healthy adults, dairy intake was not associated with GI inflammation.

Keywords: dairy intake; gastrointestinal inflammation

1. Introduction

The Dietary Guidelines for Americans recommend three servings of dairy each day as a source of essential nutrients, especially for under-consumed nutrients of concern such as calcium, potassium, and vitamin D [1]. Dairy consumption is known to be beneficial for bone health, to reduce the risk of cardiovascular disease and diabetes, and is associated with lower mortality [2–5]. Systematic reviews of randomized controlled trials report a neutral to positive, anti-inflammatory effect of dairy intake on biomarkers of inflammation [6–11]. Individuals with commonly experienced gastrointestinal symptoms such as abdominal pain, bloating, or diarrhea often avoid dairy on their own or are advised to do so by their health practitioners [12]. However, the effect of dairy products on gastrointestinal health in adults is largely understudied.

Very few studies of fecal markers of gastrointestinal inflammation in response to dairy products have been conducted with healthy adults. Fecal calprotectin, a clinical diagnostic for gastrointestinal inflammation, was measured in three studies: an intervention with whipping cream [13], a comparison of A1 and A2 milk [14], and a tolerance study for casein glycomacropeptide [15]. None of these studies have relevance for the Dietary Guidelines which recommend low-fat milk, cheese, and yogurt (but not whipping cream, ice cream, etc.). The association between short- or long-term recommended dairy intake and fecal calprotectin levels in healthy people remains unknown.

The healthy gastrointestinal tract absorbs nutrients while maintaining a protective barrier between gut bacteria and the bloodstream. Even fewer studies have investigated the effects of dairy intake with respect to gastrointestinal barrier function in healthy individuals. In an intervention study with healthy men, whipping cream intake resulted in no significant change in gut permeability as directly measured with non-metabolizable sugars [13]. Gastrointestinal barrier function is often indirectly measured by quantitating the abundance in plasma of lipopolysaccharide-binding protein (LBP), which increases when lipopolysaccharide, a component of gram-negative bacteria, bypasses the GI tract and enters the blood stream. A study of yogurt consumption compared with a soy control had ambiguous findings: individual markers of endotoxin exposure, such as LBP, did not change, but the ratio of the markers improved [16]. In vitro experiments suggest that dairy and dairy-derived products can improve intestinal barrier function [17,18].

A systematic review of yogurt and/or fermented dairy consumption and health identified associations of fermented dairy intake with improvements in GI symptoms, diarrhea, and constipation, as well as a causal relationship with lactose digestion [19]. Studies of yogurt intervention in patients with irritable bowel syndrome show mixed results with some improving symptoms relative to placebo [20,21], but no worsening symptoms [22–24]. We, therefore, hypothesized that yogurt consumption would be negatively associated with markers of GI inflammation and intestinal permeability in healthy adults.

Given the paucity of studies of dairy and gastrointestinal status in healthy adults, the objective of the current study was to examine the relationship of dairy intake with fecal markers of gastrointestinal inflammation and with plasma LBP in a multi-ethnic cohort of normal to moderately obese men and women, ages 18 to 65 years, for whom both recent and habitual dietary intake was assessed. Gastrointestinal inflammation was measured using fecal calprotectin, fecal myeloperoxidase, and fecal neopterin. While fecal calprotectin is a generic and commonly used clinical measure, fecal myeloperoxidase specifically increases with the involvement of neutrophils while fecal neopterin increases with the involvement of macrophages.

2. Materials and Methods

2.1. Participants

Study participants were healthy adults aged 18–65 years, with a BMI (kg/m^2) of 18.5–45.0 (normal to obese), living near Davis, California. Participants were recruited in the cross-sectional USDA Nutritional Phenotyping Study as stratified by 18 categories defined by age, sex, and BMI to obtain a diverse sample population (NCT02367287) [25]. The purpose of the study was to characterize immunologic and physiologic phenotypes of healthy adults to identify factors that may be intervention targets to improve metabolic flexibility. Primary hypotheses included that higher diet quality would be associated with lower GI inflammation. Volunteers were excluded if they had been diagnosed with a chronic disease or if their blood pressure readings indicated hypertension at either of the two visits. A total of 393 participants were enrolled in the study, and 348 with complete dietary data, fasting plasma, and stool samples were included in the analyses.

2.2. Dietary Intake Assessment

Recent dietary intake in the form of three 24-h recalls was collected and analyzed using the Automated Self-Administered 24-h (ASA24) Dietary Assessment Tool, version (2016), developed by the National Cancer Institute, Bethesda, MD, USA (https://epi.grants.cancer.gov/asa24, accessed on 4 December 2020). Manual data cleaning was previously described [26]. The 24-h recalls were conducted in the 10-day period prior to the stool collection. There was a training recall (with staff present to assist the participant) followed by three prompts for at-home recalls, two weekdays and one weekend day. Total Energy Expenditure (TEE) was independently calculated using resting metabolic rate (measured using a metabolic cart) and physical activity levels (measured over the 10-days with an accelerometer). Calories reported via the training recall were lower, on average, than reported in the at-home recalls. Calories reported in the at-home recalls were more highly correlated with calculated TEE. We, therefore, used only the at-home recalls for the assessment of dairy intake. Habitual dietary intake was completed using the 2014 Block food frequency questionnaire (FFQ) with which participants were asked to report consumption of foods over the previous 12 months.

2.3. Stool Collection

Stool collection and processing procedures were described previously [27,28]. Briefly, volunteers collected a single stool sample at home, which was stored on ice immediately and brought to the Western Human Nutrition Research Center (WHNRC) as soon as possible. Fecal samples were homogenized, flash frozen and aliquoted by a technician, and stored at $-70\ °C$ until analyses.

2.4. Plasma Collection

Plasma was processed from fasting blood collected in either EDTA or heparin tubes immediately after the blood draw [28]. Plasma aliquots were stored at $-80\ °C$ until use.

2.5. Quantification of Gut Inflammation Markers

We measured the abundance of fecal calprotectin, myeloperoxidase, and neopterin via ELISA. We also used ELISA to measure the abundance of LPS-binding protein (LBP) in plasma collected at fasting.

2.6. Fecal Calprotectin and MPO

Calprotectin (Immundiagnostik, Bensheim, Germany; catalog [cat] number K6927) and MPO (Immundiagnostik; cat number KR6630) enzyme-linked immunosorbent assays (ELISAs) were used per kit instructions to analyze frozen homogenized stool samples, which were thawed slowly prior to extraction with the IDK Extract Stool Sample Preparation System (Immundiagnostik) as described in detail before [28].

2.7. Fecal Neopterin

Stool aliquots were extracted into a saline solution as published previously [29] and fecal neopterin was quantified from the extracts with ELISAs (B·R·A·H·M·S/ThermoFisher, Hennigsdorf, Germany; cat number 14-HD-99.1).

2.8. Plasma Lipopolysaccharide-Binding Protein (LBP)

LBP was quantified from clarified and 800-fold diluted fasting heparin plasma with ELISAs (Abnova, Taipei City, Taiwan; cat number KA0448) as described elsewhere [28].

2.9. Statistical Methods

R was used for statistical analysis and visualizations. Linear regression was used to examine associations between total dairy, fluid milk, cheese, and yogurt intake and stool calprotectin, myeloperoxidase, neopterin, and plasma LBP. Distributions for fecal calprotectin, and fecal myeloperoxidase were transformed with $\ln(x + 3)$ and $\ln(x + 1)$ transformations, respectively. Fecal neopterin was transformed using the Box Cox transformation. Plasma LBP distribution was transformed with an $\ln(x + 1)$ transformation. Age, sex, and BMI were included in the models to account for covariates when examining associations between dairy intake variables and markers of GI inflammation. Since yogurt is episodically consumed, the distributions for recent intake were zero-inflated. Therefore, we characterized yogurt consumers as those with any amount reported in averages of their 24-h recalls and ran similar regression models. Distributions for markers of GI inflammation were transformed using suggestions from the BestNormalize package when assessing associations with yogurt consumption: calprotectin (orderNorm), myeloperoxidase (Box Cox), neopterin (orderNorm), and LBP remained with the original $\ln(x + 1)$ transformation as residuals were normal when checked by Shapiro test. Student's t-tests were also used to test differences in mean levels of GI inflammation markers between recent yogurt consumers and non-consumers.

3. Results

3.1. Participant Characteristics

Of the 348 participants included in this study, 164 were male and 184 were female. Mean age was 40.51 ± 13.7 years with a range of 18 to 66 years. Mean BMI was 27.28 ± 4.9 kg/m^2 with a range of 18.04 to 43.87 kg/m^2.

Participants reported recent total dairy intake, as an average across 24 h recalls as 1.60 ± 1.05 cup equivalents per day, range 0 to 6.71. They reported habitual consumption of 1.48 ± 1.09 cup equivalents of total dairy per day with a range of 0.21 to 8.06 (per the FFQ). As some dairy intake is aggregated from mixed dishes (e.g., scrambled eggs) in which a consumer may not have consumed dairy (e.g., scrambled eggs made without milk), some amount of dairy consumption may be incidental; if one conservatively (to minimize false positives at the expense of false negatives) defines those who consume more than 0.25 cups/day as a dairy consumer, then at least 92% of participants in this cohort would be defined as dairy consumers. Recent fluid milk consumption was 0.56 ± 0.65 cup equivalents per day, range 0 to 5.73. Habitual fluid milk consumption was 0.64 ± 0.72 cup equivalents per day, range 0.05 to 5.20. Recent cheese intake was 0.84 ± 0.79 cup equivalents per day, range 0 to 4.60. Habitual cheese intake was 0.84 ± 0.58 cup equivalents per day, range 0.09 to 4.00. Recent yogurt intake was 0.13 ± 0.25 cup equivalents per day, range 0 to 1.84. 57% of participants reported no recent yogurt intake. Habitual yogurt intake was 0.19 ± 0.25 cup equivalents per day, range 0 to 2.01. As yogurt is an episodically consumed food, yogurt consumers were defined as those who consumed more than 0 cup equivalents per day.

Mean calprotectin was 65.09 ± 136.43 µg/g with a range from 0 to 1878.79. Mean myeloperoxidase was 606.48 ± 1619.45 ng/g with a range from 13.75 to 21,668.50. Mean neopterin was 20.19 ± 27.98 ng/g with a range from 4.33 to 228.71. Mean LBP was 10.65 ± 6.00 µg/mL with range 1.00 to 38.27.

3.2. Association of Dairy Intake with Fecal Markers of GI Inflammation

Given that age, sex, or BMI may influence inflammation, we adjusted all analyses for these three covariates. We found no associations between recent intake of total dairy, fluid milk, or cheese, as measured via ASA24 recalls, with any fecal markers of inflammation (Tables 1–3, Figures 1–3). There was also no association between habitual intake, as measured with an FFQ, of total dairy, fluid milk, or cheese with any fecal markers (Supplementary Tables S1–S3, Supplementary Figures S1–S3).

Table 1. Results from linear regression between total dairy intake from 24-h recall (ASA24) and markers of GI inflammation adjusted for age, sex, and BMI. Results from linear regression between age, sex, or BMI vs. GI inflammation markers are also shown.

Predictors	Transformed Calprotectin Estimates (95% CI)	p-Value	Transformed Myeloperoxidase Estimates (95% CI)	p-Value	Transformed Neopterin Estimates (95% CI)	p-Value	Transformed LPS-Binding Protein Estimates (95% CI)	p-Value
Total Dairy	0.02 (−0.08–0.13)	0.678	−0.06 (−0.18–0.07)	0.374	−0.05 (−0.16–0.06)	0.380	−0.02 (−0.07–0.02)	0.358
Age	−0.01 (−0.01–0.00)	0.215	0.00 (−0.01–0.01)	0.860	−0.00 (−0.01–0.00)	0.353	0.00 (−0.00–0.01)	0.195
Sex	0.15 (−0.07–0.38)	0.175	0.11 (−0.15–0.37)	0.414	0.34 (0.10–0.57)	**0.005**	0.13 (0.04–0.23)	**0.005**
BMI	0.00 (−0.02–0.02)	0.846	0.00 (−0.03–0.03)	0.993	0.02 (−0.01–0.04)	0.166	0.04 (0.03–0.05)	**<0.001**
R^2/R^2 adjusted	0.011/−0.002		0.007/−0.007		0.044/0.030		0.226/0.217	

Bold indicates statistically significant p-values (alpha = 0.05).

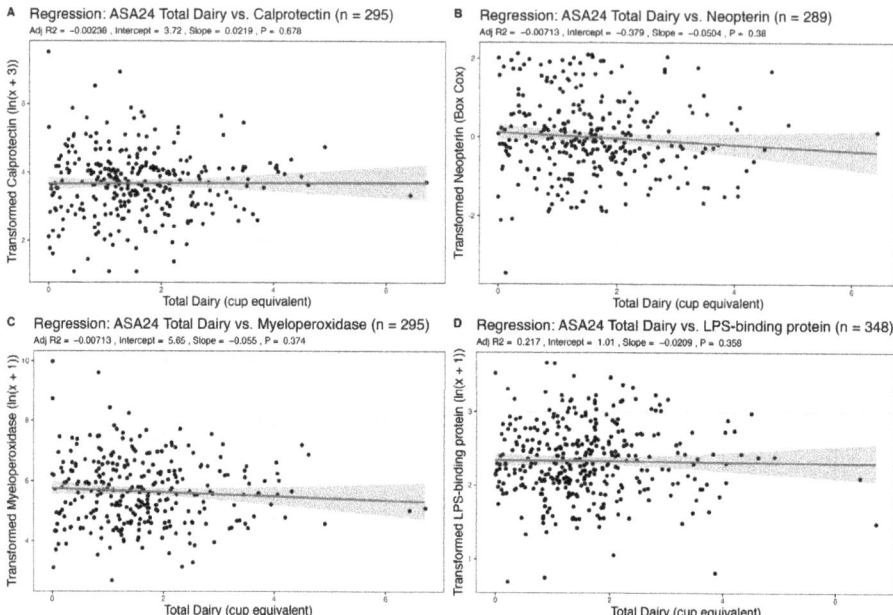

Figure 1. Association of recent total dairy intake (cup equivalent per day) with markers of GI inflammation adjusted for sex, age, and BMI.

Table 2. Results from linear regression between fluid milk from 24-h recall (ASA24) and markers of GI inflammation adjusted for age, sex, and BMI. Results from linear regression between age, sex, or BMI vs. GI inflammation markers are also shown.

Predictors	Transformed Calprotectin Estimates (95% CI)	p-Value	Transformed Myeloperoxidase Estimates (95% CI)	p-Value	Transformed Neopterin Estimates (95% CI)	p-Value	Transformed LPS-Binding Protein Estimates (95% CI)	p-Value
Fluid Milk	−0.00 (−0.17–0.16)	0.961	−0.06 (−0.26–0.13)	0.515	−0.04 (−0.21–0.14)	0.692	−0.05 (−0.12–0.02)	0.129
Age	−0.00 (−0.01–0.00)	0.226	0.00 (−0.01–0.01)	0.860	−0.00 (−0.01–0.00)	0.338	0.00 (−0.00–0.01)	0.169
Sex	0.14 (−0.08–0.36)	0.199	0.13 (−0.13–0.38)	0.332	0.35 (0.12–0.58)	**0.003**	0.13 (0.04–0.23)	**0.004**
BMI	0.00 (−0.02–0.02)	0.799	−0.00 (−0.03–0.02)	0.914	0.02 (−0.01–0.04)	0.202	0.04 (0.03–0.05)	**<0.001**
R^2/R^2 adjusted	0.011/−0.003		0.005/−0.008		0.042/0.028		0.229/0.220	

Bold indicates statistically significant p-values (alpha = 0.05).

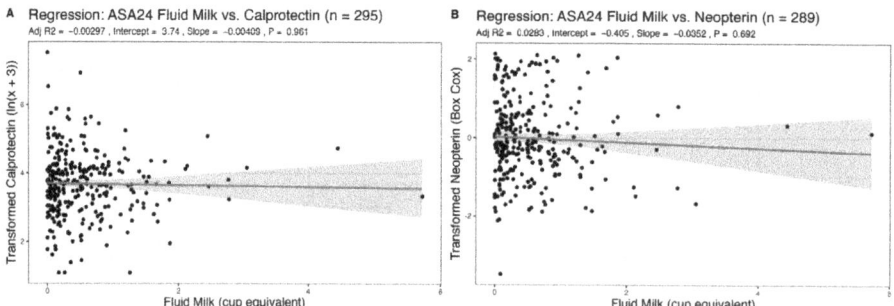

Figure 2. *Cont.*

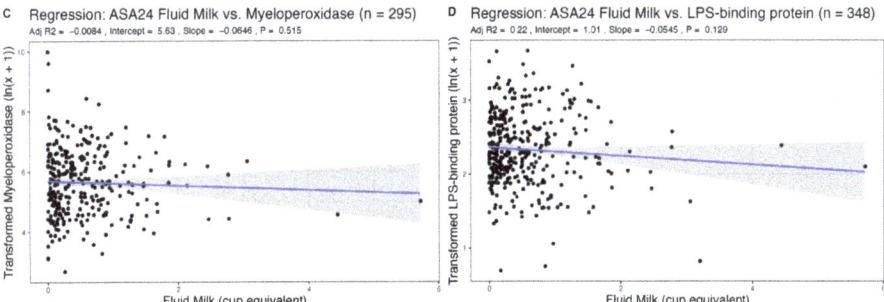

Figure 2. Association of recent fluid milk intake (cup equivalents per day) with markers of GI Inflammation adjusted for sex, age, and BMI.

Table 3. Results from linear regression between cheese intake from ASA24 and markers of GI inflammation adjusted for age, sex, and BMI. Results from linear regression between age, sex, or BMI vs. GI inflammation markers are also shown.

Predictors	Transformed Calprotectin Estimates (95% CI)	p-Value	Transformed Myeloperoxidase Estimates (95% CI)	p-Value	Transformed Neopterin Estimates (95% CI)	p-Value	Transformed LPS-Binding Protein Estimates (95% CI)	p-Value
Cheese	0.03 (−0.11–0.17)	0.686	−0.03 (−0.19–0.13)	0.711	−0.07 (−0.22–0.08)	0.366	−0.00 (−0.06–0.06)	0.952
Age	−0.00 (−0.01–0.00)	0.227	0.00 (−0.01–0.01)	0.908	−0.00 (−0.01–0.00)	0.312	0.00 (−0.00–0.01)	0.216
Sex	0.15 (−0.07–0.37)	0.178	0.13 (−0.13–0.39)	0.333	0.34 (0.11–0.57)	**0.004**	0.14 (0.05–0.23)	**0.003**
BMI	0.00 (−0.02–0.02)	0.869	−0.00 (−0.03–0.03)	0.972	0.02 (−0.01–0.04)	0.151	0.04 (0.03–0.05)	**<0.001**
R^2/R^2 adjusted	0.011/−0.002		0.004/−0.009		0.044/0.031		0.224/0.215	

Bold indicates statistically significant p-values (alpha = 0.05).

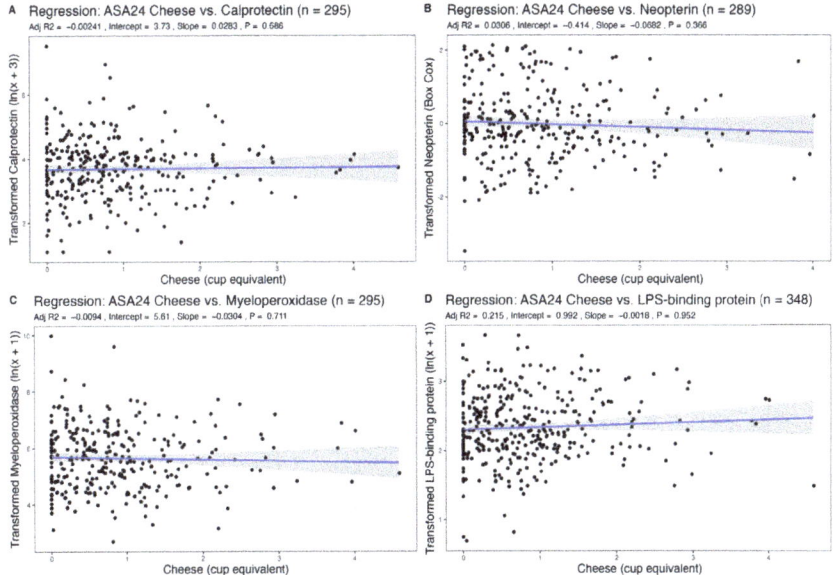

Figure 3. Association of recent cheese intake (cup equivalents per day) with markers of GI inflammation after adjustment for sex, age, and BMI.

Table 4. Results from linear regression between yogurt from ASA24 (consumers only) and markers of GI inflammation adjusted for age, sex, and BMI. Results from linear regression between age, sex, or BMI vs. GI inflammation markers are also shown.

Predictors	Transformed Calprotectin Estimates (95% CI)	p-Value	Transformed Myeloperoxidase Estimates (95% CI)	p-Value	Transformed Neopterin Estimates (95% CI)	p-Value	Transformed LPS-Binding Protein Estimates (95% CI)	p-Value
Yogurt	0.32 (−0.34–0.97)	0.339	0.42 (−0.27–1.11)	0.235	−0.06 (−0.71–0.59)	0.856	0.05 (−0.18–0.29)	0.659
Age	−0.01 (−0.03–−0.00)	**0.026**	0.00 (−0.01–0.02)	0.711	0.01 (−0.00–0.02)	0.155	0.00 (−0.00–0.01)	0.120
Sex	0.10 (−0.24–0.43)	0.570	0.19 (−0.16–0.55)	0.283	0.46 (0.12–0.79)	**0.008**	0.18 (0.04–0.31)	**0.011**
BMI	−0.01 (−0.05–0.03)	0.622	−0.04 (−0.08–0.00)	0.061	0.02 (−0.02–0.06)	0.278	0.04 (0.03–0.06)	**<0.001**
R^2/R^2 adjusted	0.049/0.015		0.058/0.025		0.093/0.060		0.240/0.218	

Bold indicates statistically significant p-values (alpha = 0.05).

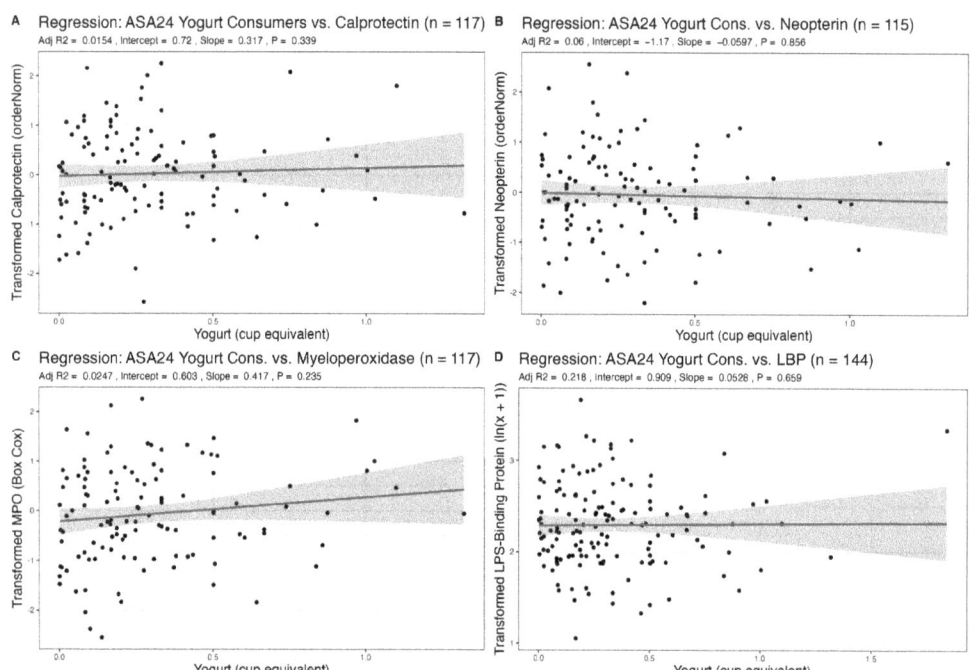

Figure 4. Association of recent yogurt intake (consumers only, >0 cup eq.) with markers of GI inflammation after adjustment for sex, age, and BMI.

Yogurt intake was a zero-inflated variable, particularly for ASA24 recalls. Therefore, we stratified subjects as non-consumers and consumers (>0 cup equivalents yogurt reported in their averaged recalls). We found no significant differences in fecal markers of inflammation between non-consumers and consumers of yogurt. When analyzing relationships only among consumers of yogurt, we found no association between the amount of yogurt recently consumed and markers of GI inflammation (Table 4, Figure 4). Using the FFQs, there was also no relationship between habitual consumption of yogurt and GI inflammation (Supplementary Table S4, Figure S4).

3.3. Association of Dairy Intake with Plasma LBP, a Marker of Endotoxin Exposure

The distribution for plasma LPS-binding protein (LBP), an indirect marker of endotoxin exposure, was transformed with an $\ln(x + 1)$ transformation. We found no associations between total dairy, fluid milk, cheese, and yogurt intake from ASA24 recalls (a measure of recent dietary intake) with plasma LBP (Tables 1–4, Figures 1–4). Using FFQ data (as a measure of habitual intake), we also found no significant association of dairy consumption with LBP levels (Supplementary Tables S1–S4, Supplementary Figures S1–S4). We also found no significant differences in plasma LBP between non-consumers and consumers of yogurt. There were no significant differences between mean GI inflammation markers by t-test (Figure 5).

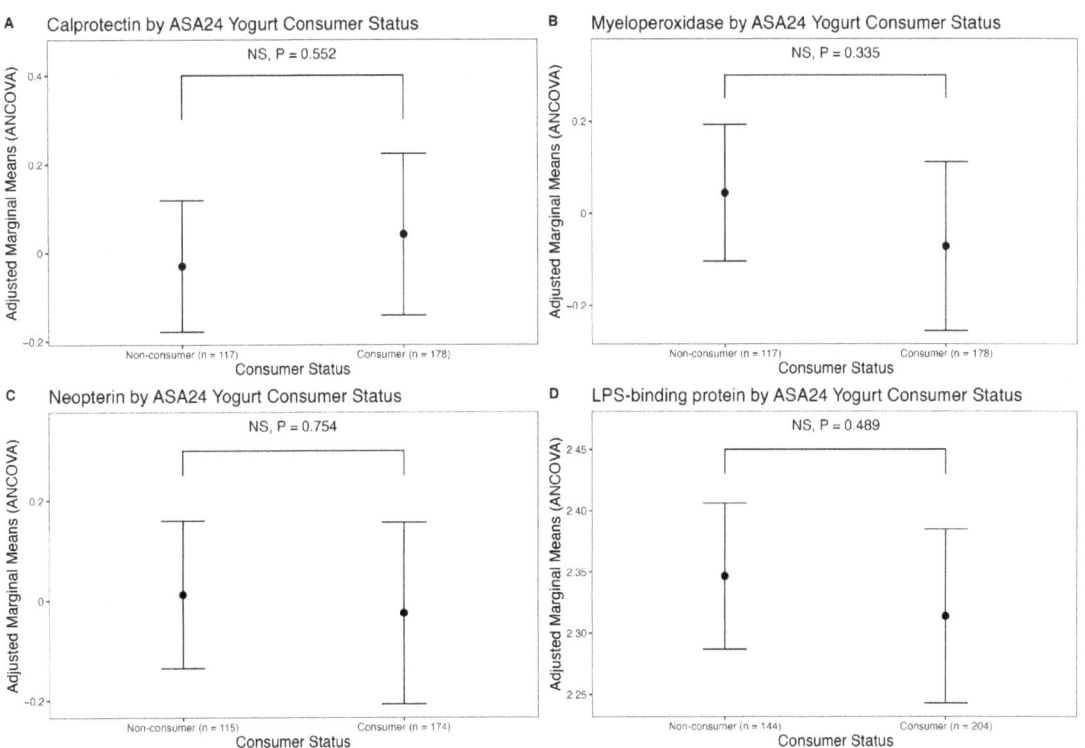

Figure 5. Points show adjusted marginal means from ANCOVA analysis for calprotectin (**A**), neopterin (**B**), myeloperoxidase (**C**), and LBP (**D**) based on consumer status. Error bars represent 95% confidence intervals. NS indicates p-values not significant.

4. Discussion

Previous studies have examined the association of dairy intake with systemic inflammation and found no or beneficial effects of dairy consumption (reviewed in [10]). An analysis of data from 35,352 postmenopausal women in the Women's Health Initiative demonstrated that higher total dairy intake, cheese, and yogurt were associated with lower concentrations of C-reactive protein [30]. However, as large national surveys do not measure gastrointestinal inflammation, this has been a gap in the scientific literature. In our cohort of 348 multi-ethnic U.S. adults, we found no significant associations between dairy intake, fluid milk intake, cheese intake, or yogurt intake with fecal markers of gastrointestinal inflammation. We also found no association between dairy intake, fluid milk intake, cheese intake, or yogurt intake with plasma LBP, an indirect measure of gastrointestinal permeability.

Some adults avoid dairy consumption due to real or perceived lactose intolerance. We previously showed that the multi-ethnic participants in our cohort included more than 40% of participants with lactase non-persistent genotypes [31]. Despite the high incidence of genetic lactose intolerance in this cohort, we found no association of total dairy, fluid milk, or cheese intake with gastrointestinal inflammation.

Beta-casein, an abundant protein in milk, appears in different forms, such as A1 and A2, depending on the genetic variants present in the cow's genome [32]. A randomized crossover double-blinded trial found that A2 milk reduced digestive symptoms in 600 Chinese adults [33]. However, a randomized crossover blinded clinical trial of 40 women in New Zealand showed that while lactose-intolerant participants experienced reduced symptoms with A2 milk, dairy tolerant participants had increased diarrhea [34]. The impact of A2 milk, relative to regular milk, which contains both A1 and A2 protein, remains controversial with more studies needed. In the current study, as A2 milk was not generally available in the U.S. during most of the years that participants were enrolled (2015–2019), it is a reasonable assumption that all or most of the fluid milk consumed by participants was not A2 milk. Nevertheless, we saw no association of fluid milk intake with GI inflammation.

Fermented dairy products have been shown to improve stool frequency or consistency in patients with constipation in small clinical trials [35,36]. In the EPIC-Italy cohort ($n > 45,000$) adults, yogurt consumption was association with reduced colon cancer risk [37] and it is known that chronic GI inflammation increases the risk of developing colon cancer [38]. Interventions with fermented milk products, which contain lactic acid bacteria (LAB), have been shown to attenuate GI inflammation in a mouse model of colitis though various mechanisms such as altering the gut microbiome to reduce colitogenic microbes [39], reducing production of Th1-type cytokines [40], reducing IL-6 by a polysaccharide peptidoglycan component of LAB [41], reducing IL-6 and TNF-α expression by fatty acids produced during LAB fermentation of milk [42], and activation of epidermal growth factor receptor on intestinal epithelial cells [43]. Therefore, we had hypothesized that increased yogurt consumption would be associated with a decrease in GI inflammation. However, we found no association between yogurt consumption and GI inflammation in healthy adults. It is possible that participants in our study may not have consumed enough yogurt with 57% of the cohort reporting no yogurt consumption in their 24 h recalls and with a median of 0.25 cups/day even among consumers.

The effect of yogurt consumption on intestinal permeability is not well-studied in humans, likely due to the invasiveness of such study. In a double-blind controlled trial, participants who were to undergo endoscopy and treated with low-dose aspirin for one month were randomized to consume either yogurt (220 mL/day) or placebo daily [44]. The patients consuming yogurt had fewer mucosal breaks and improvement in GI symptoms. In our study, we found no association between yogurt intake and plasma LBP, an indirect measure of gastrointestinal permeability, but our participants did not undergo a challenge such as low-dose aspirin.

A major limitation of our study is its observational nature. However, observational analyses are low-cost first steps prior to designing an intervention study and no previous observational study with GI endpoints had been conducted for dairy consumption. Another limitation is the exclusion of participants with GI disease. We, therefore, cannot infer an association beyond healthy people. However, as we did find associations of our GI endpoints with age, sex, and BMI in this cohort, the negative findings are not due to all participants having unremarkable GI outcomes. LBP was elevated in obese individuals (Tables 1–4) and both age and sex were significant in some models of fecal GI markers (Table 4) with older individuals and females associated with higher inflammation, compared with those younger than 50 years and males, respectively. Another limitation is generalizability around the world as recommendations for dairy intake vary internationally with some countries grouping dairy under protein foods instead of a separate food group [45].

In summary, we found no association of dairy intake of any type with GI inflammation or with GI permeability in a multi-ethnic healthy U.S. cohort of adults who were heterogenous for lactose intolerance. Future studies are warranted, particularly for interventions with daily doses of yogurt to define effects on GI inflammation and/or GI permeability, perhaps with older (>50 y), obese females, and incorporating a gastrointestinal challenge.

Supplementary Materials: The following supporting information can be downloaded at: https://www.mdpi.com/article/10.3390/nu15163504/s1, Table S1: Results from linear regression between total dairy intake (cup equivalents per day) from food frequency questionnaire (FFQ) and markers of GI inflammation adjusted for age, sex, and BMI; Figure S1: Association of habitual total dairy intake with markers of GI inflammation adjusted for sex, age, BMI; Table S2: Results from linear regression between fluid milk intake (cup equivalents per day) from FFQ and markers of GI inflammation adjusted for age, sex, and BMI; Figure S2: Association of habitual fluid milk intake with markers of GI inflammation after adjustment for sex, age, BMI; Table S3: Results from linear regression between cheese intake (cup equivalents per day) from FFQ and markers of GI inflammation adjusted for age, sex, and BMI; Figure S3: Association of habitual cheese intake with markers of GI inflammation after adjustment for sex, age, BMI; Table S4: Results from linear regression between yogurt intake (cup equivalents per day) from FFQ and markers of GI inflammation adjusted for age, sex, and BMI; Figure S4: Association of habitual yogurt intake with markers of GI inflammation after adjustment for sex, age, BMI.

Author Contributions: Conceptualization, D.G.L.; methodology, D.G.L., Y.Y.B., E.L.C., Z.A. and C.B.S.; formal analysis, Y.Y.B. and E.L.C.; investigation, S.S.S. and Z.A.; writing—original draft preparation, D.G.L., Y.Y.B., S.S.S. and Z.A.; writing—review and editing, E.L.C., Z.A., S.S.S. and C.B.S.; visualization, Y.Y.B.; supervision, D.G.L. and C.B.S.; funding acquisition, D.G.L. and C.B.S. All authors have read and agreed to the published version of the manuscript.

Funding: The California Dairy Research Foundation, TCFA 58-2032-9-018, and the United States Department of Agriculture, Agricultural Research Service, 2032-51530-026-00D. The USDA is an equal opportunity provider and employer.

Institutional Review Board Statement: Ethical approval for this study was received from the University of California Davis Institutional Review Board on 20 February 2015, under identification number 691654.

Informed Consent Statement: Written informed consent for study participation is obtained in compliance with the IRB guidelines.

Data Availability Statement: Not applicable.

Acknowledgments: We acknowledge Ellen Bonnel for human studies management; Eduardo Cervantes, Evelyn Holguin, Annie Kan, Barbara Gale, Danna Juarez Rios, Justin Waller, Ashley Tovar, Christine Bowlus, Yanhua "Eva" Li, and Diane Han for human studies and physiology assessment in the USDA Nutritional Phenotyping Study; Jerome Crawford, Debra Standridge, Joe Domek, and Connor Osato for stool and plasma processing; Joanne Arsenault for dietary quality control; and the Western Human Nutrition Research Center Bioanalytical Support Lab.

Conflicts of Interest: The authors declare no conflict of interest.

References

1. U.S. Department of Agriculture; U.S. Department of Health and Human Services. *Dietary Guidelines for Americans, 2020–2025*, 9th ed.; U.S. Department of Agriculture: Washington, DC, USA, 2020. Available online: https://www.dietaryguidelines.gov/sites/default/files/2020-12/Dietary_Guidelines_for_Americans_2020-2025.pdf (accessed on 19 July 2022).
2. Mazidi, M.; Mikhailidis, D.P.; Sattar, N.; Howard, G.; Graham, I.; Banach, M. Consumption of Dairy Product and Its Association with Total and Cause Specific Mortality—A Population-Based Cohort Study and Meta-Analysis. *Clin. Nutr.* **2018**, *38*, 2833–2845. [CrossRef] [PubMed]
3. Dehghan, M.; Mente, A.; Rangarajan, S.; Sheridan, P.; Mohan, V.; Iqbal, R.; Gupta, R.; Lear, S.; Wentzel-Viljoen, E.; Avezum, A.; et al. Association of Dairy Intake with Cardiovascular Disease and Mortality in 21 Countries from Five Continents (PURE): A Prospective Cohort Study. *Lancet* **2018**, *392*, 2288–2297. [CrossRef] [PubMed]
4. Sahni, S.; Tucker, K.L.; Kiel, D.P.; Quach, L.; Casey, V.A.; Hannan, M.T. Milk and Yogurt Consumption Are Linked with Higher Bone Mineral Density but Not with Hip Fracture: The Framingham Offspring Study. *Arch. Osteoporos.* **2013**, *8*, 119. [CrossRef]
5. Gijsbers, L.; Ding, E.L.; Malik, V.S.; de Goede, J.; Geleijnse, J.M.; Soedamah-Muthu, S.S. Consumption of Dairy Foods and Diabetes Incidence: A Dose-Response Meta-Analysis of Observational Studies. *Am. J. Clin. Nutr.* **2016**, *103*, 1111–1124. [CrossRef]

6. Ulven, S.M.; Holven, K.B.; Gil, A.; Rangel-Huerta, O.D. Milk and Dairy Product Consumption and Inflammatory Biomarkers: An Updated Systematic Review of Randomized Clinical Trials. *Adv. Nutr.* **2019**, *10*, S239–S250. [CrossRef] [PubMed]
7. Moosavian, S.P.; Rahimlou, M.; Saneei, P.; Esmaillzadeh, A. Effects of Dairy Products Consumption on Inflammatory Biomarkers among Adults: A Systematic Review and Meta-Analysis of Randomized Controlled Trials. *Nutr. Metab. Cardiovasc. Dis.* **2020**, *30*, 872–888. [CrossRef]
8. Labonté, M.-È.; Couture, P.; Richard, C.; Desroches, S.; Lamarche, B. Impact of Dairy Products on Biomarkers of Inflammation: A Systematic Review of Randomized Controlled Nutritional Intervention Studies in Overweight and Obese Adults. *Am. J. Clin. Nutr.* **2013**, *97*, 706–717. [CrossRef]
9. Hess, J.M.; Stephensen, C.B.; Kratz, M.; Bolling, B.W. Exploring the Links between Diet and Inflammation: Dairy Foods as Case Studies. *Adv. Nutr.* **2021**, *12*, 1S–13S. [CrossRef]
10. Nieman, K.M.; Anderson, B.D.; Cifelli, C.J. The Effects of Dairy Product and Dairy Protein Intake on Inflammation: A Systematic Review of the Literature. *J. Am. Coll. Nutr.* **2021**, *40*, 571–582. [CrossRef]
11. Bordoni, A.; Danesi, F.; Dardevet, D.; Dupont, D.; Fernandez, A.S.; Gille, D.; Nunes dos Santos, C.; Pinto, P.; Re, R.; Rémond, D.; et al. Dairy Products and Inflammation: A Review of the Clinical Evidence. *Crit. Rev. Food Sci. Nutr.* **2017**, *57*, 2497–2525. [CrossRef]
12. Pearlman, M.; Akpotaire, O. Diet and the Role of Food in Common Gastrointestinal Diseases. *Med. Clin. N. Am.* **2019**, *103*, 101–110. [CrossRef]
13. Ott, B.; Skurk, T.; Lagkouvardos, L.; Fischer, S.; Büttner, J.; Lichtenegger, M.; Clavel, T.; Lechner,, A.; Rychlik, M.; Haller, D.; et al. Short-Term Overfeeding with Dairy Cream Does Not Modify Gut Permeability, the Fecal Microbiota, or Glucose Metabolism in Young Healthy Men. *J. Nutr.* **2018**, *148*, 77–85. [CrossRef]
14. Ho, S.; Woodford, K.; Kukuljan, S.; Pal, S. Comparative Effects of A1 versus A2 Beta-Casein on Gastrointestinal Measures: A Blinded Randomised Cross-over Pilot Study. *Eur. J. Clin. Nutr.* **2014**, *68*, 994–1000. [CrossRef] [PubMed]
15. Wernlund, P.G.; Hvas, C.L.; Dahlerup, J.F.; Bahl, M.I.; Licht, T.R.; Knudsen, K.E.B.; Agnholt, J.S. Casein Glycomacropeptide Is Well Tolerated in Healthy Adults and Changes Neither High-Sensitive C-Reactive Protein, Gut Microbiota nor Faecal Butyrate: A Restricted Randomised Trial. *Br. J. Nutr.* **2021**, *125*, 1374–1385. [CrossRef] [PubMed]
16. Pei, R.; DiMarco, D.M.; Putt, K.K.; Martin, D.A.; Gu, Q.; Chitchumroonchokchai, C.; White, H.M.; Scarlett, C.O.; Bruno, R.S.; Bolling, B.W. Low-Fat Yogurt Consumption Reduces Biomarkers of Chronic Inflammation and Inhibits Markers of Endotoxin Exposure in Healthy Premenopausal Women: A Randomised Controlled Trial. *Br. J. Nutr.* **2017**, *118*, 1043–1051. [CrossRef] [PubMed]
17. Calatayud, M.; Börner, R.A.; Ghyselinck, J.; Verstrepen, L.; Medts, J.D.; Abbeele, P.V.; Boulangé, C.L.; Priour, S.; Marzorati, M.; Damak, S. Water Kefir and Derived Pasteurized Beverages Modulate Gut Microbiota, Intestinal Permeability and Cytokine Production In Vitro. *Nutrients* **2021**, *13*, 3897. [CrossRef] [PubMed]
18. Zhao, X.; Xu, X.-X.; Liu, Y.; Xi, E.-Z.; An, J.; Tabys, D.; Liu, N. The In Vitro Protective Role of Bovine Lactoferrin on Intestinal Epithelial Barrier. *Molecules* **2019**, *24*, 148. [CrossRef]
19. Savaiano, D.A.; Hutkins, R.W. Yogurt, Cultured Fermented Milk, and Health: A Systematic Review. *Nutr. Rev.* **2021**, *79*, 599–614. [CrossRef]
20. Zeng, J.; Li, Y.-Q.; Zuo, X.-L.; Zhen, Y.-B.; Yang, J.; Liu, C.-H. Clinical Trial: Effect of Active Lactic Acid Bacteria on Mucosal Barrier Function in Patients with Diarrhoea-Predominant Irritable Bowel Syndrome. *Aliment. Pharm.. Ther.* **2008**, *28*, 994–1002. [CrossRef] [PubMed]
21. Agrawal, A.; Houghton, L.A.; Morris, J.; Reilly, B.; Guyonnet, D.; Goupil Feuillerat, N.; Schlumberger, A.; Jakob, S.; Whorwell, P.J. Clinical Trial: The Effects of a Fermented Milk Product Containing *Bifidobacterium lactis* DN-173 010 on Abdominal Distension and Gastrointestinal Transit in Irritable Bowel Syndrome with Constipation. *Aliment. Pharm. Ther.* **2009**, *29*, 104–114. [CrossRef]
22. Simrén, M.; Öhman, L.; Olsson, J.; Svensson, U.; Ohlson, K.; Posserud, I.; Strid, H. Clinical Trial: The Effects of a Fermented Milk Containing Three Probiotic Bacteria in Patients with Irritable Bowel Syndrome—A Randomized, Double-Blind, Controlled Study. *Aliment. Pharm. Ther.* **2010**, *31*, 218–227. [CrossRef] [PubMed]
23. Søndergaard, B.; Olsson, J.; Ohlson, K.; Svensson, U.; Bytzer, P.; Ekesbo, R. Effects of Probiotic Fermented Milk on Symptoms and Intestinal Flora in Patients with Irritable Bowel Syndrome: A Randomized, Placebo-Controlled Trial. *Scand. J. Gastroenterol.* **2011**, *46*, 663–672. [CrossRef] [PubMed]
24. Roberts, L.M.; McCahon, D.; Holder, R.; Wilson, S.; Hobbs, F.D.R. A Randomised Controlled Trial of a Probiotic 'Functional Food' in the Management of Irritable Bowel Syndrome. *BMC Gastroenterol.* **2013**, *13*, 45. [CrossRef] [PubMed]
25. Baldiviez, L.M.; Keim, N.L.; Laugero, K.D.; Hwang, D.H.; Huang, L.; Woodhouse, L.R.; Burnett, D.J.; Zerofsky, M.S.; Bonnel, E.L.; Allen, L.H.; et al. Design and Implementation of a Cross-Sectional Nutritional Phenotyping Study in Healthy US Adults. *BMC Nutr.* **2017**, *3*, 79. [CrossRef]
26. Bouzid, Y.Y.; Arsenault, J.E.; Bonnel, E.L.; Cervantes, E.; Kan, A.; Keim, N.L.; Lemay, D.G.; Stephensen, C.B. Effect of Manual Data Cleaning on Nutrient Intakes Using the Automated Self-Administered 24-Hour Dietary Assessment Tool (ASA24). *Curr. Dev. Nutr.* **2021**, *5*, nzab005. [CrossRef]
27. Lemay, D.G.; Baldiviez, L.M.; Chin, E.L.; Spearman, S.S.; Cervantes, E.; Woodhouse, L.R.; Keim, N.L.; Stephensen, C.B.; Laugero, K.D. Technician-Scored Stool Consistency Spans the Full Range of the Bristol Scale in a Healthy US Population and Differs by Diet and Chronic Stress Load. *J. Nutr.* **2021**, *151*, 1443–1452. [CrossRef]

28. Oliver, A.; Xue, Z.; Villanueva, Y.T.; Durbin-Johnson, B.; Alkan, Z.; Taft, D.H.; Liu, J.; Korf, I.; Laugero, K.D.; Stephensen, C.B.; et al. Association of Diet and Antimicrobial Resistance in Healthy U.S. Adults. *mBio* **2022**, *13*, e00101-22. [CrossRef]
29. Larke, J.A.; Bacalzo, N.; Castillo, J.J.; Couture, G.; Chen, Y.; Xue, Z.; Alkan, Z.; Kable, M.E.; Lebrilla, C.B.; Stephensen, C.B.; et al. Dietary Intake of Monosaccharides from Foods Is Associated with Characteristics of the Gut Microbiota and Gastrointestinal Inflammation in Healthy US Adults. *J. Nutr.* **2023**, *153*, 106–119. [CrossRef]
30. Shi, N.; Olivo-Marston, S.; Jin, Q.; Aroke, D.; Joseph, J.J.; Clinton, S.K.; Manson, J.E.; Rexrode, K.M.; Mossavar-Rahmani, Y.; Fels Tinker, L.; et al. Associations of Dairy Intake with Circulating Biomarkers of Inflammation, Insulin Response, and Dyslipidemia among Postmenopausal Women. *J. Acad. Nutr. Diet.* **2021**, *121*, 1984–2002. [CrossRef]
31. Chin, E.L.; Huang, L.; Bouzid, Y.Y.; Kirschke, C.P.; Durbin-Johnson, B.; Baldiviez, L.M.; Bonnel, E.L.; Keim, N.L.; Korf, I.; Stephensen, C.B.; et al. Association of Lactase Persistence Genotypes (Rs4988235) and Ethnicity with Dairy Intake in a Healthy U.S. Population. *Nutrients* **2019**, *11*, 1860. [CrossRef]
32. Farrell, H.M., Jr.; Jimenez-Flores, R.; Bleck, G.T.; Brown, E.M.; Butler, J.E.; Creamer, L.K.; Hicks, C.L.; Hollar, C.M.; Ng-Kwai-Hang, K.F.; Swaisgood, H.E. Nomenclature of the Proteins of Cows & Milk; Sixth Revision. *J. Dairy Sci.* **2004**, *87*, 1641–1674. [CrossRef]
33. He, M.; Sun, J.; Jiang, Z.Q.; Yang, Y.X. Effects of Cow's Milk Beta-Casein Variants on Symptoms of Milk Intolerance in Chinese Adults: A Multicentre, Randomised Controlled Study. *Nutr. J.* **2017**, *16*, 72. [CrossRef]
34. Milan, A.M.; Shrestha, A.; Karlström, H.J.; Martinsson, J.A.; Nilsson, N.J.; Perry, J.K.; Day, L.; Barnett, M.P.G.; Cameron-Smith, D. Comparison of the Impact of Bovine Milk β-Casein Variants on Digestive Comfort in Females Self-Reporting Dairy Intolerance: A Randomized Controlled Trial. *Am. J. Clin. Nutr.* **2020**, *111*, 149–160. [CrossRef] [PubMed]
35. Mirghafourvand, M.; Homayouni Rad, A.; Mohammad Alizadeh Charandabi, S.; Fardiazar, Z.; Shokri, K. The Effect of Probiotic Yogurt on Constipation in Pregnant Women: A Randomized Controlled Clinical Trial. *Iran. Red Crescent Med. J.* **2016**, *18*, e39870. [CrossRef] [PubMed]
36. Turan, İ.; Dedeli, Ö.; Bor, S.; İlter, T. Effects of a Kefir Supplement on Symptoms, Colonic Transit, and Bowel Satisfaction Score in Patients with Chronic Constipation: A Pilot Study. *Turk. J. Gastroenterol.* **2014**, *25*, 650–656. [CrossRef] [PubMed]
37. Sieri, S.; Agnoli, C.; Pala, V.; Mattiello, A.; Panico, S.; Masala, G.; Assedi, M.; Tumino, R.; Frasca, G.; Sacerdote, C.; et al. Dietary Habits and Cancer: The Experience of EPIC-Italy. *Epidemiol. Prev.* **2015**, *39*, 333–338.
38. Hu, T.; Li, F.L.; Shen, J.; Zhang, L.; Cho, H.C. Chronic Inflammation and Colorectal Cancer: The Role of Vascular Endothelial Growth Factor. *Curr. Pharm. Des.* **2015**, *21*, 2960–2967. [CrossRef]
39. Veiga, P.; Gallini, C.A.; Beal, C.; Michaud, M.; Delaney, M.L.; DuBois, A.; Khlebnikov, A.; van Hylckama Vlieg, J.E.T.; Punit, S.; Glickman, J.N.; et al. Bifidobacterium Animalis Subsp. Lactis Fermented Milk Product Reduces Inflammation by Altering a Niche for Colitogenic Microbes. *Proc. Natl. Acad. Sci. USA* **2010**, *107*, 18132–18137. [CrossRef] [PubMed]
40. Qian, Z.R.; Rubinson, D.A.; Nowak, J.A.; Morales-Oyarvide, V.; Dunne, R.F.; Kozak, M.M.; Welch, M.W.; Brais, L.K.; Da Silva, A.; Li, T.; et al. Association of Alterations in Main Driver Genes With Outcomes of Patients With Resected Pancreatic Ductal Adenocarcinoma. *JAMA Oncol.* **2018**, *4*, e173420. [CrossRef]
41. Matsumoto, S.; Hara, T.; Nagaoka, M.; Mike, A.; Mitsuyama, K.; Sako, T.; Yamamoto, M.; Kado, S.; Takada, T. A Component of Polysaccharide Peptidoglycan Complex on Lactobacillus Induced an Improvement of Murine Model of Inflammatory Bowel Disease and Colitis-Associated Cancer. *Immunology* **2009**, *128*, e170–e180. [CrossRef]
42. Lao, L.; Yang, G.; Zhang, A.; Liu, L.; Guo, Y.; Lian, L.; Pan, D.; Wu, Z. Anti-Inflammation and Gut Microbiota Regulation Properties of Fatty Acids Derived from Fermented Milk in Mice with Dextran Sulfate Sodium-Induced Colitis. *J. Dairy Sci.* **2022**, *105*, 7865–7877. [CrossRef] [PubMed]
43. Yoda, K.; Miyazawa, K.; Hosoda, M.; Hiramatsu, M.; Yan, F.; He, F. Lactobacillus GG-Fermented Milk Prevents DSS-Induced Colitis and Regulates Intestinal Epithelial Homeostasis through Activation of Epidermal Growth Factor Receptor. *Eur. J. Nutr.* **2014**, *53*, 105–115. [CrossRef] [PubMed]
44. Suzuki, T.; Masui, A.; Nakamura, J.; Shiozawa, H.; Aoki, J.; Nakae, H.; Tsuda, S.; Imai, J.; Hideki, O.; Matsushima, M.; et al. Yogurt Containing Lactobacillus Gasseri Mitigates Aspirin-Induced Small Bowel Injuries: A Prospective, Randomized, Double-Blind, Placebo-Controlled Trial. *Gastroenterologia* **2017**, *95*, 49–54. [CrossRef] [PubMed]
45. Comerford, K.B.; Miller, G.D.; Boileau, A.C.; Masiello Schuette, S.N.; Giddens, J.C.; Brown, K.A. Global Review of Dairy Recommendations in Food-Based Dietary Guidelines. *Front. Nutr.* **2021**, *8*, 671999. [CrossRef]

Disclaimer/Publisher's Note: The statements, opinions and data contained in all publications are solely those of the individual author(s) and contributor(s) and not of MDPI and/or the editor(s). MDPI and/or the editor(s) disclaim responsibility for any injury to people or property resulting from any ideas, methods, instructions or products referred to in the content.

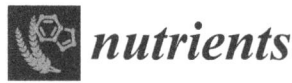

Article

The Role of Polyunsaturated Fatty Acids in Osteoarthritis: Insights from a Mendelian Randomization Study

Xuefei Li [1,†], Zhengjie Lu [2,†], Yongjian Qi [3], Biao Chen [2] and Bin Li [2,*]

[1] Department of Pathology, Union Hospital, Tongji Medical College, Huazhong University of Science and Technology, Wuhan 430022, China; lixfwurm@163.com
[2] Division of Joint Surgery and Sports Medicine, Department of Orthopedic Surgery, Zhongnan Hospital of Wuhan University, Wuhan 430071, China; chenbiao20030701@163.com (B.C.)
[3] Department of Spine Surgery and Musculoskeletal Tumor, Department of Orthopedic Surgery, Zhongnan Hospital of Wuhan University, Wuhan 430071, China
* Correspondence: libin16@whu.edu.cn
† These authors contributed equally to this work and shared first authorship.

Abstract: The prior observational research on the impact of polyunsaturated fatty acid (PUFA) supplementation on osteoarthritis (OA) patients had yielded inclusive outcomes. This study utilized the Mendelian randomization (MR) approach to explore potential causal relationships between PUFAs and OA. The MR study was performed using GWAS summary statistics for PUFAs, encompassing omega-3 and omega-6 fatty acids, and for knee OA (KOA) and hip OA (HOA). The primary inverse-variance-weighted (IVW) method and two supplementary MR approaches were used to establish robust causality. Heterogeneity and horizontal pleiotropy were assessed using Cochrane's Q and MR-Egger intercept tests. Additionally, a range of sensitivity analyses were conducted to strengthen the precision and reliability of the results. The IVW method indicated a potential genetic association between omega-3 fatty acids and KOA risk (odd ratio (OR) = 0.94, 95% confidence interval (CI): 0.89–1.00, p = 0.048). No significant correlation was found between omega-3 levels and HOA. Moreover, genetically predicted higher levels of omega-6 fatty acids were associated with a decreased risk of KOA (OR = 0.93, 95% CI: 0.86–1.00, p = 0.041) and HOA (OR = 0.89, 95% CI: 0.82–0.96, p = 0.003). The MR-Egger intercept evaluation showed no horizontal pleiotropy affecting the MR analysis (all p > 0.05). Our findings supported the causal relationship between PUFAs and OA susceptibility and offered a novel insight that high omega-6 fatty acids may reduce the risk of KOA and HOA. These results underscore the importance of maintaining optimal levels of PUFAs, particularly omega-6 fatty acids, in individuals with a genetic predisposition to OA. Future research is necessary to validate these findings and elucidate the underlying mechanisms involved.

Keywords: polyunsaturated fatty acids; omega-3 fatty acids; omega-6 fatty acids; osteoarthritis; Mendelian randomization

Citation: Li, X.; Lu, Z.; Qi, Y.; Chen, B.; Li, B. The Role of Polyunsaturated Fatty Acids in Osteoarthritis: Insights from a Mendelian Randomization Study. *Nutrients* 2023, 15, 4787. https://doi.org/10.3390/nu15224787

Academic Editors: Maria Luz Fernandez and Tyler Barker

Received: 27 September 2023
Revised: 4 November 2023
Accepted: 13 November 2023
Published: 15 November 2023

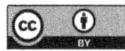

Copyright: © 2023 by the authors. Licensee MDPI, Basel, Switzerland. This article is an open access article distributed under the terms and conditions of the Creative Commons Attribution (CC BY) license (https://creativecommons.org/licenses/by/4.0/).

1. Introduction

Osteoarthritis (OA), a chronic degenerative joint disease, primarily targets the knee and hip joints. The global prevalence of this condition is estimated to exceed 500 million individuals, accounting for approximately 7% of the world's population [1]. Projections by the United Nations suggest that this percentage is expected to rise to 15–20% by the year 2050 [2]. In light of the high occurrence of OA, the search for effective treatments beyond end-stage surgeries such as total joint arthroplasty continues. Additionally, the increasing expenses related to surgical interventions [3] and the significant impact of OA on individuals, economies, and societies mean that it is imperative to investigate alternative and complementary strategies that can alleviate symptoms and improve functional outcomes. While various medications have been employed in OA patients with an improved understanding of its pathogenesis, none have demonstrated significant efficacy in symptom relief [4,5]. Given these medications' potential long-term adverse effects in OA patients, there is a pressing need to identify alternative therapeutic agents.

Nutritional interventions targeting osteoarthritis (OA) have gained attention, as including anti-inflammatory nutrients holds potential benefits [6]. Polyunsaturated fatty acids (PUFAs), including omega-3 and omega-6 fatty acids, are obtained from various sources and can be incorporated into routine diet to maintain health. Omega-3 fatty acids, abundant in fatty fish, seafood, cereals, seeds, nuts, and vegetables, are widely consumed; however, Western diets are rich in omega-6 fatty acids [7]. Omega-3 fatty acids have demonstrated efficacy in benefiting OA patients [8]. Conversely, omega-6 fatty acids were previously believed to stimulate the secretion of pro-inflammatory cytokines [9]. These two pivotal nutritional bioactive compounds are often regarded as having divergent physiological functions [10]. However, the results of previous randomized controlled trials (RCTs) assessing the efficacy of omega-3 fatty acid supplementation in individuals with OA have shown inconsistent findings. While certain studies have indicated that additional supplementation of omega-3 fatty acids may alleviate arthritis pain in individuals with OA [11–13], others have not corroborated these findings [14,15]. Notably, no RCTs to date have examined the impact of omega-6 fatty acids on OA.

As an alternative research method, Mendelian randomization (MR) has emerged as a valuable analytical approach that utilizes genetic variants, specifically single-nucleotide polymorphisms (SNPs), as instrumental variables to emulate the random allocation commonly seen in randomized controlled trials (RCTs) [16,17]. In situations where reliable RCTs are lacking, or initiating new RCTs may be impractical, MR serves as an ideal strategy to elucidate causal relationships between exposures and outcomes [18]. Moreover, MR effectively avoids reverse causality, as the formation of genotypes precedes disease onset and remains unaffected by disease progression [19,20]. Notably, to our knowledge, no MR studies have been conducted to explore the relationship between PUFAs and OA. Therefore, this study employed the MR method to investigate potential causal associations between PUFAs and the risk of developing OA. We aimed for the outcomes of this investigation to enhance our comprehension of the underlying pathophysiology of OA and offer substantial evidence for establishing effective treatment and prevention strategies in clinical practice.

2. Materials and Methods

2.1. Study Design

In this study, we employed an MR approach utilizing summary statistics derived from genome-wide association studies (GWASs) to examine the associations between polyunsaturated fatty acids (PUFAs), specifically omega-3 fatty acids and omega-6 fatty acids, and osteoarthritis (OA), including knee OA (KOA) and hip OA (HOA). To ensure the robustness of our MR analysis, we adhered to three fundamental assumptions: (i) the selected genetic variants should exhibit significant associations with the exposure of interest; (ii) the genetic variants employed should not exert any influence on the outcome, except through the chosen exposure; and (iii) the genetic variants should not be correlated with any confounding factors that may impact the relationship between the exposure and the outcome. The detailed study design is illustrated in Figure 1.

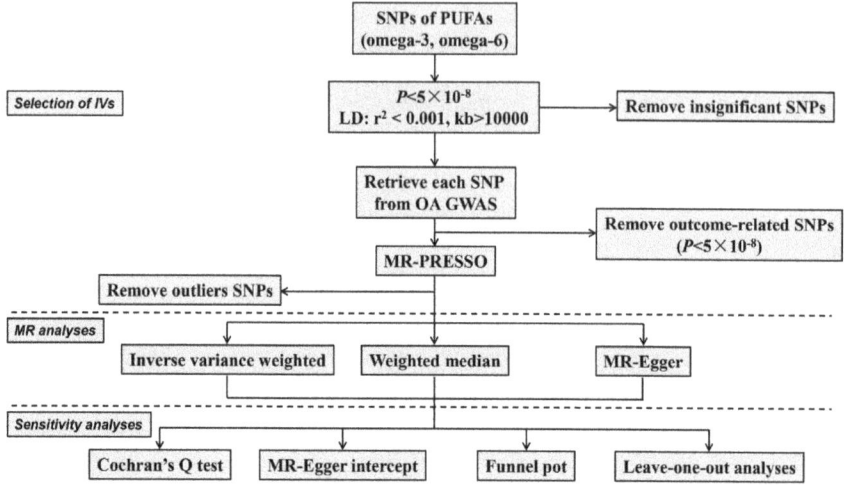

Figure 1. Study flame chart of the MR study evaluating the causality between PUFAs and osteoarthritis. SNPs, single-nucleotide polymorphisms; PUFAs, polyunsaturated fatty acids; IVs, instrumental variables; LD, linkage disequilibrium; OA, osteoarthritis; IVW, inverse-variance-weighted; GWAS, genome-wide association study; MR, Mendelian randomization.

2.2. Data Sources

The SNP summary data associated with polyunsaturated fatty acids (PUFAs) were obtained from the Nightingale Health UK Biobank Initiative, which provided access to information on both omega-3 and omega-6 fatty acids for our investigation [20]. The genetic instrumental variables for omega-3 and omega-6 were sourced from the Metabolic Biomarkers in the UK Biobank study—the GWAS associated with omega-3 and omega-6 fatty acids involved 114,999 European individuals [20]. The UK Biobank initiative aims to explore the genetic and environmental factors contributing to disease, with a participant pool of over 500,000 individuals of European descent. For this project, the circulating concentrations of omega-3 and omega-6 fatty acids were assessed in randomly selected EDTA plasma samples using a targeted high-throughput nuclear magnetic resonance (NMR) metabolomics platform provided by Nightingale Health Ltd. The initial sample collection comprised 121,577 samples, with duplicates and observations not meeting the quality control criteria in the non-fasting plasma samples collected at baseline being excluded. This platform's measurement technology and applications for epidemiological studies have been previously evaluated [21,22].

Summary-level data for the SNP associated with KOA and HOA were obtained from the UK Biobank study [23]. The datasets of KOA and HOA comprised many individuals of European ancestry, respectively, including 403,124 individuals and 393,873 individuals. The OA cases were sourced from the Arthritis Research UK Osteoarthritis Genetics (arcOGEN) project, which comprises unrelated individuals of European descent with knee or hip osteoarthritis from the arcOGEN Consortium. These cases were identified based on either clinical evidence of disease necessitating joint replacement or radiographic evidence of disease with a Kellgren–Lawrence grade of 2 or higher. The controls were obtained from the United Kingdom Household Longitudinal Study (UKHLS), a longitudinal panel survey representing 40,000 households across England, Scotland, Wales, and Northern Ireland and representative of the UK population. The genetic associations between polyunsaturated fatty acids (PUFAs) and OA are presented in Table 1.

Table 1. Details of the GWAS summary-level data.

Trait	Dataset	Sample Size	GWAS ID	Population
Omega-3	UK Biobank	114,999	met-d-Omega_3	European
Omega-6	UK Biobank	114,999	met-d-Omega_6	European
KOA	UK Biobank	403,124	ebi-a-GCST007090	European
HOA	UK Biobank	393,873	ebi-a-GCST007091	European

GWAS, genome-wide association study; KOA, knee osteoarthritis; HOA, hip osteoarthritis.

2.3. Selection of Instrumental Variables (IVs)

When selecting IVs for our MR analysis, we strictly followed three well-established assumptions: (i) IVs should exhibit strong associations with the exposure of interest; (ii) IVs should be independent of any confounding factors; and (iii) IVs should solely influence the outcomes through the chosen exposure, without having any direct associations with the outcomes themselves [24]. We first applied a genome-wide significance threshold ($p < 5 \times 10^{-8}$) to initiate the IV screening process for our MR study. Subsequently, we implemented SNP pruning within a window size of 10,000 kb, ensuring that the linkage disequilibrium (LD) between SNPs remained below the threshold of $r^2 < 0.001$. Furthermore, the selected SNPs related to Omega-3 and Omega-6 fatty acids were retrieved from the GWAS data of the outcomes (KOA and HOA), and any SNPs significantly associated with the outcomes ($p < 5 \times 10^{-8}$) were excluded. In addition, we carefully assessed the IVs selected through the above process for any indications of weak instrument bias by using the F-statistic [25,26]. To mitigate bias stemming from weak IVs, we exclusively retained IVs with an F value surpassing 10, while those with an F value of less than 10 were discarded due to weak instrument bias [27].

2.4. MR Analysis

The causal effects of PUFAs (omega-3 and omega-6 fatty acids) on knee and hip OA were systematically examined using the R package TwoSample MR (version 0.5.7), adhering to established methodologies [28]. The primary technique for estimating causal effects was the random-effects inverse-variance weighted (IVW) method [29]. Alongside the IVW method, we utilized two additional MR methods (MR-Egger and weighted median) to evaluate causal associations. The IVW method operates under the assumption that all SNPs included in the analysis are valid instrumental variables [30]. The weighted median approach presupposes that a minimum of 50% of genetic variants are valid, satisfying the three fundamental assumptions. It is applicable in situations where the majority of IVs do not demonstrate horizontal pleiotropy [31]. In contrast, the MR-Egger regression method assumes that more than 50% of genetic variants are invalid (do not adhere to the three fundamental assumptions), which may result in a slightly lower estimation accuracy being achieved with this approach [32,33]. The MR estimates were presented as beta or odds ratios (ORs) with 95% confidence intervals (CIs). The Bonferroni correction is a method for selecting a threshold p-value due to the assumption that every variant tested is independent of the rest. The statistical calculation via the Bonferroni correction method is $p = 0.05/$(number of exposures $\times$ number of outcomes), widely used to evaluate the significance of causal relationship between exposures and outcomes in MR studies [34–36]. To account for multiple tests in our MR study, we applied a Bonferroni correction with 4 tests, setting a significance threshold of $p < 0.0125$ ($0.05/2 \times 2$).

Significant associations ($p < 0.05$) before but not after Bonferroni correction ($p < 0.005$) were considered as suggestive association results [24]. If the IVW method result is significant and no pleiotropy is detected, despite the insignificant results of other methods, it can be considered a positive result, provided that the beta values of the other methods are in the same direction [37].

We conducted a series of sensitivity analyses in our study, including Cochran's Q test, MR-Egger intercept, funnel plots, and leave-one-out analyses, so as to explore potential heterogeneity and pleiotropy and ensure the robustness of the results. Heterogeneity was assessed via implementing IVW and MR-Egger regressions, with Cochran's Q statistic utilized for evaluation [38]. If the p values of Cochran's Q test for IVW and MR-Egger are greater than 0.05, it does not indicate significant heterogeneity. To ascertain the absence of pleiotropy in our MR results, we examined the intercept in the MR-Egger regression, with a p value exceeding 0.05, indicating no presence of pleiotropy [39]. To evaluate directional pleiotropy, we visually analyzed MR-Egger intercepts and funnel plots. A leave-one-SNP-out analysis was conducted to further investigate causal relationships, to prevent the MR analysis results from being driven by a single SNP [40].

3. Results

3.1. Causal Effects of Omega-3 Fatty Acids on KOA and HOA

Figure 2 depicts the MR methods to ascertain the causal relationships between omega-3 fatty acids and OA. A total of 49 LD-independent and suitable IVs were chosen from GWASs for KOA and HOA (Supplementary Table S1). The primary IVW analysis suggested a potential association between omega-3 fatty acids and a reduced risk of KOA (p = 0.048). A 1 SD increase in omega-3 fatty acids corresponded to an OR and 95% (CI) for KOA of OR = 0.94 (95% CI: 0.89–1.00). However, other MR methods, including MR-Egger (OR = 0.99, 95% CI: 0.91–1.09; p = 0.887) and weighted median (OR = 0.94, 95% CI: 0.87–1.01; p = 0.092), indicated a consistent but non-significant direction (Figure 2). Given the significant results of the IVW and the consistent direction of beta values from other methods, this can be interpreted as a positive result [22,37]. Consequently, omega-3 fatty acids were deemed to have a causal association with a decreased risk of KOA. However, no significant associations were observed between omega-3 fatty acids and HOA risk (p = 0.051).

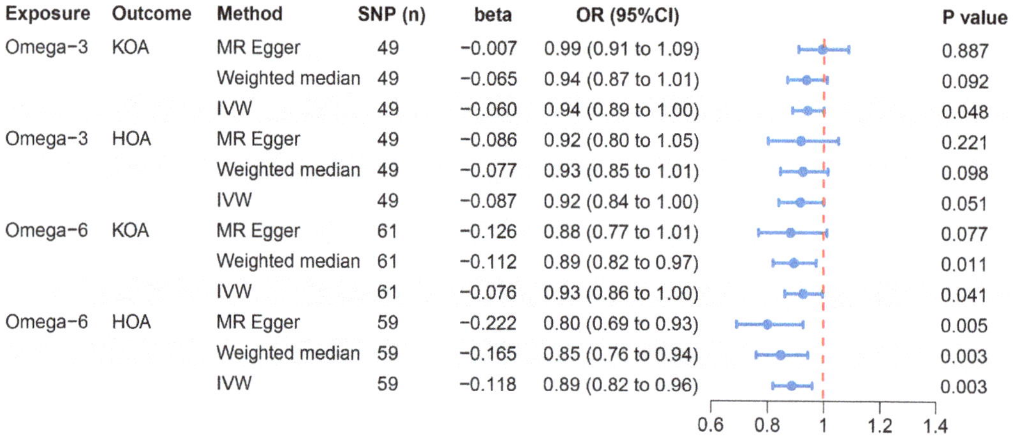

Exposure	Outcome	Method	SNP (n)	beta	OR (95%CI)	P value
Omega-3	KOA	MR Egger	49	−0.007	0.99 (0.91 to 1.09)	0.887
		Weighted median	49	−0.065	0.94 (0.87 to 1.01)	0.092
		IVW	49	−0.060	0.94 (0.89 to 1.00)	0.048
Omega-3	HOA	MR Egger	49	−0.086	0.92 (0.80 to 1.05)	0.221
		Weighted median	49	−0.077	0.93 (0.85 to 1.01)	0.098
		IVW	49	−0.087	0.92 (0.84 to 1.00)	0.051
Omega-6	KOA	MR Egger	61	−0.126	0.88 (0.77 to 1.01)	0.077
		Weighted median	61	−0.112	0.89 (0.82 to 0.97)	0.011
		IVW	61	−0.076	0.93 (0.86 to 1.00)	0.041
Omega-6	HOA	MR Egger	59	−0.222	0.80 (0.69 to 0.93)	0.005
		Weighted median	59	−0.165	0.85 (0.76 to 0.94)	0.003
		IVW	59	−0.118	0.89 (0.82 to 0.96)	0.003

Figure 2. Estimation of the causal relationship between PUFAs and OA using different MR methods. SNPs, single-nucleotide polymorphisms; KOA, knee osteoarthritis; HOA, hip osteoarthritis; IVW, inverse-variance-weighted; PUFAs, polyunsaturated fatty acids; MR, Mendelian randomization.

MR-Egger regression and IVW analyses were conducted to assess heterogeneity. Heterogeneity was observed in the MR analyses of omega-3 fatty acids for KOA (MR-Egger: p = 0.009; IVW: p = 0.005) and HOA (MR-Egger: p = 1.498 × 10^{-6}; IVW: p = 2.304 × 10^{-6}) (Table 2). Given the heterogeneity, using random-effects IVW estimation was appropriate in evaluating causality under these circumstances [41]. Nevertheless, the IVW results consistently supported the causal relationship between omega-3 fatty acids and KOA risk (Figure 2). Additionally, the MR-Egger intercept tests indicated no horizontal pleiotropy in any of the analyses, as all p values exceeded 0.05 (Table 2). The scatter plot illustrated the estimated impact of SNPs on omega-3 fatty acids and KOA/HOA (Figure 3A,B). Furthermore, the leave-one-out analysis demonstrated that no outlier instrumental variables significantly influenced the overall results (Figure 4A,B). The funnel plot of the omega-3 fatty acids and KOA/HOA analysis indicated no apparent horizontal pleiotropy, as the variation in effect size around the point estimate was symmetrical (Figure 5A,B).

Table 2. Heterogeneity and pleiotropy test of MR studies.

Exposure	Outcome	MR-Egger (p Value)	IVW (p Value)	MR-Egger Intercept (p Value)
Omega-3	KOA	0.009	0.005	0.131
Omega-3	HOA	1.498×10^{-6}	2.304×10^{-6}	0.979
Omega-6	KOA	5.993×10^{-5}	6.037×10^{-5}	0.404
Omega-6	HOA	0.052	0.035	0.110

MR, Mendelian randomization; KOA, knee osteoarthritis; HOA, hip osteoarthritis; IVW, inverse-variance-weighted.

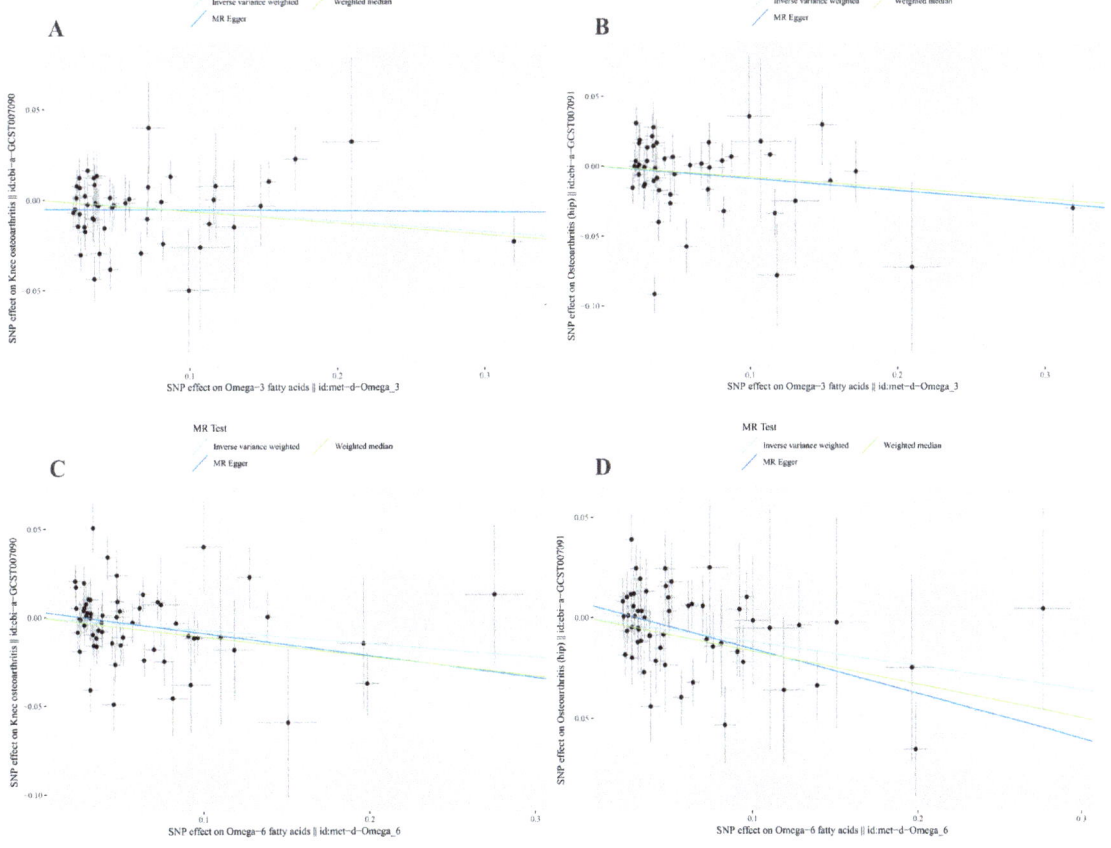

Figure 3. Scatter plots of genetic correlations of omega-3/omega-6 fatty acids and KOA/HOA using different MR methods. (**A**) Scatter plot of genetic correlations of omega-3 fatty acids with KOA. (**B**) Scatter plot of genetic correlations of omega-3 fatty acids with HOA. (**C**) Scatter plot of genetic correlations of omega-6 fatty acids with KOA. (**D**) Scatter plot of genetic correlations of omega-6 fatty acids with HOA. SNPs, single-nucleotide polymorphisms; KOA, knee osteoarthritis; HOA, hip osteoarthritis; MR, Mendelian randomization.

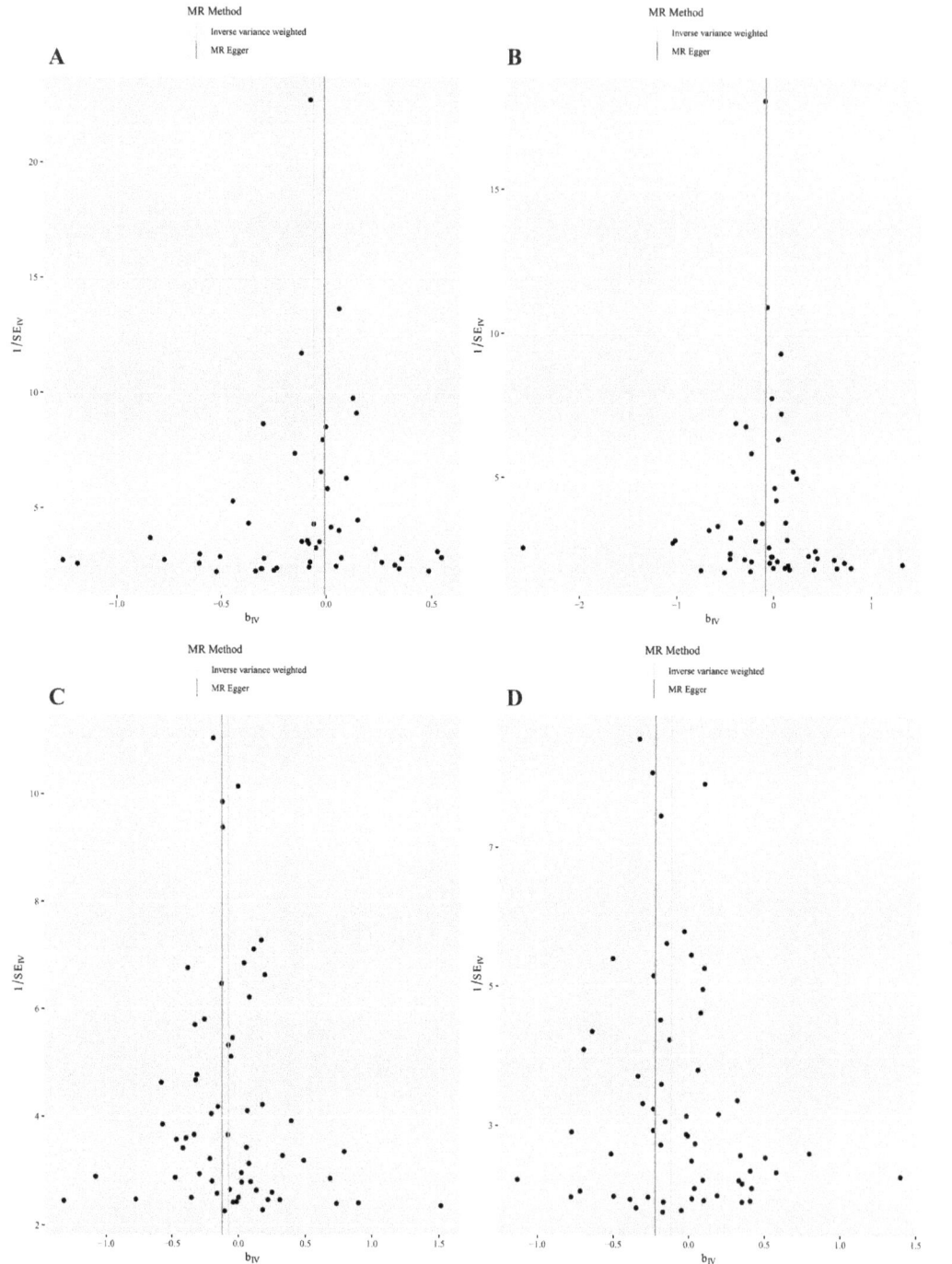

Figure 4. Funnel plots of SNPs associated with omega-3/omega-6 fatty acids and KOA/HOA. (**A**) Funnel plot for omega-3 fatty acids with KOA. (**B**) Funnel plot for omega-3 fatty acids with HOA. (**C**) Funnel plot for omega-6 fatty acids with KOA. (**D**) Funnel plot for omega-6 fatty acids with HOA. SNPs, single-nucleotide polymorphisms; KOA, knee osteoarthritis; HOA, hip osteoarthritis.

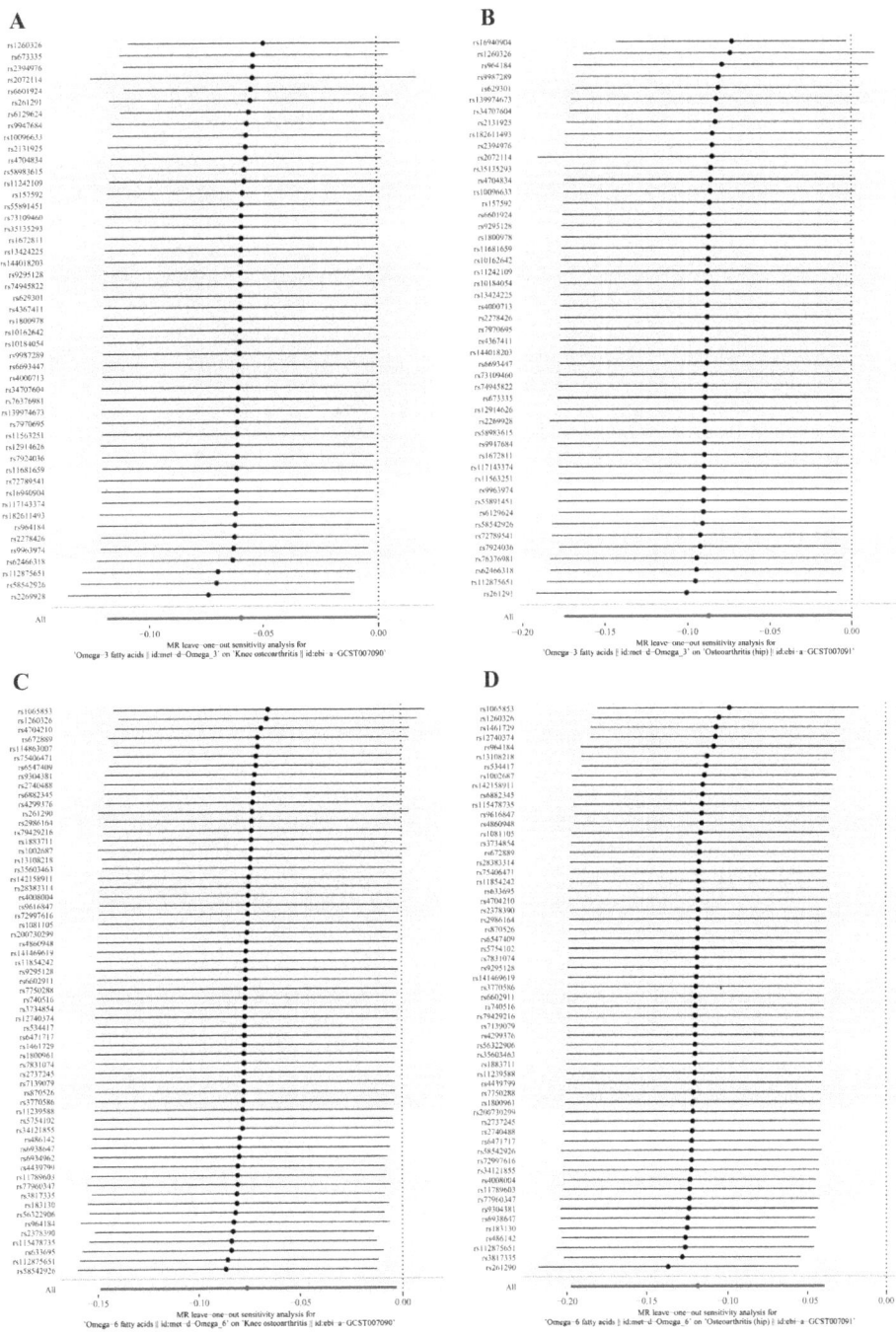

Figure 5. Leave-one-out plots to visualize the causal effects of omega-3/omega-6 fatty acids on KOA/HOA. (**A**) Leave-one-out analysis for omega-3 fatty acids with KOA. (**B**) Leave-one-out analysis for omega-3 fatty acids with HOA. (**C**) Leave-one-out analysis for omega-6 fatty acids with KOA. (**D**) Leave-one-out analysis for omega-6 fatty acids with HOA. KOA, knee osteoarthritis; HOA, hip osteoarthritis.

3.2. Causal Effects of Omega-6 on KOA and HOA

Figure 2 depicts the MR analyses examining the causal relationships between omega-6 fatty acids and OA risk. In total, 61 and 59 LD-independent and suitable IVs were chosen from GWASs for KOA and HOA (Supplementary Tables S2 and S3). The IVW method suggested that genetically predicted omega-6 fatty acids might be associated with a reduced risk of KOA (OR = 0.93, 95% CI: 0.86–1.00; p = 0.041). The weighted median analysis yielded similar significant results (OR = 0.89, 95% CI: 0.82–0.97; p = 0.011), while the MR-Egger analysis showed consistent but non-significant results (OR = 0.88, 95% CI: 0.77–1.01; p = 0.077). Given the significant results of the IVW and the consistent direction of beta values from the other two methods [22,37], these findings suggest that omega-3 fatty acids may have a causal association with a decreased risk of KOA. Simultaneously, our IVW method provided evidence of genetically predicted omega-6 fatty acids being associated with a reduced risk of HOA (OR = 0.89, 95% CI: 0.82–0.96; p = 0.003). Significant results were observed using both the MR-Egger (OR = 0.80, 95% CI: 0.69–0.93; p = 0.005) and weighted median (OR = 0.85, 95% CI: 0.76–0.94; p = 0.003) methods, aligning with the findings obtained through the IVW approach.

Considering the potential heterogeneity observed in the MR analyses of omega-6 for KOA (MR-Egger: $p = 5.993 \times 10^{-5}$; IVW: $p = 6.037 \times 10^{-5}$) and HOA (MR-Egger: $p = 0.052$; IVW: $p = 0.035$) (Table 2), we employed the random-effects IVW method to further support the causal relationship between omega-6 and KOA/HOA (Figure 2). No evidence of horizontal pleiotropy was found in this analysis, as indicated by both intercepts having p values greater than 0.05 (Table 2). The scatter plots displaying the individual causal estimates were presented (Figure 3C,D). The results remained consistent even after removing one SNP, as shown by the leave-one-out test (Figure 4C,D). The funnel plots illustrated the analyses of omega-6 and KOA/HOA (Figure 5C,D).

4. Discussion

In this MR study, we employed extensive GWAS summary data to examine the potential causal association between PUFAs and the risk of OA in individuals of European ancestry. Our analysis involved a sizable cohort of individuals with European heritage, comprising 114,999 individuals for PUFAs and OA, 450,243 individuals for KOA, and 256,523 individuals for HOA. The findings demonstrated that genetically predicted omega-3 fatty acids were linked to a decreased risk of KOA, while no significant association was observed with HOA. Furthermore, our results revealed an innovative association between genetically predicted omega-6 fatty acids and a decreased risk of both KOA and HOA. Significantly, this study endeavours to investigate the causal association between PUFAs and OA risk using an MR method. By elucidating the impact of PUFAs on OA risk, our findings effectively bridge a critical research gap and present promising prospects for personalized treatment strategies.

Omega-3 fatty acids encompass alpha linolenic acid (ALA), eicosapentaenoic acid (EPA), and docosahexaenoic acid (DHA). ALA is primarily sourced from flaxseed oil, tahini, certain nuts, and seeds, while EPA and DHA are predominantly present in oily marine fish and certain seaweed. Unlike plant cells, the human body lacks the necessary enzymes to synthesize ALA, making dietary intake the sole means of obtaining this fatty acid. However, the accumulation of ALA at significant levels is uncommon, even when consumed in relatively high dietary quantities. This limited accumulation is primarily attributed to the β-oxidation of dietary ALA within the mitochondria hampering its conversion to EPA and DHA, which occurs at a minimal rate of less than 1% [42,43]. The level of EPA and DHA in the tissues and cells can be increased through their direct dietary consumption. Therefore, omega-3 fatty acids, mainly referring to EPA and DHA, should be consumed in the diet from fish oil or functional foods fortified with them [44]. Omega-3 fatty acids have been proposed as potential therapeutic agents for individuals with OA due to their ability to mitigate the systemic inflammatory response and create an environment that counteracts cartilage degradation [8]. However, previous observational studies investigating the efficacy of omega-3 fatty acids in OA patients have produced inconsistent outcomes. In one study, 86 participants diagnosed with OA were randomly allocated to receive either a cod liver oil supplement (786 mg EPA) or a placebo (olive oil) in conjunction with their existing non-steroidal anti-inflammatory drug regimen for 24 weeks. The utilization of cod liver oil did not yield significant differences in reported pain or disability compared to the placebo group [45]. Similarly, another study revealed that omega-3 fatty acids did not substantially improve functional scores [14]. Additionally, an early meta-analysis suggested that marine oil supplementation with a high content of EPA and DHA could potentially alleviate arthritis-related pain. However, it is worth noting that most of the studies included in the analysis focused on patients with rheumatoid arthritis. When subgroup analysis was conducted on five studies involving individuals with OA, the potential effectiveness of marine oil in managing arthritis pain was not substantiated [46].

Nevertheless, there is also substantiated evidence supporting the utilization of omega-3 fatty acids in the management of OA. One RCT trial that enrolled 202 patients indicated that low-dose fish oil containing EPA and DHA led to greater improvement in pain and function scores in KOA at 2 years [47]. Recently, Stonehouse et al. reported that krill oil containing EPA and DHA could improve pain, stiffness, and physical function for individuals with mild-to-moderate KOA [12]. Moreover, a recent systematic review and meta-analysis, encompassing data from nine RCTs involving 2070 individuals with OA, demonstrated that supplementation with omega-3 fatty acids resulted in a significant reduction in arthritis pain and improvement in joint function [48]. Our study outcomes establish a causal association between omega-3 fatty acids and the risk of KOA, consistent with recent meta-analysis findings [48]. The potential mechanisms underlying the beneficial effects of omega-3 fatty acids on KOA are multifactorial, which might include the inhibition of inflammatory markers such as interleukin-1 beta (IL-1β) and inducible nitric oxide synthase (iNOS), the suppression of metalloproteinase 13 expression and chondrocyte apoptosis, and the restraining of bone remodelling and vessel formation within the osteochondral unit [46,49,50]. It is imperative to acknowledge that EPA and DHA exhibit distinct effects. EPA can convert into DHA within the liver and primarily functions to reduce cellular inflammation. It exerts anti-inflammatory actions by inhibiting the enzyme delta-5-desaturase (D5D), responsible for synthesizing arachidonic acid (AA), an omega-6 fatty acid known to mediate cellular inflammation. Moreover, EPA competes with AA for the enzyme phospholipase A2, essential for liberating AA from membrane phospholipids. This synergetic interaction aids in diminishing the generation of inflammatory eicosanoids [44]. Nevertheless, the literature on the optimal concentration ratio of EPA and DHA for individuals with OA is still limited. Further research in this domain is warranted.

Omega-6 fatty acids mainly comprise AA and linoleic acid (LA). AA is a precursor to various potent pro-inflammatory mediators, such as prostaglandins and leukotrienes, which have been extensively studied. Biochemically, AA derived from LA leads to the production of pro-inflammatory molecules. Consequently, an increased intake of omega-6 fatty acids, either AA or its precursor LA, is widely believed to promote inflammation [51]. However, the human studies available to date do not support this assumption. This discrepancy may be attributed to the previously mentioned low in vivo conversion rate of dietary LA to AA [52]. Moreover, the available data essentially refute the idea that high intakes of omega-6 fatty acids result in systemic inflammation. A notable example is a cross-sectional study that scrutinized the dietary levels of PUFAs in 364 individuals with confirmed cardiovascular disease. The findings revealed that omega-6 fatty acids had an inverse association with c-reactive protein (CRP) levels and IL-1β [53]. Another epidemiological study reported that individuals in the highest quintiles of omega-6 fatty acids exhibited lower concentrations of CRP and reduced incidences of cardiovascular disease, cancer, and all-cause mortality [54]. Several additional studies have consistently showcased an inverse correlation between circulating levels of omega-6 fatty acids and inflammatory biomarkers [55–57]. A comprehensive meta-analysis concluded that randomized controlled intervention studies fail to furnish evidence supporting a causal link between heightened consumption of LA and elevated concentrations of inflammatory markers [58]. Up to date, no RCTs or MR studies have been undertaken to elucidate the impact of omega-6 fatty acids on susceptibility to OA. Our study effectively addressed this research void by presenting compelling evidence of the advantageous effects of omega-6 fatty acids on KOA and HOA. It has been reported that some oxylipins produced by AA exhibit pro-inflammatory properties, while other eicosanoids derived from AA show anti-inflammatory activities [51]. However, the administration of AA (which is challenging due to its limited availability) at relatively high doses has not altered circulating inflammation biomarkers, at least in healthy volunteers [59,60]. Hence, these beneficial effects of omega-6 fatty acids might be attributed to the inherent anti-inflammatory properties associated with LA [52]. One intervention trial showed that an increased intake of LA does not increase circulating concentrations of AA and AA-derived lipid mediators [61]. Therefore, the supplementation of LA may be a more practical and promising strategy in the future.

The implications of these findings are of significant clinical importance. Our results unequivocally demonstrate that maintaining optimal levels of PUFAs, specifically omega-6 fatty acids, may effectively mitigate the risk of both KOA and HOA. These findings align with the outcomes of a prospective study, wherein 2029 participants diagnosed with KOA exhibited less joint space loss over 4 years when they consumed higher quantities of PUFAs [62]. Consequently, healthcare professionals may consider an augmented intake of PUFA-rich foods or supplements for individuals afflicted with OA, particularly those with a genetic predisposition. However, it is essential to note that a global study has reported suboptimal omega-6 fatty acids intake worldwide [63]. According to the Global Burden of Disease 2017 group, a lack of adequate dietary intake of omega-6 fatty acids is considered one of the critical factors associated with diet-related cardiovascular disease [64]. Given that nutritional recommendations and guidelines play a crucial role in shaping health policies, it is essential to carefully analyze and evaluate the quantity and quality of dietary fats within the context of a healthy diet. Seed oils, mainly vegetable oils, are rich sources of omega-6 fatty acids, with LA comprising more than 50% of their lipid content. Other significant sources of LA include nuts, while lower levels can be found in whole grains, legumes, non-ruminant meats, eggs, and dairy products [52]. The recommended limits for total and saturated fat intake, as established by authoritative societies, typically fall below 30–35% and 10% of the total energy, respectively. The recommended intake for total PUFAs, including omega-3 and omega-6 fatty acids, typically falls within 5% to 10% of energy intake. However, recommendations for omega-6 fatty acids, especially LA, are less consistent across societies, with most suggesting intakes between 2.5% and 5% of total energy [52]. Nonetheless, it is vital to conduct further research to substantiate the clinical viability of these recommendations.

This MR research features four major noteworthy strengths. Firstly, this study employed genetic variants as IVs to evaluate the causal impacts of PUFAs (omega-3 and omega-6 fatty acids) on the risk of knee and hip OA. Through the utilization of the MR approach, concerns regarding confounding factors and reverse causation, commonly encountered in conventional observational investigations, were mitigated to the greatest extent. Secondly, the study made use of large-scale genomic data obtained from the UK Biobank, thereby bolstering the universality and robustness of our innovative discoveries. Thirdly, the utilization of publicly accessible datasets and open-source software in this study contributes to the transparency and repeatability of our MR research. Lastly, the MR analysis strategy facilitates the estimation of causal effect sizes, which carries both theoretical and practical implications for sensible clinical or public health decision making.

Several considerations should be acknowledged regarding our study. Firstly, it is worth noting that the dataset utilized in our GWAS analysis solely consisted of individuals of European descent. Consequently, the generalizability of our findings to other ethnic groups is limited, hindering the exploration of cultural diversity. Secondly, heterogeneity was observed in our results. However, we effectively addressed this issue by employing the random-effect IVW method as our primary analytical approach, successfully controlling for pooled heterogeneity. Thirdly, it is essential to highlight that, due to the constraints imposed by GWAS summary data, a stratified analysis based on crucial factors such as age and gender could not be conducted. Therefore, future studies should encompass more extensive and diverse populations, incorporating individuals with varied ancestries and cultural backgrounds. Additionally, these studies should adopt a combination of observational and genetic approaches to further investigate the causal effects of PUFAs on OA, while concurrently considering stratified factors, such as age and gender.

5. Conclusions

To sum up, our study has provided compelling evidence of a genetic causal relationship between PUFAs and OA risk, as demonstrated through the two-sample MR analysis. Specifically, our findings indicate that increased levels of omega-3 fatty acids were associated with a decreased risk of KOA. Intriguingly, our results challenged the traditional belief regarding the detrimental impact of omega-6 fatty acids on OA, as higher levels of omega-6 fatty acids decreased the risk of both KOA and HOA. These findings suggest that targeted dietary interventions aimed at modulating omega-6 fatty acid levels might serve as an effective preventive strategy for mitigating the burden of OA. However, it is essential to note that further research is indispensable to validate these findings, preferably through large-scale longitudinal studies or RCTs. Additionally, exploring the underlying mechanisms behind these observed associations could provide valuable insights into the pathogenesis of OA.

Supplementary Materials: The following supporting information can be downloaded at: https://www.mdpi.com/article/10.3390/nu15224787/s1, Table S1: Instrumental variables of Omega-3 fatty acids for knee osteoarthritis and hip osteoarthritis; Table S2: Instrumental variables of Omega-6 fatty acids for knee osteoarthritis; Table S3: Instrumental variables of Omega-6 fatty acids for hip osteoarthritis.

Author Contributions: X.L., B.C. and B.L. designed the study; X.L. conducted the analysis with help from Z.L., B.C. and Y.Q.; Z.L. and B.L. wrote the manuscript and had primary responsibility for the final content. All authors have read and agreed to the published version of the manuscript.

Funding: This work was supported by grants from the National Natural Science Foundation of China (No. 82304643, 82000324).

Institutional Review Board Statement: Not applicable.

Informed Consent Statement: Not applicable.

Data Availability Statement: The summary statistics used and/or analyzed in the current study are available from the corresponding authors upon reasonable request.

Acknowledgments: The authors thank all the investigators of UK Biobank for providing the data publicly.

Conflicts of Interest: The authors declare no conflict of interest.

References

1. Hunter, D.J.; March, L.; Chew, M. Osteoarthritis in 2020 and beyond: A lancet commission. *Lancet* **2020**, *396*, 1711–1712. [CrossRef] [PubMed]
2. Papathanasiou, I.; Anastasopoulou, L.; Tsezou, A. Cholesterol metabolism related genes in osteoarthritis. *Bone* **2021**, *152*, 116076. [CrossRef] [PubMed]
3. Delanois, R.E.; Mistry, J.B.; Gwam, C.U.; Mohamed, N.S.; Choksi, U.S.; Mont, M.A. Current epidemiology of revision total knee arthroplasty in the United States. *J. Arthroplast.* **2017**, *32*, 2663–2668. [CrossRef] [PubMed]
4. Kolasinski, S.L.; Neogi, T.; Hochberg, M.C.; Oatis, C.; Guyatt, G.; Block, J.; Callahan, L.; Copenhaver, C.; Dodge, C.; Felson, D.; et al. 2019 American college of rheumatology/arthritis foundation guideline for the management of osteoarthritis of the hand, hip, and knee. *Arthritis Rheumatol.* **2020**, *72*, 220–233. [CrossRef]
5. Bannuru, R.R.; Osani, M.C.; Vaysbrot, E.E.; Arden, N.K.; Bennell, K.; Bierma-Zeinstra, S.M.A.; Kraus, V.B.; Lohmander, L.S.; Abbott, J.H.; Bhandari, M.; et al. OARSI guidelines for the non-surgical management of knee, hip, and polyarticular osteoarthritis. *Osteoarthr. Cartil.* **2019**, *27*, 1578–1589. [CrossRef] [PubMed]

6. Mathieu, S.; Soubrier, M.; Peirs, C.; Monfoulet, L.E.; Boirie, Y.; Tournadre, A. A meta-analysis of the impact of nutritional supplementation on osteoarthritis symptoms. *Nutrients* **2022**, *14*, 1607. [CrossRef] [PubMed]
7. Cholewski, M.; Tomczykowa, M.; Tomczyk, M. A comprehensive review of chemistry, sources and bioavailability of omega-3 fatty acids. *Nutrients* **2018**, *10*, 1662. [CrossRef]
8. Cordingley, D.M.; Cornish, S.M. Omega-3 fatty acids for the management of osteoarthritis: A narrative review. *Nutrients* **2022**, *14*, 3362. [CrossRef]
9. Calder, P.C.; Grimble, R.F. Polyunsaturated fatty acids, inflammation and immunity. *Eur. J. Clin. Nutr.* **2002**, *56* (Suppl. S3), S14–S19. [CrossRef]
10. DiNicolantonio, J.J.; OKeefe, J. Importance of maintaining a low omega-6/omega-3 ratio for reducing platelet aggregation, coagulation and thrombosis. *Open Heart* **2019**, *6*, e001011. [CrossRef]
11. Jacquet, A.; Girodet, P.O.; Pariente, A.; Forest, K.; Mallet, L.; Moore, N. Phytalgic, a food supplement, vs placebo in patients with osteoarthritis of the knee or hip: A randomised double-blind placebo-controlled clinical trial. *Arthritis Res. Ther.* **2009**, *11*, R192. [CrossRef] [PubMed]
12. Stonehouse, W.; Benassi-Evans, B.; Bednarz, J.; Vincent, A.D.; Hall, S.; Hill, C.L. Krill oil improved osteoarthritic knee pain in adults with mild to moderate knee osteoarthritis: A 6-month multicenter, randomized, double-blind, placebo-controlled trial. *Am. J. Clin. Nutr.* **2022**, *116*, 672–685. [CrossRef]
13. Kuszewski, J.C.; Wong, R.H.X.; Howe, P.R.C. Fish oil supplementation reduces osteoarthritis-specific pain in older adults with overweight/obesity. *Rheumatol. Adv. Pract.* **2020**, *4*, rkaa036. [CrossRef] [PubMed]
14. Gruenwald, J.; Petzold, E.; Busch, R.; Petzold, H.P.; Graubaum, H.J. Effect of glucosamine sulfate with or without omega-3 fatty acids in patients with osteoarthritis. *Adv. Ther.* **2009**, *26*, 858–871. [CrossRef] [PubMed]
15. Stebbings, S.; Gray, A.; Schneiders, A.G.; Sansom, A. A randomized double-blind placebo-controlled trial to investigate the effectiveness and safety of a novel green-lipped mussel extract -BioLex(R) -for managing pain in moderate to severe osteoarthritis of the hip and knee. *BMC Complement. Altern. Med.* **2017**, *17*, 416. [CrossRef] [PubMed]
16. Holmes, M.V.; Ala-Korpela, M.; Smith, G.D. Mendelian randomization in cardiometabolic disease: Challenges in evaluating causality. *Nat. Rev. Cardiol.* **2017**, *14*, 577–590. [CrossRef]
17. Sekula, P.; Del Greco, M.F.; Pattaro, C.; Kottgen, A. Mendelian randomization as an approach to assess causality using observational data. *J. Am. Soc. Nephrol.* **2016**, *27*, 3253–3265. [CrossRef] [PubMed]
18. Burgess, S.; Small, D.S.; Thompson, S.G. A review of instrumental variable estimators for Mendelian randomization. *Stat. Metod. Med. Res.* **2017**, *26*, 2333–2355. [CrossRef]
19. Emdin, C.A.; Khera, A.V.; Kathiresan, S. Mendelian Randomization. *JAMA* **2017**, *318*, 1925–1926. [CrossRef]
20. Burgess, S.; Foley, C.N.; Allara, E.; Staley, J.R.; Howson, J.M.M. A robust and efficient method for Mendelian randomization with hundreds of genetic variants. *Nat. Commun.* **2020**, *11*, 376. [CrossRef]
21. Julkunen, H.; Cichonska, A.; Slagboom, P.E.; Wurtz, P.; Nightingale Health UKBI. Metabolic biomarker profiling for identification of susceptibility to severe pneumonia and COVID-19 in the general population. *eLife* **2021**, *10*, e63033. [CrossRef] [PubMed]
22. Lei, P.; Xu, W.; Wang, C.; Lin, G.; Yu, S.; Guo, Y. Mendelian randomization analysis reveals causal associations of polyunsaturated fatty acids with sepsis and mortality risk. *Infect. Dis. Ther.* **2023**, *12*, 1797–1808. [CrossRef] [PubMed]
23. Tachmazidou, I.; Hatzikotoulas, K.; Southam, L.; Esparza-Gordillo, J.; Haberland, V.; Zheng, J.; Johnson, T.; Koprulu, M.; Zengini, E.; Steinberg, J.; et al. Identification of new therapeutic targets for osteoarthritis through genome-wide analyses of UK Biobank data. *Nat. Genet.* **2019**, *51*, 230–236. [CrossRef]
24. Meng, H.; Jiang, L.; Song, Z.; Wang, F. Causal associations of circulating lipids with osteoarthritis: A bidirectional mendelian randomization study. *Nutrients* **2022**, *14*, 1327. [CrossRef]
25. Zhao, G.; Lu, Z.; Sun, Y.; Kang, Z.; Feng, X.; Liao, Y.; Sun, J.; Zhang, Y.; Huang, Y.; Yue, W. Dissecting the causal association between social or physical inactivity and depression: A bidirectional two-sample Mendelian Randomization study. *Transl. Psychiatry* **2023**, *13*, 194. [CrossRef]
26. Burgess, S.; Thompson, S.G.; Collaboration CCG. Avoiding bias from weak instruments in Mendelian randomization studies. *Int. J. Epidemiol.* **2011**, *40*, 755–764. [CrossRef]
27. Pierce, B.L.; Ahsan, H.; Vanderweele, T.J. Power and instrument strength requirements for Mendelian randomization studies using multiple genetic variants. *Int. J. Epidemiol.* **2011**, *40*, 740–752. [CrossRef] [PubMed]
28. Hemani, G.; Zheng, J.; Elsworth, B.; Wade, K.H.; Haberland, V.; Baird, D.; Laurin, C.; Burgess, S.; Bowden, J.; Langdon, R.; et al. The MR-Base platform supports systematic causal inference across the human phenome. *eLife* **2018**, *7*, e34408. [CrossRef]
29. Pagoni, P.; Dimou, N.L.; Murphy, N.; Stergiakouli, E. Using Mendelian randomisation to assess causality in observational studies. *Evid. Based Ment. Health* **2019**, *22*, 67–71. [CrossRef] [PubMed]
30. Davey Smith, G.; Hemani, G. Mendelian randomization: Genetic anchors for causal inference in epidemiological studies. *Hum. Mol. Genet.* **2014**, *23*, R89–R98. [CrossRef]
31. Bowden, J.; Davey Smith, G.; Haycock, P.C.; Burgess, S. Consistent estimation in mendelian randomization with some invalid instruments using a weighted median estimator. *Genet. Epidemiol.* **2016**, *40*, 304–314. [CrossRef] [PubMed]
32. Burgess, S.; Thompson, S.G. Interpreting findings from Mendelian randomization using the MR-Egger method. *Eur. J. Epidemiol.* **2017**, *32*, 377–389. [CrossRef] [PubMed]

3. Bowden, J.; Davey Smith, G.; Burgess, S. Mendelian randomization with invalid instruments: Effect estimation and bias detection through Egger regression. *Int. J. Epidemiol.* **2015**, *44*, 512–525. [CrossRef] [PubMed]
4. Lin, J.; Zhou, J.; Xu, Y. Potential drug targets for multiple sclerosis identified through Mendelian randomization analysis. *Brain* **2023**, *146*, 3364–3372. [CrossRef] [PubMed]
5. Chong, R.S.; Li, H.; Cheong, A.J.Y.; Fan, Q.; Koh, V.; Raghavan, L.; Nongpiur, M.E.; Cheng, C.Y. Mendelian randomization implicates bidirectional association between myopia and primary open-angle glaucoma or intraocular pressure. *Ophthalmology* **2023**, *130*, 394–403. [CrossRef] [PubMed]
6. Yoshiji, S.; Butler-Laporte, G.; Lu, T.; Willett, J.D.S.; Su, C.Y.; Nakanishi, T.; Morrison, D.R.; Chen, Y.; Liang, K.; Hultström, M.; et al. Proteome-wide Mendelian randomization implicates nephronectin as an actionable mediator of the effect of obesity on COVID-19 severity. *Nat. Metab.* **2023**, *5*, 248–264. [CrossRef] [PubMed]
7. Chen, X.; Kong, J.; Diao, X.; Cai, J.; Zheng, J.; Xie, W.; Qin, H.; Huang, J.; Lin, T. Depression and prostate cancer risk: A Mendelian randomization study. *Cancer Med.* **2020**, *9*, 9160–9167. [CrossRef]
8. Gao, R.C.; Sang, N.; Jia, C.Z.; Zhang, M.Y.; Li, B.H.; Wei, M.; Wu, G.C. Association between sleep traits and rheumatoid arthritis: A mendelian randomization study. *Front. Public Health* **2022**, *10*, 940161. [CrossRef]
9. Chen, D.; Zhang, Y.; Yidilisi, A.; Xu, Y.; Dong, Q.; Jiang, J. Causal associations between circulating adipokines and cardiovascular disease: A mendelian randomization study. *J. Clin. Endocrinol. Metab.* **2022**, *107*, e2572–e2580. [CrossRef]
10. Luo, Q.; Chen, J.; Qin, L.; Luo, Y.; Zhang, Y.; Yang, X.; Wang, H. Psoriasis may increase the risk of lung cancer: A two-sample Mendelian randomization study. *J. Eur. Acad. Dermatol. Venereol.* **2022**, *36*, 2113–2119. [CrossRef]
11. Burgess, S.; Davey Smith, G.; Davies, N.M.; Dudbridge, F.; Gill, D.; Glymour, M.M.; Hartwig, F.P.; Kutalik, Z.; Holmes, M.V.; Minelli, C.; et al. Guidelines for performing Mendelian randomization investigations. *Wellcome Open Res.* **2019**, *4*, 186. [CrossRef] [PubMed]
12. Pawlosky, R.J.; Hibbeln, J.R.; Lin, Y.; Goodson, S.; Riggs, P.; Sebring, N.; Brown, G.L.; Salem, N., Jr. Effects of beef- and fish-based diets on the kinetics of n-3 fatty acid metabolism in human subjects. *Am. J. Clin. Nutr.* **2003**, *77*, 565–572. [CrossRef] [PubMed]
13. Brenna, J.T. Efficiency of conversion of alpha-linolenic acid to long chain n-3 fatty acids in man. *Curr. Opin. Clin. Nutr. Metab. Care* **2002**, *5*, 127–132. [CrossRef] [PubMed]
14. Kaur, N.; Chugh, V.; Gupta, A.K. Essential fatty acids as functional components of foods—A review. *J. Food Sci. Technol.* **2014**, *51*, 2289–2303. [CrossRef]
15. So, J.; Wu, D.; Lichtenstein, A.H.; Tai, A.K.; Matthan, N.R.; Maddipati, K.R.; Lamon-Fava, S. EPA and DHA differentially modulate monocyte inflammatory response in subjects with chronic inflammation in part via plasma specialized pro-resolving lipid mediators: A randomized, double-blind, crossover study. *Atherosclerosis* **2021**, *316*, 90–98. [CrossRef]
16. Senftleber, N.K.; Nielsen, S.M.; Andersen, J.R.; Bliddal, H.; Tarp, S.; Lauritzen, L.; Furst, D.E.; Suarez-Almazor, M.E.; Lyddiatt, A.; Christensen, R. Marine oil supplements for arthritis pain: A systematic review and meta-analysis of randomized trials. *Nutrients* **2017**, *9*, 42. [CrossRef]
17. Hill, C.L.; March, L.M.; Aitken, D.; Lester, S.E.; Battersby, R.; Hynes, K.; Fedorova, T.; Proudman, S.M.; James, M.; Cleland, L.G.; et al. Fish oil in knee osteoarthritis: A randomised clinical trial of low dose versus high dose. *Ann. Rheum. Dis.* **2016**, *75*, 23–29. [CrossRef]
18. Deng, W.; Yi, Z.; Yin, E.; Lu, R.; You, H.; Yuan, X. Effect of omega-3 polyunsaturated fatty acids supplementation for patients with osteoarthritis: A meta-analysis. *J. Orthop. Surg. Res.* **2023**, *18*, 381. [CrossRef]
19. Phitak, T.; Boonmaleerat, K.; Pothacharoen, P.; Pruksakorn, D.; Kongtawelert, P. Leptin alone and in combination with interleukin-1-beta induced cartilage degradation potentially inhibited by EPA and DHA. *Connect. Tissue Res.* **2018**, *59*, 316–331. [CrossRef]
20. Sakata, S.; Hayashi, S.; Fujishiro, T.; Kawakita, K.; Kanzaki, N.; Hashimoto, S.; Iwasa, K.; Chinzei, N.; Kihara, S.; Haneda, M.; et al. Oxidative stress-induced apoptosis and matrix loss of chondrocytes is inhibited by eicosapentaenoic acid. *J. Orthop. Res.* **2015**, *33*, 359–365. [CrossRef]
21. Innes, J.K.; Calder, P.C. Omega-6 fatty acids and inflammation. *Prostaglandins Leukot. Essent. Fat. Acids* **2018**, *132*, 41–48. [CrossRef] [PubMed]
22. Poli, A.; Agostoni, C.; Visioli, F. Dietary fatty acids and inflammation: Focus on the n-6 series. *Int. J. Mol. Sci.* **2023**, *24*, 4567. [CrossRef] [PubMed]
23. Bersch-Ferreira, A.C.; Sampaio, G.R.; Gehringer, M.O.; Ross-Fernandes, M.B.; Kovacs, C.; Alves, R.; Pereira, J.L.; Magnoni, C.D.; Weber, B.; Rogero, M.M. Association between polyunsaturated fatty acids and inflammatory markers in patients in secondary prevention of cardiovascular disease. *Nutrition* **2017**, *37*, 30–36. [CrossRef] [PubMed]
24. Virtanen, J.K.; Mursu, J.; Voutilainen, S.; Tuomainen, T.P. The associations of serum n-6 polyunsaturated fatty acids with serum C-reactive protein in men: The Kuopio Ischaemic Heart Disease Risk Factor Study. *Eur. J. Clin. Nutr.* **2018**, *72*, 342–348. [CrossRef]
25. Gonzalez-Gil, E.M.; Santabarbara, J.; Siani, A.; Ahrens, W.; Sioen, I.; Eiben, G.; Günther, K.; Iacoviello, L.; Molnar, D.; Rise, P.; et al. Whole-blood fatty acids and inflammation in European children: The IDEFICS Study. *Eur. J. Clin. Nutr.* **2016**, *70*, 819–823. [CrossRef]
26. Poudel-Tandukar, K.; Nanri, A.; Matsushita, Y.; Sasaki, S.; Ohta, M.; Sato, M.; Mizoue, T. Dietary intakes of alpha-linolenic and linoleic acids are inversely associated with serum C-reactive protein levels among Japanese men. *Nutr. Res.* **2009**, *29*, 363–370. [CrossRef]

57. Muka, T.; Kiefte-de Jong, J.C.; Hofman, A.; Dehghan, A.; Rivadeneira, F.; Franco, O.H. Polyunsaturated fatty acids and serum C-reactive protein: The Rotterdam study. *Am. J. Epidemiol.* **2015**, *181*, 846–856. [CrossRef]
58. Johnson, G.H.; Fritsche, K. Effect of dietary linoleic acid on markers of inflammation in healthy persons: A systematic review of randomized controlled trials. *J. Acad. Nutr. Diet.* **2012**, *112*, 1029–1041.e15. [CrossRef]
59. Kelley, D.S.; Taylor, P.C.; Nelson, G.J.; Mackey, B.E. Arachidonic acid supplementation enhances synthesis of eicosanoids without suppressing immune functions in young healthy men. *Lipids* **1998**, *33*, 125–130. [CrossRef]
60. Kakutani, S.; Ishikura, Y.; Tateishi, N.; Horikawa, C.; Tokuda, H.; Kontani, M.; Kawashima, H.; Sakabibara, Y.; Kiso, Y.; Shibata, H.; et al. Supplementation of arachidonic acid-enriched oil increases arachidonic acid contents in plasma phospholipids, but does not increase their metabolites and clinical parameters in Japanese healthy elderly individuals: A randomized controlled study. *Lipids Health Dis.* **2011**, *10*, 241. [CrossRef]
61. Meuronen, T.; Lankinen, M.A.; Kolmert, J.; de Mello, V.D.; Sallinen, T.; Agren, J.; Virtanen, K.A.; Laakso, M.; Wheelock, C.E.; Pihlajamäki, J.; et al. The fads1 rs174550 genotype modifies the n-3 and n-6 pufa and lipid mediator responses to a high alpha-linolenic acid and high linoleic acid diets. *Mol. Nutr. Food Res.* **2022**, *66*, e2200351. [CrossRef] [PubMed]
62. Lu, B.; Driban, J.B.; Xu, C.; Lapane, K.L.; McAlindon, T.E.; Eaton, C.B. Dietary fat intake and radiographic progression of knee osteoarthritis: Data from the osteoarthritis initiative. *Arthritis Care Res.* **2017**, *69*, 368–375. [CrossRef] [PubMed]
63. Wang, Q.; Afshin, A.; Yakoob, M.Y.; Singh, G.M.; Rehm, C.D.; Khatibzadeh, S.; Micha, R.; Shi, P.; Mozaffarian, D.; Global Burden of Diseases Nutrition and Chronic Diseases Expert Group (NutriCoDE). Impact of nonoptimal intakes of saturated, polyunsaturated, and trans fat on global burdens of coronary heart disease. *J. Am. Heart Assoc.* **2016**, *5*, e002891. [CrossRef] [PubMed]
64. Collaborators GBDD. Health effects of dietary risks in 195 countries, 1990–2017: A systematic analysis for the Global Burden of Disease Study 2017. *Lancet* **2019**, *393*, 1958–1972. [CrossRef] [PubMed]

Disclaimer/Publisher's Note: The statements, opinions and data contained in all publications are solely those of the individual author(s) and contributor(s) and not of MDPI and/or the editor(s). MDPI and/or the editor(s) disclaim responsibility for any injury to people or property resulting from any ideas, methods, instructions or products referred to in the content.

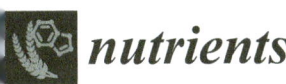

Article

Elephantopus scaber L. Polysaccharides Alleviate Heat Stress-Induced Systemic Inflammation in Mice via Modulation of Characteristic Gut Microbiota and Metabolites

Chen Wang [1,†], Dongfang Sun [1,2,†], Qi Deng [1,*], Lijun Sun [1], Lianhua Hu [1], Zhijia Fang [1], Jian Zhao [3] and Ravi Gooneratne [4]

1. Guangdong Provincial Key Laboratory of Aquatic Product Processing and Safety, College of Food Science and Technology, Guangdong Ocean University, Zhanjiang 524088, China; 18642326533@163.com (C.W.); dfsun@stu.njau.edu.cn (D.S.); suncamt@126.com (L.S.); lianhuashipin@126.com (L.H.); fzj4437549@163.com (Z.F.)
2. College of Food Science and Technology, Nanjing Agricultural University, Nanjing 210095, China
3. School of Chemical Engineering, The University of New South Wales, Sydney, NSW 2052, Australia; jian.zhao@unsw.edu.au
4. Department of Wine, Food and Molecular Biosciences, Faculty of Agriculture and Life Sciences, Lincoln University, P.O. Box 85084, Lincoln 7647, New Zealand; ravi.gooneratne@lincoln.ac.nz
* Correspondence: gdoudengqi@163.com; Tel./Fax: +86-0759-2396027
† These authors have contributed equally to this work.

Abstract: *Elephantopus scaber* L. (ESL) is a Chinese herb that is used both as a food and medicine, often being added to soups in summer in south China to relieve heat stress (HS), but its exact mechanism of action is unknown. In this study, heat-stressed mice were gavaged with ESL polysaccharides (ESLP) at 0, 150, 300, and 450 mg/kg/d^{-1} (*n* = 5) for seven days. The gut microbiota composition, short-chain fatty acids (SCFAs), seven neurotransmitters in faeces, expression of intestinal epithelial tight junction (TJ) proteins (Claudin-1, Occludin), and serum inflammatory cytokines were measured. The low dose of ESLP (ESLL) improved the adverse physiological conditions; significantly reduced the cytokines (TNF-α, IL-1β, IL-6) and lipopolysaccharide (LPS) levels ($p < 0.05$); upregulated the expression of Claudin-1; restored the gut microbiota composition including *Achromobacter* and *Oscillospira*, which were at similar levels to those in the normal control group; significantly increased beneficial SCFAs like butyric acid and 5-HT levels in the faeces of heat-stressed mice; and significantly decreased the valeric acid and glutamic acid level. The level of inflammatory markers significantly correlated with the above-mentioned indicators ($p < 0.05$). Thus, ESLL reduced the HS-induced systemic inflammation by optimizing gut microbiota (*Achromobacter*, *Oscillospira*) abundance, increasing gut beneficial SCFAs like butyric acid and 5-HT levels, and reducing gut valeric and glutamic acid levels.

Keywords: *Elephantopus scaber* L. polysaccharides; heat stress; systemic inflammation; gut microbiota; short chain fatty acids; neurotransmitters

Citation: Wang, C.; Sun, D.; Deng, Q.; Sun, L.; Hu, L.; Fang, Z.; Zhao, J.; Gooneratne, R. *Elephantopus scaber* L. Polysaccharides Alleviate Heat Stress-Induced Systemic Inflammation in Mice via Modulation of Characteristic Gut Microbiota and Metabolites. *Nutrients* **2024**, *16*, 262. https://doi.org/10.3390/nu16020262

Academic Editor: Ana Valdes

Received: 9 December 2023
Revised: 7 January 2024
Accepted: 12 January 2024
Published: 16 January 2024

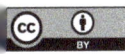

Copyright: © 2024 by the authors. Licensee MDPI, Basel, Switzerland. This article is an open access article distributed under the terms and conditions of the Creative Commons Attribution (CC BY) license (https://creativecommons.org/licenses/by/4.0/).

1. Introduction

Excessive exposure to high temperatures causes heat stress (HS) [1]. HS can result in restlessness, poor concentration and anorexia [2]. In severe cases, it can lead to heat stroke, heat exhaustion and intestinal diseases [3]. A series of adverse reactions during HS are closely related to systemic inflammation [1,4]. Therefore, systemic inflammation is often used as a key indicator to evaluate the effectiveness of measures to protect against HS. The current mainstay treatment approaches for HS (such as physical cooling and antibiotics) [5] have various adverse side effects and cannot fundamentally relieve the HS response. Therefore, there is an urgent need to explore safer and more effective intervention methods.

In the subtropical and tropical areas of Southern China and Southeast Asia, *Elephantopus scaber* L. (ESL), a perennial herb [6], is often added to soup and consumed in summer to relieve the physical discomfort caused by high temperatures [7]. Therefore, ESL may have a good intervention effect on systemic inflammation caused by high temperatures. However, there are no scientific studies on the effective components and mechanism of action of ESL in alleviating HS-induced systemic inflammation, limiting its further development and application.

Research has demonstrated that plant polysaccharides can reduce the negative effects of HS on the body. Liu et al. [8] reported that alfalfa polysaccharides improve the growth performance of heat-stressed rabbits. Sohail et al. [9] showed that mannan oligosaccharides improve the relative weight of immune organs in heat-stressed broilers. Similarly, atractylodes polysaccharides are reported to alleviate the splenic inflammatory response induced by HS in broiler chickens [10,11]. These findings suggest that plant polysaccharides may effectively reduce systemic inflammation to protect against HS. Our previous study revealed that ESL extract contains many polysaccharides. Thus, the polysaccharides in ESL may be the effective components underlying the HS-reducing effects of ESL. However, at present, there is a lack of direct evidence, and the mechanism of action requires exploration.

Plant polysaccharides, especially heteropolysaccharides, are generally difficult for the human body to digest and absorb [12]. They can be fermented by the gut microbiota in the large intestine and thus exert their nutritional or pharmacological effects [13]. Plant polysaccharides can improve the health of the body by regulating the composition of the gut microbiota [14]. Research has indicated that fructan (inulin) can improve the diabetic phenotype by enriching *Lactobacillus* and/or *Bifidobacterium* spp. [15]. In another study, fucoidan selectively increased the proportion of *Bacteroides* spp., *Akkermansia muciniphila*, *Blautia* spp. and *Alloprevotella* spp. to ameliorate metabolic syndrome and intestinal malnutrition in mice [16]. However, it is unclear whether *Elephantopus scaber* L. polysaccharides (ESLP) can protect against HS-induced systemic inflammation by regulating the abundance of the particular target gut microbes.

Recent research has demonstrated that polysaccharides can be degraded into short-chain fatty acids (SCFAs) by the intestinal microbiota and that SCFAs play a crucial role in maintaining the health of the body [17]. One study found that *Zizyphus Jujuba* cv. *Muzao* polysaccharides can significantly increase butyrate and acetate, reducing the risk of colitis-related colon cancer [18]. In another study, *Cyclocarya paliurus* polysaccharides alleviated type 2 diabetes mellitus (T2DM) by increasing the levels of SCFAs (acetic acid, propionic acid, butyric acid, isobutyric acid, valeric acid and isovaleric acid) [19]. It is clear that different polysaccharides can increase the total amount of SCFAs; however, the levels of the increases in specific SCFAs are different, and different SCFAs play different roles. Thus, the effects of ESLP on SCFA production require further clarification.

In addition, it appears that neurotransmitters produced by the gut microbiota also play a role in inflammation. Feng et al. [20] reported that *Atractylodes macrocephala* Koidz. polysaccharides alleviate dextran sulphate sodium salt-induced ulcerative colitis inflammation by changing the gut microbiota and reversing the reduction in tryptophan. Polysaccharides from the leaves of *Ginkgo biloba* have been found to upregulate the abundance of *Lactobacillus* species and increase the levels of 5-HT in the gut, thus producing anti-inflammatory and antidepressant effects [21]. This suggests that neurotransmitters produced by the intestinal flora are very important in the development of inflammation. However, it is not clear if ESLP can reduce HS-induced systemic inflammation by controlling the neurotransmitters produced by the gut microbiota.

In this study, ESLP was orally administered to heat-stressed mice to investigate the (a) relationships between exposure to HS, systemic inflammation, the gut microbiome, and related SCFAs and neurotransmitters, and (b) the potential mechanism of action underlying the effect of ESLP on systemic inflammation caused by HS.

2. Materials and Methods

2.1. Extraction of Crude Polysaccharides

Polysaccharides were isolated from *Elephantopus scaber* L. (Product No. PB20200505, a dry powder) purchased from Shaanxi Pioneer Biotech Co., Ltd., Tongchuan, China, according to Zhou's method with some modifications [22]. Briefly, the crude polysaccharide was extracted via water extraction and ethanol precipitation. The crude polysaccharide solution underwent treatment with a 5% trichloroacetic acid solution to eliminate any remaining protein residues. The supernatant was followed by dialysis using a dialysis bag, then concentrated using a rotary evaporator. After that, lyophilization was used on the concentrated solution, which made *Elephantopus scaber* L. polysaccharides (ESLP).

2.2. Composition Analysis

Total carbohydrates were quantified via the phenol-sulfuric acid method, using glucose as the standard [23]. The reducing sugar content was evaluated via the dinitro salicylic acid (DNS) method [24]. The meta-hydroxy diphenyl technique was used to determine the concentration of uronic acid [25].

2.3. Animal Ethics Statement

The Animal Ethics Committee of Guangdong Ocean University approved all animal tests and methods conducted in this study (file number: GDOU-LAE-2020-015, 18 October 2020). All procedures and experiments were carried out at the laboratory animal centre at Guangdong Ocean University (License No. SYXK 2019-0204) in strict accordance with the university's laws on animal experimentation.

2.4. Animals and Study Design

The experimental conditions for feeding mice were the same as previously described [26], with some modifications. In total, 25 6-week-old male C57BL/6J mice of average weight (18 ± 2 g) were purchased from Beijing Huafukang Biotechnology Co., Ltd., (Beijing, China). All mice had unlimited access to distilled water and feed pellets sterilised with Co60. High-pressure steam was used to sanitise the materials used for the water bottles, cage, and pads. Three times every week, the water bottles and pad fillings were changed. After a week of acclimatisation, all mice were randomly divided into five groups [Normal Control (NC), HS model (HSS), HS + Low-dose ESLP gavage (150 mg/kg/d^{-1}; ESLL), HS + Medium dose ESLP gavage (300 mg/kg/d^{-1}; ESLM), HS + High-dose ESLP gavage (450 mg/kg/d^{-1}; ESLH)] and housed in different cages ($n = 5$). The NC and HSS group mice were given a normal saline gavage. The NC group was kept in a normal rearing environment (temperature: 22 ± 3 °C, humidity: $60 \pm 10\%$) without HS treatment. The rest of the groups were subjected to HS in an artificial environment simulation cabin to maintain a core temperature of 38 ± 0.5 °C and a humidity of 90–95% [27,28]. The experimental period was 7 days, and the mice were subjected to HS once a day for 4 h. The three ESLP group mice received normal diet plus the ESLP after each HS exposure.

2.5. Temperature-Humidity Index (THI) Measurements

The experimental conditions for constructing the HS model mice were the same as previously described [29], with some modifications. The experimental room ambient temperature (Td, °C) and relative humidity (RH, %) were measured three times each day at 07:00, 13:00, and 20:00. The THI was calculated using the formula below: THI = (1.8 × Td + 32) − (0.55 − 0.55 × RH × 0.01) × (1.8 × Td − 26).

2.6. Physiological Variables and Sample Collection

During the experiment, the physiological parameters (body weight, feed intake, body surface temperature, physiological behaviours) of the mice were recorded daily. At the end of the experiment, before dissecting, the mice were massaged on the belly to collect faecal particles, which were placed in sterile centrifuge tubes in an ice bath. The samples were stored at −80 °C. The mice were dissected immediately after 1 mL of eyeball blood was taken. The blood was centrifuged at 1200× g and 4 °C for 5 min. The serum samples were separated from the supernatant and kept at −80 °C until required. The organs were collected and weighed. The ileum was immediately collected, and some were washed with precooled phosphate-buffered saline (PBS), frozen in liquid nitrogen, and then stored at −80 °C; others were immediately stored in 10% formalin until analysis.

2.7. Measurement of Inflammatory Markers and Lipopolysaccharide (LPS)

A few modifications were made to previous work [26] regarding the measurement of serum inflammatory cytokines and LPS levels. The following mouse ELISA kits, TNF-α (Cat no. M190408-102a), IL-10 (M190408-005a), IL-1β (M190408-001a) and IL-6 (M190408-004a), were purchased from Neobioscience Technology Co., Ltd., Shenzhen, China. The microplate quantitative chromogenic matrix Limulus kit (Cat no. 18030067) was purchased from Xiamen Limulus Reagent Biotechnology Co., Ltd., Xiamen, Fujian Province, China. They were used according to the manufacturer's instructions.

2.8. Haematoxylin and Eosin (H&E) Staining of Intestinal Tissue

Tissues were processed and stained as reported in [26]. Then, 5 μm sections (n = 3/animal) were light-microscopically examined for histological damage. The numbers of goblet cells, the villi length and the crypt depth were measured. A total of 5 areas were selected for each sample and an average for each sample and each group was calculated.

2.9. Western Blot (WB) Analysis

The experimental conditions for WB were the same as previously described [30], with some modifications. The separated proteins were transferred onto PVDF membranes (Cat no. G6015-0.45, Servicebio, Wuhan, China) using protein extracts (50 μg) from each sample in 10% SDS-PAGE gels. After washing with Tris-Buffered Saline with Tween 20 (TBS-T), the protein bands were detected by chemiluminescence using ECL Western Blot Substrate (Cat no. G2019, Servicebio). β-actin was used as the internal standard. The signals were recorded with a chemiluminescence imager (Cat no. 6300, CLINX, Shanghai, China) and analysed using Alpha Innotech (AlphaEaseFC 4.1.0) and Adobe (Adobe PhotoShop 20.0) software.

2.10. Gut Microbiota Analysis

2.10.1. DNA Extraction

Following the manufacturer's instructions, total gut bacterial genomic DNA samples were obtained using the Metagenomic DNA isolation kit GHFDE100 (Zhejiang Hangzhou Equipment Preparation 20190952) from GUHE Laboratories in Hangzhou, China.

2.10.2. 16S rRNA Amplicon Pyrosequencing and Sequence Analysis

We used 515F (5′-GTGCCAGCMGCCGCGGTAA-3′) as the forward primer and 806R 5′-GGACTACHVGGGTWTCTAAT-3′ as the reverse primer. Details are in a previous publication [26].

2.10.3. Bioinformatics and Statistical Analysis

The experimental bioinformatics and statistical analysis were as described previously [26]. Using the default parameters, linear discriminant analysis effect size (LEfSe) was performed to identify differentially abundant species across groups.

2.11. SCFA Analysis

SCFAs in mouse faeces were measured as described previously using GC-MS [26].

2.12. Neurotransmitter Analysis

Seven neurotransmitter standards were used. Acetylcholine and Adrenaline were purchased from Sigma, St. Louis, MO, USA. The 5-Hydroxytryptamine (5-HT), Dopamine, γ-aminobutyric acid (GABA), Noradrenaline and Glutamic acid used were from Beijing Suolaibao Technology Co., Ltd. (Beijing, China). The standards were weighed, dissolved in methanol containing 0.2% formic acid and dissolved in acetonitrile/water (2:8) to nine standard concentration gradient mixtures. Faecal samples were thawed on ice prior to extracting polar metabolites for LC-MS analysis. Then, 50 mg of each faecal sample was added into cold water containing 0.2% formic acid. The homogenate was sonicated in an ice bath for 15 min. Next, 1 mL of the homogenate was added to 1 mL of ice-cold 0.2% formic acid in acetonitrile and centrifuged at 4 °C, 12,000× g for 3 min. The solution was filtered using an organic microporous membrane of 0.22 μm pore size, and the supernatant was collected and examined using an LC-MS1000 device. The quantitative measurement of faecal neurotransmitters was carried out using a calibration curve. The peak-area integration was assessed based on the retention time.

The neurotransmitters in the faeces of mice were determined via LC-MS. The LC conditions were as follows: Column (TSK-GEL amide-80 column; 4.5 × 150 mm, 5 μm; Tosoh, Tokyo, Japan). The column temperature was 40 °C. Mobile phase A: 100% acetonitrile, Mobile phase B: 0.1% formic acid-water solution (20%:80%). Flow rate: 0.3 mL/min. The MS conditions were as follows: the EI ion source was heated to 450 °C and an ion spray voltage of 4500 V was applied. Data were collected using the ion MRM method.

2.13. Pro-Inflammatory Experiment of Valeric and Glutamic Acid In Vitro

2.13.1. Cytotoxicity Test of Valeric and Glutamic Acid

The experimental conditions for the RAW264.7 cells were the same as previously described [31], with some modifications. The DMEM medium was changed to DMEM medium supplemented with 0, 10, 25, 50, 100, and 200 μg/mL valeric and glutamic acid, respectively.

2.13.2. Pro-Inflammatory Test of Valeric and Glutamic Acid

The experimental conditions for the RAW264.7 cells were the same as previously described [31] with some modifications. The culture medium was changed into DMEM culture medium containing 0, 10, 25, 50, 100, 200 μg/mL valeric and glutamic acid, respectively. After 24 h of cultivation, the concentrations of IL-1β and IL-6 were measured using ELISA kits (Neobioscience Technology Co., Ltd., Shenzhen, China), according to the manufacturer's instructions.

2.14. Statistical Analysis

The mean and standard error of the mean (SEM) were used to represent the results. SPSS 21.0 (SPSS, Chicago, IL, USA) was used for statistical analysis. One-way analysis of variance (ANOVA) and the LSD test were used to compare the differences between groups, with $p < 0.05$ regarded as statistically significant.

3. Results

3.1. Basic Physicochemical Properties of ESLP

The crude polysaccharides of ESL were obtained via hot water extraction and ethanol precipitation. The content (%) of total carbohydrates was 84.69% (including 9.82% reducing sugars), while the uronic acid content was 31.39%.

3.2. Effect of ESLP on the Body Weight, Food Intake, Viscera Coefficients, Body Surface Temperature and Physiological Behaviour of Mice

The body weight (BW), food intake and viscera coefficients of the mice are shown in Figure 1. Compared with the NC group, the mice in the HSS group exhibited a slower rate of weight gain and decreased food intake. ESLP increased the rate of weight gain and food intake (vs. HSS group). The effect was particularly evident in the ESLL group (Figure 1A,B). Mice in the HSS group had higher spleen and intestine viscera coefficients compared to the NC group. ESLP significantly decreased the viscera indices of the spleen, stomach and intestine of the heat-stressed mice ($p < 0.05$) (Figure 1C). As shown in Table 1, the mice in the HSS group had considerably higher rectal temperatures ($p < 0.05$) than those in the NC group. The ESLL significantly reduced the rectal temperature compared to the HS mice ($p < 0.05$), somewhat similar to the NC group. Although the ESLM and ESLH groups tended to have lower rectal temperatures than the HSS group, these differences were not statistically significant. The HSS group showed increased neck and ear base temperatures compared to the mice in the NC group. Mice in the three ESLP groups exhibited slightly lower neck and ear base temperatures compared to the HS mice. ESLP induced some positive effects with regard to the regulation of the surface body temperature of HS mice, and these effects were particularly visible in the ESLL group.

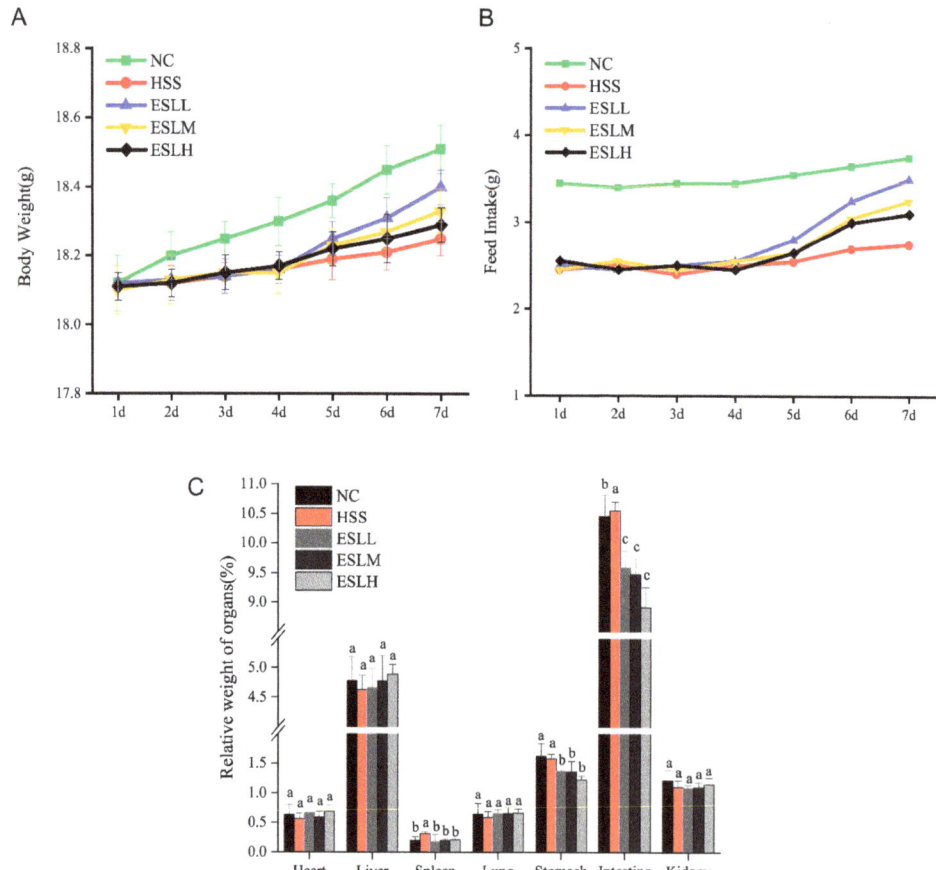

Figure 1. Effects of ESLP on the body weight, food intake and viscera coefficient in heat-stressed mice ((A): body weight, (B): food intake, (C): viscera coefficient). Data are shown as mean ± SE ($n = 5$). Based on the ANOVA statistical analysis, the different letters (a, b, and c) above the bars of each group are statistically different ($p < 0.05$). [Normal control (NC), Heat stress (HS) model (HSS), HS + Low-dose ESLP gavage (ESLL), HS + Medium dose ESLP gavage (ESLM), HS + High-dose ESLP gavage (ESLH)].

Table 1. Effect of ESLP on the body surface temperature in heat-stressed mice (Mean ± SE).

Temperature	NC	HSS	ESLL	ESLM	ESLH
ear base/°C	36.07 ± 0.29 [a]	36.20 ± 0.08 [a]	36.12 ± 0.25 [a]	36.02 ± 0.20 [a]	35.96 ± 0.23 [a]
neck/°C	36.40 ± 0.11 [a]	36.46 ± 0.19 [a]	36.44 ± 0.17 [a]	36.46 ± 0.11 [a]	36.42 ± 0.19 [a]
rectal/°C	35.62 ± 0.10 [b]	35.94 ± 0.13 [a]	35.57 ± 0.06 [b]	35.87 ± 0.05 [a]	35.70 ± 0.25 [a]

Data are shown as mean ± SE ($n = 5$). In the same row, data with different small letter (a, b) superscripts are significantly different ($p < 0.05$) based on the ANOVA statistical analysis. [Normal control (NC), Heat stress (HS) model (HSS), HS + Low-dose ESLP gavage (ESLL), HS + Medium dose ESLP gavage (ESLM), HS + High-dose ESLP gavage (ESLH)].

During the experimental period, the NC group mice were alert, active and healthy, and exhibited dense shiny hair. However, the mice in the HSS group developed the following symptoms from day two onwards: reduced activity, sleepiness, fear, anxiety, irritability, a rapid and irregular breathing rhythm, the visible trembling of legs, coarse hair and severe hair loss. There were significant improvements in these physiological parameters in the groups that received ESLP, indicating that ESLP can ameliorate adverse physiological reactions in HSS group mice.

3.3. Effects of ESLP on Inflammatory Markers and LPS on Heat-Stressed Mice

The serum concentrations of the pro-inflammatory factors (TNF-α, IL-1β, IL-6) are shown in Figure 2A–C. When compared to the NC group, the HSS group pro-inflammatory factors concentrations were significantly higher ($p < 0.05$); the TNF-α concentration was >two times the NC group. The concentrations of pro-inflammatory factors in the ESLL group were significantly lower than in the HSS group mice ($p < 0.05$), similar to the concentrations in the NC group. The serum concentration of anti-inflammatory factor IL-10 is shown in Figure 2D. The HSS group IL-10 concentration was significantly lower ($p < 0.05$ vs. NC group), whereas in the ESLH group, the IL-10 concentration was significantly higher ($p < 0.05$) than that of the HSS group. The serum LPS concentration in the HSS group was >three times higher than that of the NC group ($p < 0.01$) (Figure 2E). The ESLP treatment significantly reduced the serum LPS concentration in HS mice ($p < 0.01$). This effect was particularly noticeable in the ESLL and ESLH groups. These results indicate that ESLP inhibited inflammation in HS mice, especially in the ESLL. The key indicators that ESLL reduced the systemic inflammation caused by HS were TNF-α, IL-1β, IL-6, and LPS.

3.4. Effect of ESLP Treatment on Intestinal Tissue

In Figure 3A, the NC group displayed an ileum mucosa with regularly aligned villi, a typical crypt architecture, a large number of goblet cells, and a condensed configuration of the lamina propria. The ileum mucosa tissue in the HSS group suffered severe damage, including goblet cell depletion, crypt hyperplasia, exposed lamina propria, disrupted intestinal epithelial cell organisation, and the partial loss of villi. The HSS group exhibited a lower ratio of intestinal villi length to crypt depth ($p < 0.05$) (Figure 3B,C). The morphology of the intestinal mucosal in the ESLL and ESLH groups was improved in the HSS group mice. In the ESLL and ESLH groups, the intestinal mucosa was relatively intact, with the crypt morphology, goblet cell numbers and the arrangement of villi and intestinal epithelial cells substantially recovered from HS. In the ESLL and ESLH groups, both the mean number of goblet cells and the ratio of intestinal villi length to crypt depth increased to levels, which were nearly identical to those in the NC group. ESLP treatment affected the intestinal tissue after HS. These effects were particularly evident in the ESLL group.

The impact of ESLP on the tight junction (TJ) proteins occludin and claudin-1 expression in the intestinal tissues of HS mice was assessed via WB. The relative protein expressions of ileum claudin-1 and occludin were significantly lower in the HSS group compared to the NC group (Figure 3D,E; $p < 0.05$). ESLP treatment significantly ($p < 0.05$) increased the expression of TJ proteins to levels comparable to those observed in the NC group.

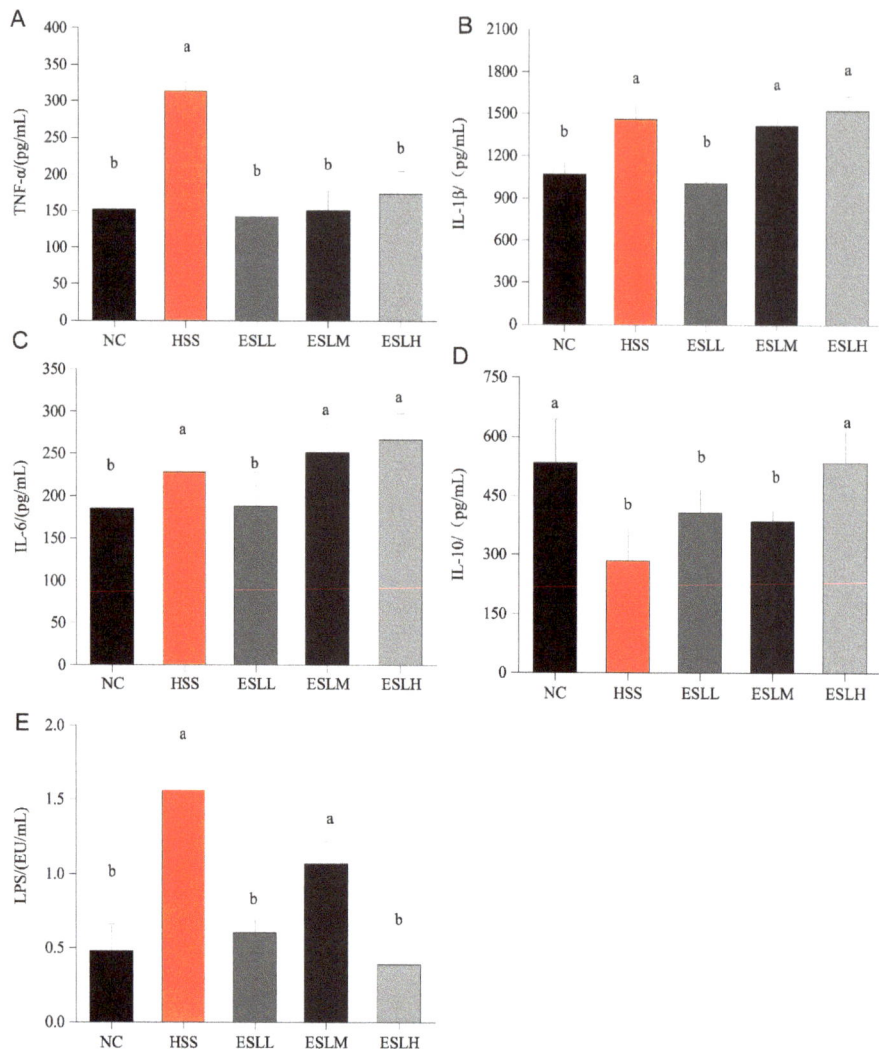

Figure 2. Changes in four serum inflammatory markers and LPS concentrations in mice. (**A**) TNF-α, (**B**) IL-1β, (**C**) IL-6, (**D**) IL-10 (**E**) LPS. Data are shown as mean ± SE (n = 5). Based on the ANOVA statistical analysis, the different letters (a, b) above the bars of each group are statistically different ($p < 0.05$). [Normal Control (NC), Heat stress (HS) model (HSS), HS + Low-dose ESLP gavage (ESLL), HS + Medium dose ESLP gavage (ESLM), HS + High-dose ESLP gavage (ESLH)].

3.5. Effect of ESLP Treatment on the Structure and Function of the Gut Microbiota in Heat-Stressed Mice

3.5.1. ESLP Maintained the Diversity of the Gut Microbiota in Heat-Stressed Mice

ESLL significantly counteracted the HS-induced decline in the species richness and α-diversity of the gut microbiota (Table 2). Unweighted UniFrac distances were used to estimate the beta diversity of the gut flora in the different mouse groups, and PCoA was used to visualise the results (Figure 4D–G). The NC group's and the HSS group's confidence ellipses differed significantly from one another (Figure 4D). After the ESLL intervention, the confidence ellipse of this group overlapped with that of the NC group (Figure 4E). However, as the ESLP dose increased, the confidence ellipse gradually deviated from that of the NC group until there was complete separation (Figure 4F,G). The intestinal flora abundance and composition of the ESLL and NC groups were similar.

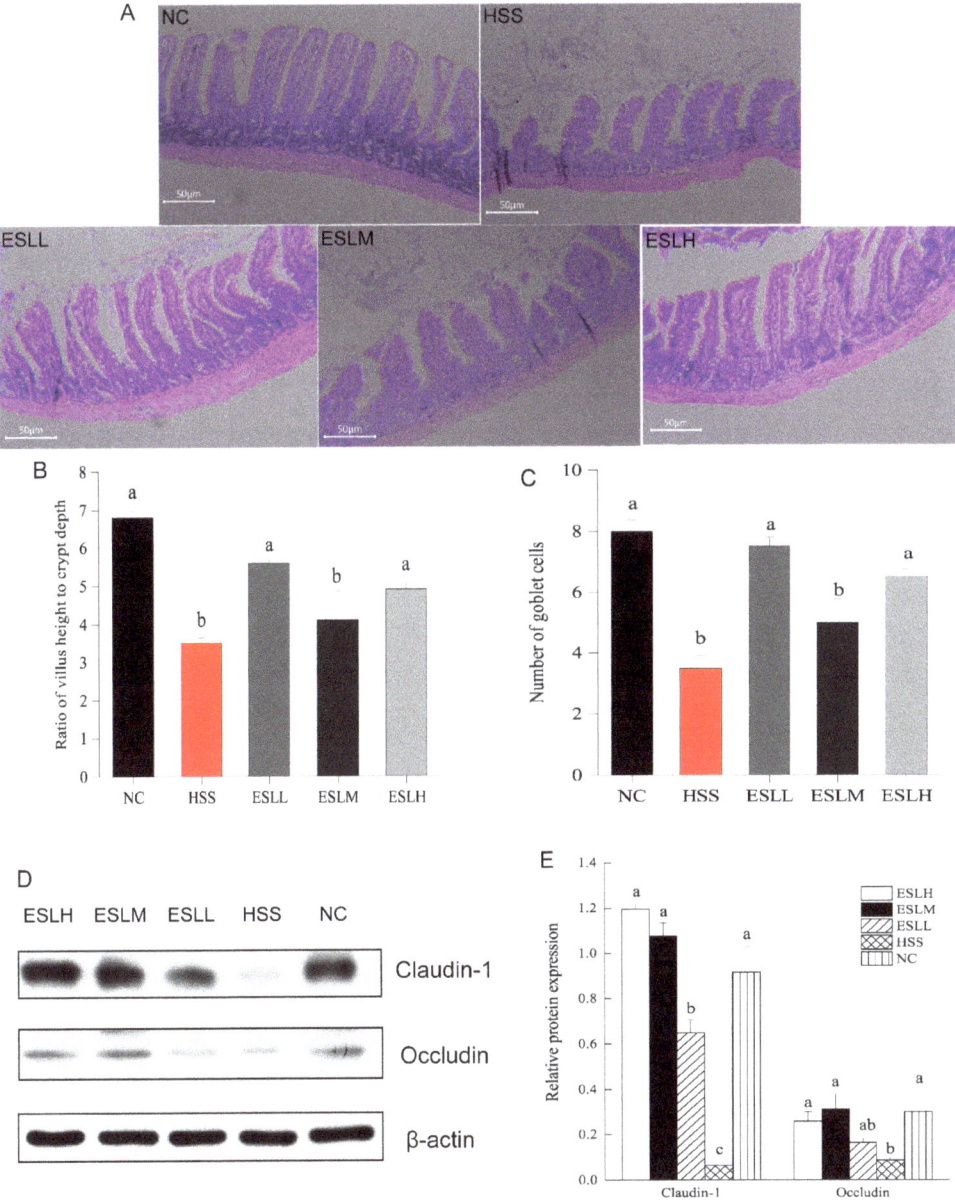

Figure 3. Effect of ESLP on intestinal tissue in HS mice. (**A**): Histological changes observed in the intestinal tissue in different groups; (**B**): Ratio of intestinal villi length to crypt depth; (**C**): mean number of goblet cells in the visual field; (**D**): Western blot of TJ protein; (**E**): Relative expression level of TJ protein. The data are shown as mean ± SE (n = 5). The ANOVA statistical analysis shows that the data with distinct letters (a, b, and c) are statistically different in each group ($p < 0.05$). [Normal control (NC), Heat stress (HS) model (HSS), HS + Low-dose ESLP gavage (ESLL), HS + Medium dose ESLP gavage (ESLM), HS + High-dose ESLP gavage (ESLH)].

Table 2. Effect of ESLP on the gut microbiota α-diversity index of the heat-stressed mice (Mean ± SE).

Groups	Shannon	Simpson	Chao1	ACE	Goods Coverage
NC	1.960 ± 0.911 [a]	0.662 ± 0.219 [a]	263.414 ± 86.015 [a]	265.013 ± 81.011 [a]	1.000 ± 0.000 [a]
HSS	1.457 ± 0.411 [ab]	0.465 ± 0.045 [a]	172.756 ± 25.611 [ab]	163.025 ± 30.418 [b]	1.000 ± 0.000 [a]
ESLL	1.847 ± 1.220 [a]	0.647 ± 0.111 [a]	212.085 ± 100.941 [ab]	203.030 ± 89.117 [a]	1.000 ± 0.000 [a]
ESLM	0.557 ± 0.139 [b]	0.126 ± 0.037 [b]	161.470 ± 42.782 [b]	168.618 ± 37.352 [b]	1.000 ± 0.000 [a]
ESLH	1.526 ± 0.323 [ab]	0.565 ± 0.028 [a]	202.863 ± 25.556 [ab]	191.318 ± 24.231 [ab]	1.000 ± 0.000 [a]

Data are shown as mean ± SE ($n = 5$). In the same column, data with different small letter (a, b) superscripts are significantly different in different groups ($p < 0.05$) based on the ANOVA statistical analysis. [Normal control (NC), Heat stress (HS) model (HSS), HS + Low-dose ESLP gavage (ESLL), HS + Medium dose ESLP gavage (ESLM), HS + High-dose ESLP gavage (ESLH)].

3.5.2. ESLP Maintained the Composition of the Gut Microbiota in Heat-Stressed Mice

The intestinal microflora was examined at two different classification levels. At the phylum level, Proteobacteria, Firmicutes, and Bacteroidetes in the HSS group differed significantly from the NC group ($p < 0.05$). Mice given ESLL showed a significant increase in the abundance of Firmicutes and a similar significant inhibitory effect on the relative abundance of Proteobacteria ($p < 0.05$ vs. HSS group) (Figure 5A). Proteobacteria and firmicutes made up >90% of the total flora. Firmicutes and Bacteroidetes were significantly less prevalent in the HSS group than in the NC group, but proteobacteria were 145% more abundant ($p < 0.05$). In contrast, mice given ESLP showed a significant increase in the abundance of Firmicutes and an equally significant inhibitory effect on the relative abundance of Proteobacteria ($p < 0.05$ vs. HSS group), with the abundances being comparable to those seen in the NC group. The recovery effect on Firmicutes and Proteobacteria did, however, eventually decline when the ESLP dose was increased. The relative abundances of Firmicutes and Proteobacteria in the ESLH group were comparable to those in the HSS group.

Stenotrophomonas, *Lactobacillus* and *Achromobacter* were the dominant bacteria of the gut microbiota of each group at the genus level (Figure 5B). Compared with the NC group, the abundances of *Lactobacillus*, *Allobaculum*, *Akkermansia*, *Bacteroides*, *Ruminococcus*, *Faecalibacterium*, *Clostridium*, *Oscillospira*, *Staphylococcus*, *Odoribacter* and *Prevotella* were significantly decreased ($p < 0.05$), while the abundances of *Stenotrophomonas*, *Achromobacter* and *Acinetobacter* were significantly increased ($p < 0.05$) in the HSS group. This imbalance was restored by the ESLP intervention, where a clear dose–response relationship was observed for *Lactobacillus*, *Akkermansia* and *Allobaculum*, and *Achromobacter*, *Oscillospira*. The abundance of *Clostridium* was restored only by the ESLL intervention. The ESLL group exhibited a similar ratio regarding the relative abundance of gut microbiota to the NC group.

In order to find species with statistically significant differences between the groups, LEfSe analysis was carried out (Figure 5C). At the genus level, *Achromobacter*, *Acinetobacter*, Lactobacillus, Akkermansia, Allobaculum, Verrucomjcrobia and Oscillospira in the ESLL treatment groups were quite distinct from the HSS group. In the HSS group compared to the NC group, the abundances of gram-negative, potentially pathogenic, and stress-tolerant bacteria were considerably higher ($p < 0.05$) (Figure 5E). When the ESLL group was compared with the HSS group, the abundances of gram-negative, potentially pathogenic, and stress-tolerant bacteria were reduced by 58%, 49% and 40%, respectively, and were comparable to those seen in the NC group. Of note, ESLM did not affect gram-negative bacteria.

These findings show that the HS-induced gut flora imbalance in mice could be controlled by the ESLP. The effect of ESLL was the most significant ($p < 0.01$), but at higher doses, the effect was lower. The key gut bacteria that ESLL regulated during HS were *Achromobacter*, *Acinetobacter*, *Lactobacillus*, *Akkermansia*, *Allobaculum* and *Oscillospira*.

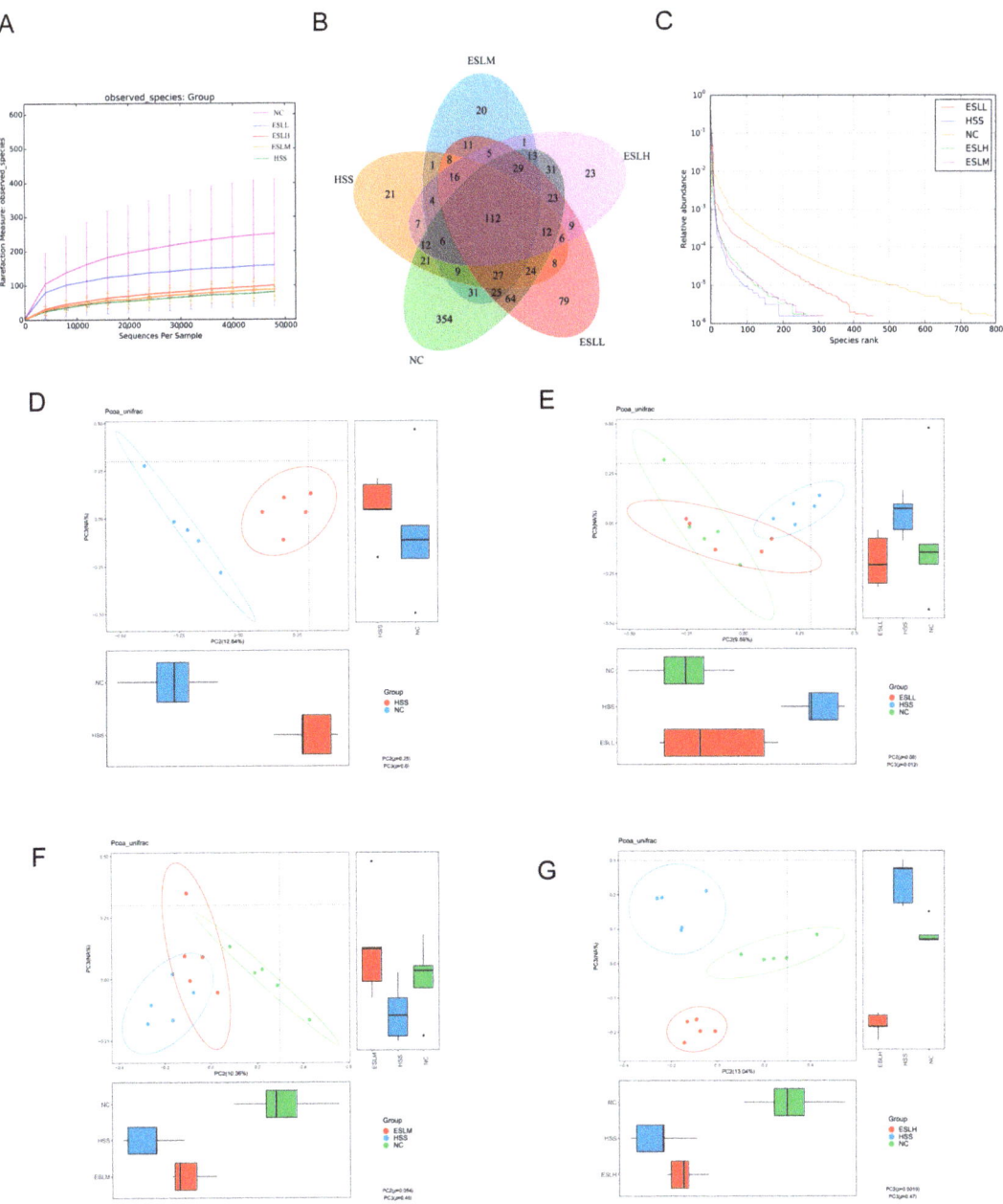

Figure 4. Effects of HS modelling and ESLP treatment on the diversity of gut microbiota in mice. (**A**) Rarefaction Curve; (**B**) Venn diagram based on OTU; (**C**) Rank Abundance curve; (**D**–**G**) PCoA analysis of the gut microbiota of mice. Data are expressed as the mean ± SE (n = 5).

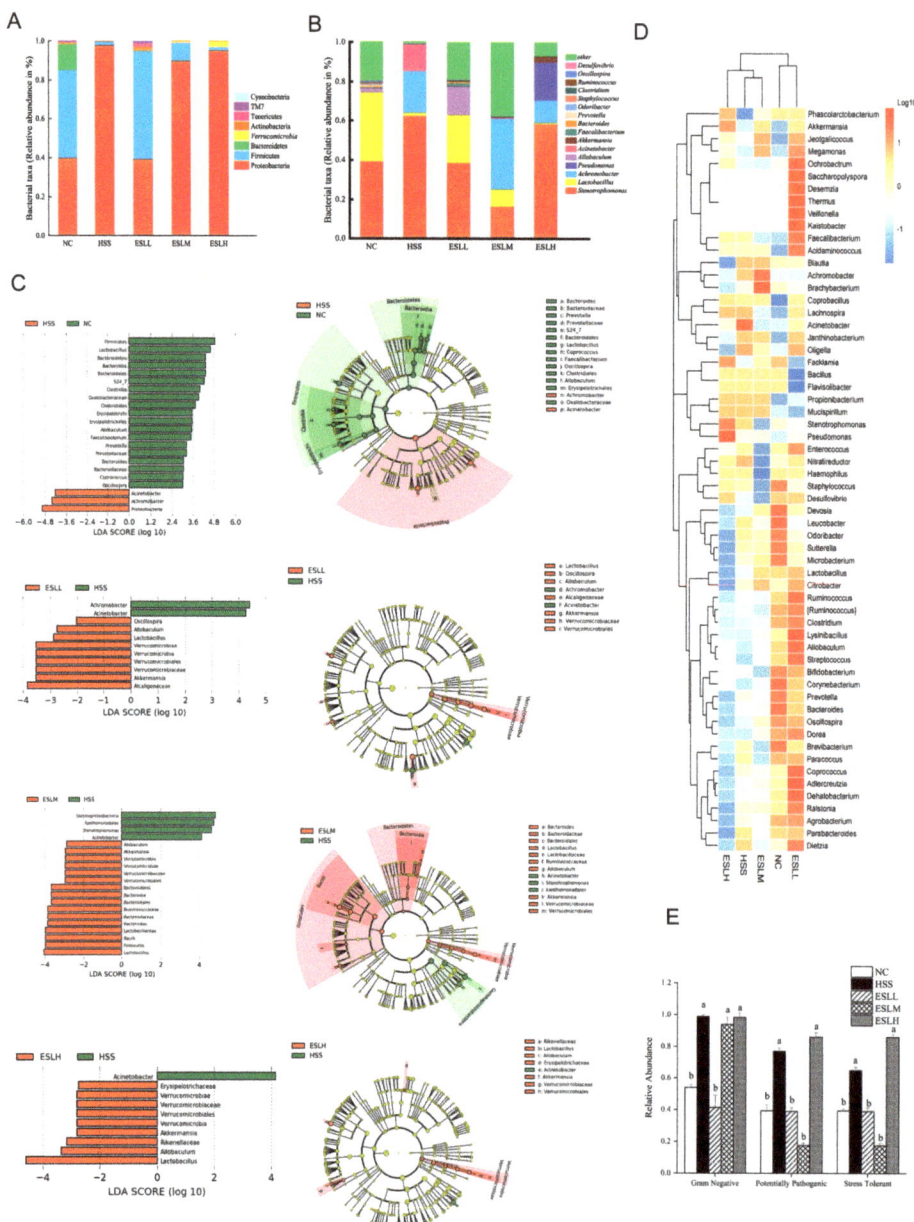

Figure 5. Modelling of the experimental data of the mice gut microbiota. Gut microbiota changes at the phylum (**A**) and genus (**B**) levels. The numerous classification units across groups based on the classification hierarchy tree based on the LEfSe and LDA histograms for taxa showed a significant difference between groups ($p < 0.05$) (**C**). Horizontal clustering heat map of gut microbiota (**D**). Comparison of the relative abundance of gram-negative, potential pathogenic, and stress-tolerant bacteria in each group (**E**). Data are shown as mean ± SE ($n = 5$). Based on the ANOVA statistical analysis, the different letters (a, b) above the bars of each group are statistically different ($p < 0.05$). [Normal control (NC), Heat stress (HS) model (HSS), HS + Low-dose ESLP gavage (ESLL), HS + Medium dose ESLP gavage (ESLM), HS + High-dose ESLP gavage (ESLH)].

3.6. Effects of ESLP on SCFAs in Heat-Stressed Mice

The concentrations of acetic, propionic, n-butyric, and isobutyric acids were significantly lower ($p < 0.05$) in the HSS group compared to the NC group (Figure 6). In contrast, the n-valeric acid concentration was significantly higher ($p < 0.05$). A lower isovaleric acid concentration was also observed ($p > 0.05$). The acetic, propionic, butyric, and isobutyric acid concentrations in the ESLL, ESLM, and ESLH groups were significantly higher than those in the HSS group ($p < 0.05$), except for isovaleric acid ($p > 0.05$). When compared with the HSS group, the n-valeric acid concentration in the ESLL group was significantly lower ($p < 0.05$), similar to the NC group. As ESLL had a superior inflammation-lowering effect than that shown in the ESLM and ESLH groups, n-valeric acid could be considered an indicator of inflammation caused by HS in ESLL.

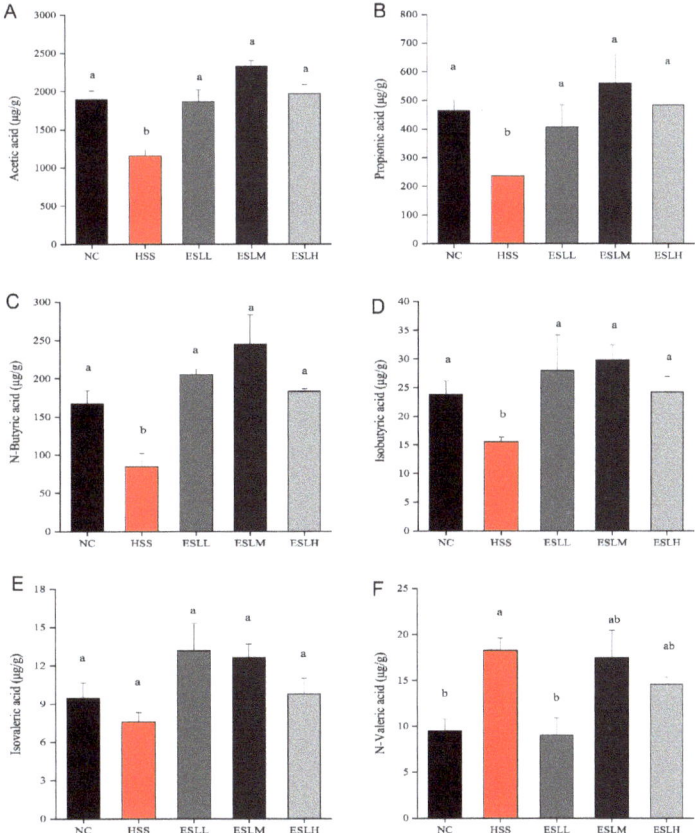

Figure 6. Mice faecal SCFA concentrations. ((**A**): Acetic acid, (**B**): Propionic acid, (**C**): N-Butyric acid, (**D**): Isobutyric acid, (**E**): Isovaleric acid, (**F**): N-Valeric acid). The data are shown as mean ± SE ($n = 5$). The ANOVA statistical analysis shows that the data with different letters a, b shown on top of each column are statistically different from each other ($p < 0.05$). [Normal control (NC), Heat stress (HS) model (HSS), HS + Low-dose ESLP gavage (ESLL), HS + Medium dose ESLP gavage (ESLM), HS + High-dose ESLP gavage (ESLH)].

3.7. Effects of ESLP on Neurotransmitters in Heat-Stressed Mice

The GABA, 5-HT, and adrenaline concentrations were significantly lower ($p < 0.05$) in the HSS group compared to the NC group, while the glutamic acid and dopamine concentrations were significantly higher ($p < 0.05$) (Figure 7). Compared with the HSS group, the concentrations of 5-HT were significantly increased ($p < 0.05$) but the glutamic acid concentration was significantly lower ($p < 0.05$) in the ESLL group. These results suggest that ESLL plays a role in regulating the concentration of neurotransmitters in HS mice.

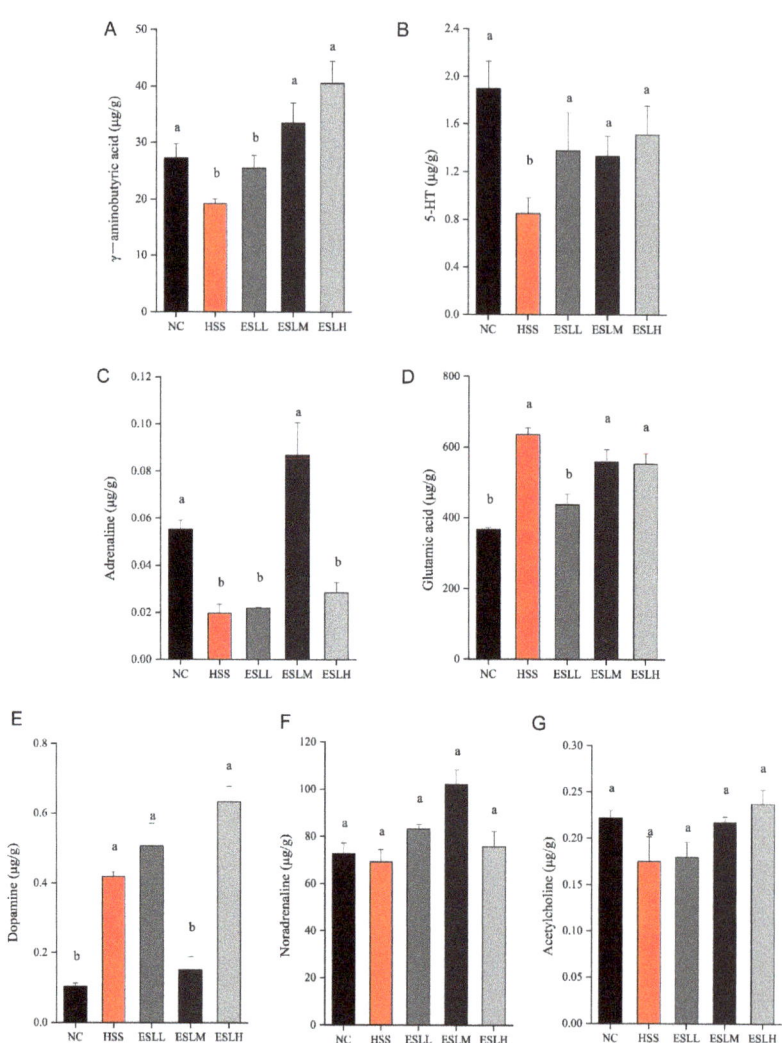

Figure 7. Faecal neurotransmitter concentrations in mice. ((**A**): γ-aminobutyric acid, (**B**): 5-HT, (**C**): Adrenaline, (**D**): Glutamic acid, (**E**): Dopamine, (**F**): Noradrenaline, (**G**): Acetylcholine). Data are shown as mean ± SE ($n = 5$). Based on the ANOVA statistical analysis, the different letters (a, b) above the bars of each group are statistically different ($p < 0.05$). [Normal control (NC), Heat stress (HS) model (HSS), HS + Low-dose ESLP gavage (ESLL), HS + Medium dose ESLP gavage (ESLM), HS + High-dose ESLP gavage (ESLH)].

3.8. Correlation Analysis of Inflammation Markers, SCFAs, Neurotransmitters and Gut Microbiota

To determine possible intrinsic associations between the serum inflammatory marker levels, faecal SCFAs levels, faecal neurotransmitters levels, and the abundance of the faecal gut microbiota, a correlation analysis between these indicators was conducted using Pearson's correlation analysis (Figure 8). The correlation between the key indicators showing that ESLL reduces systemic inflammation caused by HS was particularly analysed. *Oscillospira* positively correlated with butyric acid and negatively correlated with IL-6 and IL-1β; *Achromobacter* positively correlated with LPS, TNF-α, IL-6 and IL-1β; Acetic, propionic, butyric and isobutyric acid negatively correlated with TNF-α; Valeric acid positively correlated with IL-1β; 5-HT negatively correlated with LPS and TNF-α; and Glutamic acid positively correlated with IL-6.

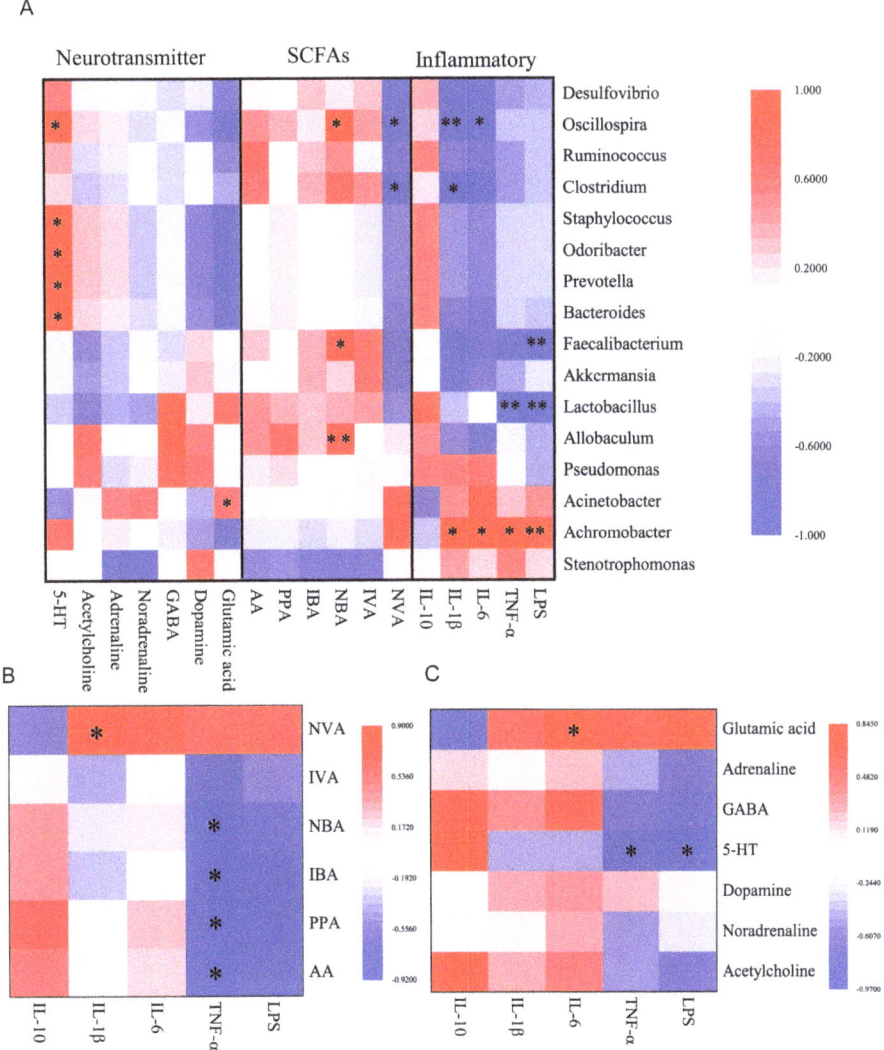

Figure 8. Correlation analysis of inflammatory markers, short-chain fatty acids (SCFAs), neurotransmitters and gut microbiota. (**A**): Relationship between the gut microbiota and inflammation, neurotransmitters, and SCFAs. (**B**): Correlation between SCFAs and inflammatory markers. (**C**): Correlation between neurotransmitters and inflammatory indicators. * $p < 0.05$, ** $p < 0.01$. AA: Acetic acid, PPA: Propionic acid, NBA: N-Butyric acid, IBA: Isobutyric acid, IVA: Isovaleric acid, NVA: N-Valeric acid. [Normal control (NC), Heat stress (HS) model (HSS), HS + Low-dose ESLP gavage (ESLL), HS + Medium dose ESLP gavage (ESLM), HS + High-dose ESLP gavage (ESLH)].

3.9. Pro-Inflammatory Activity of Valeric and Glutamic Acid In Vitro

Valeric and glutamic acid were selected for pro-inflammatory experiments in vitro. In Figure 9A,B, it can be seen that valeric and glutamic acid had no obvious cytotoxicity to RAW264.7 cells at a concentration of 10–200 μg/mL. Valeric acid significantly increased the level of IL-1β produced by RAW264.7 cells when the concentration was 50 μg/mL (Figure 9C). Glutamic acid significantly increased the level of IL-6 produced by RAW264.7 cells when the concentration was 100 μg/mL (Figure 9D). This indicates that valeric and glutamic acid have pro-inflammatory activity in vitro.

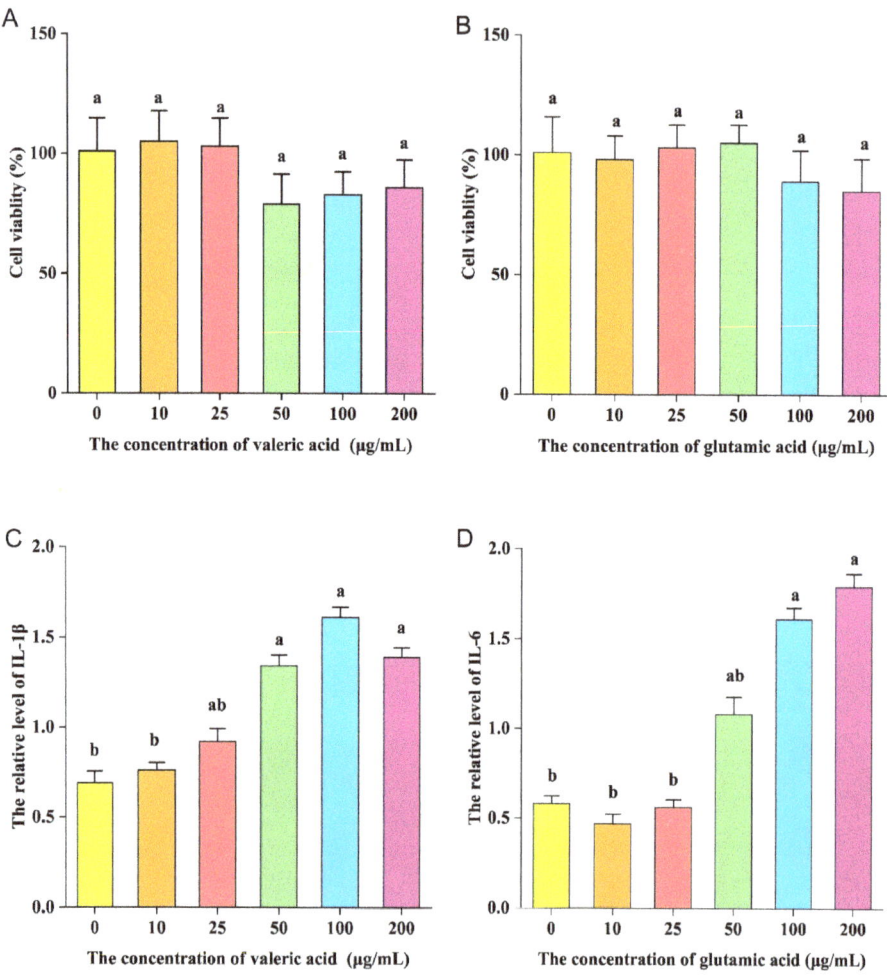

Figure 9. (**A**,**B**): The effects of different concentrations of valeric and glutamic acid on the survival rate of RAW264.7 macrophages. (**C**) The effect of different concentrations of valeric acid on IL-1β production in RAW264.7 macrophages. (**D**) The effect of different concentrations of glutamic acid on IL-6 production in RAW264.7 macrophages. The ANOVA statistical analysis shows that the data with different letters a, b shown on top of each column are statistically different from each other ($p < 0.05$).

4. Discussion

ESL is commonly added to the diet to regulate physical health [7], and has been widely studied in the scientific community [32,33]. It is known that ESL has many bioactive components, including polyphenols, flavonoids and sesquiterpene lactones [6,34]; however, the function of the polysaccharides in ESL has not yet been elucidated. In this study, the effect of ESLP on HS was investigated in heat-stressed model mice. The apparent indicators, including systemic inflammation, the gut microbiota, and related metabolites, were investigated, with the findings offering evidence of the beneficial effects of ESLP in the alleviation of systemic inflammation induced by HS and the possible targets underlying its effects.

The results of this study demonstrated that both low, medium and high doses of ESLP improved the HS-induced inflammatory response to different degrees, and that there were no significant toxic side effects on the body. A comprehensive analysis of body weight, feed intake, the serum inflammation level, intestinal tissue integrity, the gut microbiota and related metabolites, and other indicators revealed that ESLL was significantly more effective than ESLM and ESLH in improving HS. This suggests that the effect of ESLP on HS does not increase with increases in the dosage; an appropriate dosage can have a good anti-inflammatory effect. This may be because different doses of ESLP may have different effects on the gut microbiota and its metabolites; this, in turn, affects the body's immune system and leads to different levels of inflammation [35]. Other plant polysaccharides should have similar physiological effects [36]. The current findings offer a reference for future studies to investigate suitable doses of plant polysaccharide-based dietary supplements.

To date, various polysaccharides have been reported to alleviate HS. For example, alfalfa polysaccharides improve the growth performance of heat-stressed rabbits [8], atractylodes polysaccharides alleviate the splenic inflammatory response induced by HS in broiler chickens [10,11], and mannan oligosaccharides have a protective effect on HS-induced liver injury in broilers [37]. However, the above studies only focused on the local damage induced by HS and did not elucidate the mechanism by which polysaccharides alleviate HS responses in terms of key targets, such as systemic inflammation, the gut microbiota and related metabolites. Therefore, there is great potential to develop ESLP into products that resist HS responses.

Studies have shown that there are significant differences in the regulatory effects of different plant polysaccharides on the gut microbiota [15,38]. However, the role of polysaccharides in the regulation of key gut microflora during HS has rarely been reported. This study found that ESLL, like many polysaccharides, up-regulated the abundance of *Lactobacillus*, *Allobaculum* and *Akkermansia* to play a beneficial regulatory role [20]. However, inconsistent with previous findings, ESLL also significantly increased the abundance of *Oscillospira*, which was decreased due to HS, and significantly decreased the abundance of *Achromobacter*, which was increased due to HS. This suggests that *Achromobacter* and *Oscillospira* may be key target gut microbes that play a role in the regulatory effect of ESLL on HS.

Moreover, this study found, for the first time, that HS induced the massive proliferation of *Achromobacter*. However, following the ESLL intervention, the abundance of *Achromobacter* was significantly reduced. It has been reported that *Achromobacter* is an opportunistic pathogen [39], and its proliferation can induce damage to the intestinal barrier [40], leading to the entry of LPS from the gut into the bloodstream, which can trigger systemic inflammation [41]. This is consistent with the results of this study, which showed significant positive correlations between serum LPS, TNF-α, IL-6, and IL-1β levels and the abundance of *Achromobacter*. This suggests that *Achromobacter* is likely to be a key bacterium in HS-induced systemic inflammation. However, the reasons why HS triggers the proliferation of *Achromobacter* are unknown and need to be further investigated. In this study, based on the effects of the low, medium and high-dose ESLP interventions on the changes in the gut microbiota associated with HS, it is speculated that ESLL can reverse the increase in *Achromobacter*, probably because gut microbes such as *Lactobacillus*, *Akkermansia* and *Allobaculum*, which are the nutritional sources of ESLP, have the opportunity to occupy the ecological niche, resulting in a reduction in *Achromobacter*.

It is also possible that metabolites produced by the fermentative metabolism of ESLL induced by the gut flora may alter the environmental conditions in the gut, including the pH, oxygen level or other environmental parameters, to the detriment of *Achromobacter*, thus reducing systemic inflammation [42].

Oscillospira is an intestinal bacterium that can ferment complex carbohydrates and produce beneficial SCFAs such as butyric acid [43,44], which play an important role in the health of organisms. Feng et al. reported that pueraria lobata polysaccharides, like ESLL, can also significantly increase *Oscillospira* abundance, thereby attenuating antibiotic-associated diarrhoea (AAD)-induced colonic pathology and the ecological dysbiosis of mice intestinal flora [45]. However, the exact mechanism is unclear. In the current study, the correlation results revealed that the abundance of *Oscillospira* was significantly positively correlated with the butyric acid level and significantly negatively correlated with the serum inflammatory cytokine levels (IL-6 and IL-1β levels). These findings provide insight into the possible mechanism by which ESLP can alleviate HS-induced systemic inflammation. Specifically, *Oscillospira* will proliferate using ESLP as a nutrient source and will metabolise butyric acid, which is involved in the regulation of intestinal barrier integrity [46], thereby reducing the inflammatory response. Due to the relative complexity of the mechanisms by which plant polysaccharides affect the gut microbiota and the multifaceted effects of ESLP on the gut microbiota, the mechanisms of action of ESLP require further study.

SCFAs are important intestinal microbial metabolites that play a crucial role in the regulation of intestinal barrier integrity and immune factors [47]. Increases in propionate and butyrate can regulate immune homeostasis and fight against inflammation [17,19]. Increases in butyrate and acetate can reduce damage to colonic tissue and the risk of colitis [18]. This suggests that increased levels of acetic, propionic and butyric acid play a key role in reducing inflammation. This is consistent with the correlation results of this study: the serum TNF-α level was significantly negatively correlated with the acetic, propionic, butyric and isobutyric acid levels. However, in contrast to existing studies, in the current study, HS significantly increased the faecal valeric acid level and, following the ESLL intervention, this increase in the level of valeric acid was reversed. It is widely believed that valeric acid has positive effects on the body [48]. However, the results of the current study indicated that the level of the serum pro-inflammatory factor IL-1β was significantly positively correlated with the faecal valeric acid level. Further, our in vitro analysis demonstrated that valeric acid had pro-inflammatory effects on RAW264.7 cells. This suggests that valeric acid may sometimes cause inflammation. This effect may be closely linked to the amount of valeric acid present and the activation pathway of certain inflammatory cells. More research is needed to fully understand this mechanism.

Another interesting finding in this study was that ESLL restored gut barrier integrity in heat-stressed mice without maximising TJ protein expression. It is widely accepted that TJ protein expression promotes gut barrier integrity and that the two should be positively correlated. However, one study reported that valeric acid produced the biggest increase in transepithelial electrical resistance (TEER) and reduced paracellular permeability [49]. This activity was not linked to the reinforced expression of TJ-related proteins [49]. This finding also suggests that the ability of ESLL to restore gut barrier integrity in HS model mice is not only related to SCFAs such as butyric acid, which can provide energy to the gut barrier; valeric acid also appears to play an important role in this effect. Therefore, we speculate that valeric acid could be a potential indicator of HS.

Compared with the number of studies that have investigated the effects of polysaccharides on SCFAs, a smaller number of studies have investigated the effects of polysaccharides on other gut microbiota metabolites, such as neurotransmitters. Gut bacteria can produce a variety of neurotransmitters identical to those produced by the host. They can be absorbed by the gut to perform corresponding regulatory functions [50]. In this study, HS significantly reduced the faecal 5-HT concentration and, following the ESLL intervention, this effect was significantly reversed. Moreover, the faecal 5-HT level was significantly negatively correlated with the serum LPS and TNF-α levels. The available studies generally indicate that increased levels of 5-HT will affect the immune system by stimulating T-cell proliferation [51] and activating dendritic cells [52]. However, Koopman and Katsavelis [53] reported that 5-HT contributes to the strengthening of the gut barrier, which is essential for maintaining intestinal homeostasis and reducing inflammation. Thus, the role of 5-HT in inflammation is not entirely clear, as it can be either pro- or anti-inflammatory. Accordingly, the relationship between gut flora-induced changes in 5-HT levels and HS-induced systemic inflammation requires further exploration.

This study also found that the glutamic acid concentration was significantly higher in the HSS group compared to the NC group. It is widely believed that glutamic acid is a metabolite of many desirable gut bacteria, such as *Lactobacillus* and *Bifidobacterium*. Glutamic acid can assist in detoxification by removing toxic metabolic waste products [54], thus aiding in nutrient absorption and the maintenance of a healthy gut lining [55]. However, the results of this study indicated that the faecal glutamic acid level was significantly positively correlated with the serum pro-inflammatory factor IL-6 level. Further, the in vitro analysis demonstrated that glutamic acid had a pro-inflammatory effect on RAW264.7 cells. Therefore, it can be speculated that, during HS, the gut flora metabolise high levels of glutamate which, in turn, stimulates IL-6 production, thereby triggering inflammation. However, another study reported that glutamic acid decreases IL-6 production in vitro [56]. Thus, the relationship between glutamic acid and IL-6 production is complex. Further research is needed to fully understand the mechanisms and effects of glutamic acid on IL-6 production. The findings of this study also indicated that the ESLL intervention significantly reduced the glutamic acid levels. These findings imply that ESLL can alleviate HS-induced systemic inflammation by regulating the glutamic acid concentration. Thus, it can be speculated that ESLL may directly inhibit the abundance of specific gut flora involved in amino acid metabolism or that substances produced by ESLL via the metabolism of intestinal flora may inhibit glutamate synthase or glutamate metabolism for reasons that need to be further explored. Taken together, the current findings suggest that glutamic acid may also be a potential marker of HS systemic inflammation.

In summary, this study investigated the possible mechanisms by which ESLL alleviates HS-induced systemic inflammation. These findings offer a novel perspective and a viable plan for identifying potential indicators of HS inflammation and developing strategies to prevent and manage this condition. These findings also offer a theoretical basis for the ongoing development of ESLP into effective functional products that prevent and control HS, and for the safe and effective utilisation of related plant polysaccharides. This study will be followed up with a comprehensive study of ESLP, including its chemical components, molecular mass and structure, in order to fully understand the relationship between the structure and efficacy of ESLP. The ultimate goal is to develop ESLP and its structurally similar polysaccharides into functional ingredients or foods to promote health.

5. Conclusions

This study revealed that ESLL alleviates HS-induced systemic inflammation in mice by reducing serum TNF-α, IL-6 and IL-1β levels according to three main mechanisms: (a) ESLL supplementation regulates the gut microbiota, promotes the proliferation of beneficial bacteria (*Lactobacillus*, *Akkermansia* and *Allobaculum*), and inhibits the proliferation of harmful bacteria (*Achromobacter*), thus reducing the LPS level. (b) ESLL promotes the gut microbiota (*Oscillospira*), which produces beneficial SCFAs like butyric acid, provides sufficient energy for gut epithelial cells, and strengthens the intestinal barrier, making it harder for harmful substances to move into the bloodstream. (c) ESLL regulates gut microbiota metabolites, thus increasing 5-HT levels and decreasing valeric and glutamic acid levels.

Author Contributions: Conceptualization, C.W., D.S., Q.D. and L.S.; methodology, C.W., D.S., L.S., Z.F. and Q.D.; validation, C.W., D.S., Q.D. and L.H.; formal analysis, C.W.; investigation, C.W., D.S., Q.D. and L.H.; resources, C.W.; data curation, C.W., D.S. and L.S.; writing—original draft preparation, C.W.; writing—review and editing, C.W., D.S., L.S., R.G. and J.Z.; supervision, L.S. and Q.D.; project administration, Q.D. and L.S.; funding acquisition, Q.D. and L.S. All authors have read and agreed to the published version of the manuscript.

Funding: This research was funded by Guangdong Provincial Key Research and Development Programme (2021B0202060001), Guangdong Provincial Special Fund for Technological Innovation of Modern Agricultural Industry (No. 2023KJ151), Characteristic innovation project of colleges university in Guangdong Province (No. 2020KQNCX025) and Special Project for Rural Revitalization (Announcing and Leading Technology Assistance Projects) (No. 080503042201).

Institutional Review Board Statement: Animal experiments were performed according to the National Guideline for Experimental Animal Welfare and approved by the Animal Ethics Committee of Guangdong Ocean University (ethics identification number: GDOU-LAE-2020-015, 18 October 2020).

Informed Consent Statement: Not applicable.

Data Availability Statement: The corresponding author will provide the information supporting the findings upon reasonable request. The data are not publicly available due to privacy reasons.

Conflicts of Interest: The authors declare no conflict of interest.

References

1. Cantet, J.M.; Yu, Z.; Ríus, A.G. Heat Stress-Mediated Activation of Immune-Inflammatory Pathways. *Antibiotics* **2021**, *10*, 1285. [CrossRef] [PubMed]
2. Khajehnasiri, F.; Akhondzadeh, S.; Mortazavi, S.B.; Allameh, A.; Khavanin, A.; Zamanian, Z. Oxidative Stress and Depression among Male Shift Workers in Shahid Tondgouyan Refinery. *Iran. J. Psychiatry* **2014**, *4*, 11–20.
3. Tsiouris, V.; Georgopoulou, I.; Batzios, C.; Pappaioannou, N.; Ducatelle, R.; Fortomaris, P. Heat stress as a predisposing factor for necrotic enteritis in broiler chicks. *Avian Pathol.* **2018**, *47*, 616–624. [CrossRef] [PubMed]
4. Presbitero, A.; Melnikov, V.R.; Krzhizhanovskaya, V.V.; Sloot, P.M.A. A unifying model to estimate the effect of heat stress in the human innate immunity during physical activities. *Sci. Rep.* **2021**, *11*, 16688. [CrossRef] [PubMed]
5. Pease, S.; Bouadma, L.; Kermarrec, N.; Schortgen, F.; Régnier, B.; Wolff, M. Early organ dysfunction course, cooling time and outcome in classic heatstroke. *Intensive Care Med.* **2009**, *35*, 1454–1458. [CrossRef] [PubMed]
6. Hiradeve, S.M.; Rangari, V.D. Elephantopus scaber Linn.: A review on its ethnomedical, phytochemical and pharmacological profile. *J. Appl. Biomed.* **2014**, *12*, 49–61. [CrossRef]
7. Chan, C.K.; Supriady, H.; Goh, B.H.; Kadir, H.A. Elephantopus scaber induces apoptosis through ROS-dependent mitochondrial signaling pathway in HCT116 human colorectal carcinoma cells. *J. Ethnopharmacol.* **2015**, *168*, 291–304. [CrossRef]
8. Liu, H.W.; Dong, X.F.; Tong, J.M.; Zhang, Q. Alfalfa polysaccharides improve the growth performance and antioxidant status of heat-stressed rabbits. *Livest. Sci.* **2010**, *131*, 88–93. [CrossRef]
9. Sohail, M.U.; Ijaz, A.; Younus, M.; Shabbir, M.Z.; Kamran, Z.; Ahmad, S.; Anwar, H.; Yousaf, M.S.; Ashraf, K.; Shahzad, A. Effect of supplementation of mannan oligosaccharide and probiotic on growth performance, relative weights of viscera, and population of selected intestinal bacteria in cyclic heat-stressed broilers. *J. Appl. Poult. Res.* **2013**, *22*, 485–491. [CrossRef]
10. Xu, D.; Li, W.; Huang, Y.; He, J.; Tian, Y. The effect of selenium and polysaccharide of Atractylodes macrocephala Koidz.(PAMK) on immune response in chicken spleen under heat stress. *Biol. Trace Elem. Res.* **2014**, *160*, 232–237. [CrossRef]
11. Xu, D.; Li, B.; Cao, N.; Li, W.; Tian, Y.; Huang, Y. The protective effects of polysaccharide of Atractylodes macrocephala Koidz (PAMK) on the chicken spleen under heat stress via antagonizing apoptosis and restoring the immune function. *Oncotarget* **2017**, *8*, 70394. [CrossRef] [PubMed]
12. Zhang, T.; Yang, Y.; Liang, Y.; Jiao, X.; Zhao, C. Beneficial effect of intestinal fermentation of natural polysaccharides. *Nutrients* **2018**, *10*, 1055. [CrossRef]
13. Ge, Y.; Ahmed, S.; Yao, W.; You, L.; Zheng, J.; Hileuskaya, K. Regulation effects of indigestible dietary polysaccharides on intestinal microflora: An overview. *J. Food Biochem.* **2021**, *45*, e13564. [CrossRef] [PubMed]
14. Zhang, D.; Liu, J.; Cheng, H.; Wang, H.; Tan, Y.; Feng, W.; Peng, C. Interactions between polysaccharides and gut microbiota: A metabolomic and microbial review. *Food Res. Int.* **2022**, *160*, 111653. [CrossRef] [PubMed]
15. Song, Q.; Wang, Y.; Huang, L.; Shen, M.; Yu, Y.; Yu, Q.; Chen, Y.; Xie, J. Review of the relationships among polysaccharides, gut microbiota, and human health. *Food Res. Int.* **2021**, *140*, 109858. [CrossRef]
16. Shang, Q.; Song, G.; Zhang, M.; Shi, J.; Xu, C.; Hao, J.; Li, G.; Yu, G. Dietary fucoidan improves metabolic syndrome in association with increased Akkermansia population in the gut microbiota of high-fat diet-fed mice. *J. Funct. Foods* **2017**, *28*, 138–146. [CrossRef]

17. Zhang, S.; Zhao, J.; Xie, F.; He, H.; Johnston, L.J.; Dai, X.; Wu, C.; Ma, X. Dietary fiber-derived short-chain fatty acids: A potential therapeutic target to alleviate obesity-related nonalcoholic fatty liver disease. *Obes. Rev.* **2021**, *22*, e13316. [CrossRef]
18. Ji, X.; Hou, C.; Zhang, X.; Han, L.; Yin, S.; Peng, Q.; Wang, M. Microbiome-metabolomic analysis of the impact of Zizyphus jujuba cv. Muzao polysaccharides consumption on colorectal cancer mice fecal microbiota and metabolites. *Int. J. Biol. Macromol.* **2019**, *131*, 1067–1076. [CrossRef]
19. Koh, A.; De Vadder, F.; Kovatcheva-Datchary, P.; Bäckhed, F. From dietary fiber to host physiology: Short-chain fatty acids as key bacterial metabolites. *Cell* **2016**, *165*, 1332–1345. [CrossRef]
20. Feng, W.; Liu, J.; Tan, Y.; Ao, H.; Wang, J.; Peng, C. Polysaccharides from Atractylodes macrocephala Koidz. Ameliorate ulcerative colitis via extensive modification of gut microbiota and host metabolism. *Food Res. Int.* **2020**, *138*, 109777. [CrossRef]
21. Chen, P.; Hei, M.; Kong, L.; Liu, Y.; Yang, Y.; Mu, H.; Zhang, X.; Zhao, S.; Duan, J. One water-soluble polysaccharide from Ginkgo biloba leaves with antidepressant activities via modulation of the gut microbiome. *Food Funct.* **2019**, *10*, 8161–8171. [CrossRef] [PubMed]
22. Zhou, S.; Huang, G.; Chen, G. Extraction, structural analysis, derivatization and antioxidant activity of polysaccharide from Chinese yam. *Food Chem.* **2021**, *361*, 130089. [CrossRef] [PubMed]
23. Saha, S.K.; Brewer, C.F. Determination of the concentrations of oligosaccharides, complex type carbohydrates, and glycoproteins using the phenol-sulfuric acid method. *Carbohydr. Res.* **1994**, *254*, 157–167. [CrossRef] [PubMed]
24. Miller, G.L. Use of dinitrosalicylic acid reagent for determination of reducing sugar. *Anal. Chem.* **1959**, *31*, 426–428. [CrossRef]
25. Filisetti-Cozzi, T.M.; Carpita, N.C. Measurement of uronic acids without interference from neutral sugars. *Anal. Biochem.* **1991**, *197*, 157–162. [CrossRef] [PubMed]
26. Sun, D.; Wang, C.; Sun, L.; Hu, L.; Fang, Z.; Deng, Q.; Zhao, J.; Gooneratne, R. Preliminary Report on Intestinal Flora Disorder, Faecal Short-Chain Fatty Acid Level Decline and Intestinal Mucosal Tissue Weakening Caused by Litchi Extract to Induce Systemic Inflammation in HFA Mice. *Nutrients* **2022**, *14*, 776. [CrossRef]
27. Iqbal, H.; Kim, S.K.; Cha, K.M.; Jeong, M.S.; Ghosh, P.; Rhee, D.K. Korean Red Ginseng alleviates neuroinflammation and promotes cell survival in the intermittent heat stress-induced rat brain by suppressing oxidative stress via estrogen receptor beta and brain-derived neurotrophic factor upregulation. *J. Ginseng. Res.* **2020**, *44*, 593–602. [CrossRef]
28. Ducray, H.A.G.; Globa, L.; Pustovyy, O.; Morrison, E.; Vodyanoy, V.; Sorokulova, I. Yeast fermentate prebiotic improves intestinal barrier integrity during heat stress by modulation of the gut microbiota in rats. *J. Appl. Microbiol.* **2019**, *127*, 1192–1206. [CrossRef]
29. Yang, L.; Zhang, L.; Zhang, P.; Zhou, Y.; Huang, X.; Yan, Q.; Tan, Z.; Tang, S.; Wan, F. Alterations in nutrient digestibility and performance of heat-stressed dairy cows by dietary L-theanine supplementation. *Anim. Nutr. (Zhongguo Xu Mu Shou Yi Xue Hui)* **2022**, *11*, 350–358. [CrossRef]
30. Wang, L.; An, J.; Song, S.; Mei, M.; Li, W.; Ding, F.; Liu, S. Electroacupuncture preserves intestinal barrier integrity through modulating the gut microbiota in DSS-induced chronic colitis. *Life Sci.* **2020**, *261*, 118473. [CrossRef]
31. Yang, Y.; Zhang, Y.; Song, J.; Li, Y.; Zhou, L.; Xu, H.; Wu, K.; Gao, J.; Zhao, M.; Zheng, Y. Bergamot polysaccharides relieve DSS-induced ulcerative colitis via regulating the gut microbiota and metabolites. *Int. J. Biol. Macromol.* **2023**, *253*, 127335. [CrossRef] [PubMed]
32. Qi, R.; Li, X.; Zhang, X.; Huang, Y.; Fei, Q.; Han, Y.; Cai, R.; Gao, Y.; Qi, Y. Ethanol extract of Elephantopus scaber Linn. Attenuates inflammatory response via the inhibition of NF-κB signaling by dampening p65-DNA binding activity in lipopolysaccharide-activated macrophages. *J. Ethnopharmacol.* **2020**, *250*, 24–39. [CrossRef] [PubMed]
33. Doan, H.V.; Hoseinifar, S.H.; Sringarm, K.; Jaturasitha, S.; Khamlor, T.; Dawood, M.A.O.; Esteban, M.Á.; Soltani, M.; Musthafa, M.S. Effects of elephant's foot (*Elephantopus scaber*) extract on growth performance, immune response, and disease resistance of nile tilapia (*Oreochromis niloticus*) fingerlings. *Fish Shellfish Immunol.* **2019**, *93*, 328–335. [CrossRef] [PubMed]
34. Wu, Y.; Cui, H.; Cheng, B.; Fang, S.; Xu, J.; Gu, Q. Chemical constituents from the roots of *Elephantopus scaber* L. *Biochem. Syst. Ecol.* **2014**, *54*, 65–67. [CrossRef]
35. Ho Do, M.; Seo, Y.S.; Park, H.Y. Polysaccharides: Bowel health and gut microbiota. *Crit. Rev. Food Sci. Nutr.* **2021**, *61*, 1212–1224. [CrossRef]
36. Gan, L.; Wang, J.; Guo, Y. Polysaccharides influence human health via microbiota-dependent and -independent pathways. *Front. Nutr.* **2022**, *9*, 1030063. [CrossRef]
37. Chen, Y.; Cheng, Y.; Wen, C.; Zhou, Y. Protective effects of dietary mannan oligosaccharide on heat stress-induced hepatic damage in broilers. *Environ. Sci. Pollut. Res. Int.* **2020**, *27*, 29000–29008. [CrossRef]
38. Yu, W.; Zeng, D.; Xiong, Y.; Shan, S.; Yang, X.; Zhao, H.; Lu, W. Health benefits of functional plant polysaccharides in metabolic syndrome: An overview. *J. Funct. Foods* **2022**, *95*, 105154. [CrossRef]
39. Snavely, E.A.; Precit, M. It's Bordetella, It's Alcaligenes... No, It's Achromobacter! Identification, Antimicrobial Resistance, and Clinical Significance of an Understudied Gram-Negative Rod. *Clin. Microbiol. Newsl.* **2022**, *44*, 169–177. [CrossRef]
40. Xu, J.; Molin, G.; Davidson, S.; Roth, B.; Sjöberg, K. CRP in Outpatients with Inflammatory Bowel Disease Is Linked to the Blood Microbiota. *Int. J. Mol. Sci.* **2023**, *24*, 10899. [CrossRef]
41. Vicente, A.R.; Ayala-Rodriguez, C.; Colón-Núñez, C.; De Jesus, G.G.; Pabon, M.A.M. From the Gut to the Heart: Purulent Pericarditis Due to *Achromobacter* Spp. Bacteremia in a Patient with Systemic Lupus Erythematosus (Sle) and Strongyloides Stercoralis Infection. *J. Am. Coll. Cardiol.* **2023**, *81*, 3015. [CrossRef]

42. Neidhöfer, C.; Berens, C.; Parčina, M. An 18-Year Dataset on the Clinical Incidence and MICs to Antibiotics of *Achromobacter* spp. (Labeled Biochemically or by MAL-DI-TOF MS as A. xylosoxidans), Largely in Patient Groups Other than Those with CF. *Antibiotics* **2022**, *11*, 311. [CrossRef]
43. Yang, J.; Li, Y.; Wen, Z.; Liu, W.; Meng, L.; Huang, H. Oscillospira—A candidate for the next-generation probiotics. *Gut Microbes* **2021**, *13*, 1987783. [CrossRef]
44. Konikoff, T.; Gophna, U. Oscillospira: A Central, Enigmatic Component of the Human Gut Microbiota. *Trends Microbiol.* **2016**, *24*, 523–524. [CrossRef] [PubMed]
45. Feng, W.; Liu, J.; Ao, H.; Yue, S.; Peng, C. Targeting gut microbiota for precision medicine: Focusing on the efficacy and toxicity of drugs. *Theranostics* **2020**, *10*, 11278–11301. [CrossRef] [PubMed]
46. Rudiansyah, M.; Abdalkareem Jasim, S.; Azizov, B.S.; Samusenkov, V.; Kamal Abdelbasset, W.; Yasin, G.; Mohammad, H.J.; Jawad, M.A.; Mahmudiono, T.; Hosseini-Fard, S.R. The emerging microbiome-based approaches to IBD therapy: From SCFAs to urolithin A. *J. Dig. Dis.* **2022**, *23*, 412–434. [CrossRef] [PubMed]
47. Singh, R.K.; Chang, H.W.; Yan, D.; Lee, K.M.; Ucmak, D.; Wong, K.; Abrouk, M.; Farahnik, B.; Nakamura, M.; Tian, H.Z. Influence of diet on the gut microbiome and implications for human health. *J. Transl. Med.* **2017**, *15*, 11–21. [CrossRef]
48. Jayaraj, R.L.; Beiram, R.; Azimullah, S.; Mf, N.M.; Ojha, S.K.; Adem, A. Valeric Acid Protects Dopaminergic Neurons by Suppressing Oxidative Stress, Neuroinflammation and Modulating Autophagy Pathways. *Int. J. Mol. Sci.* **2020**, *21*, 7670. [CrossRef]
49. Gao, G.; Zhou, J.; Wang, H.; Ding, Y.; Zhou, J.; Chong, P.H.; Zhu, L.; Ke, L. Effects of valerate on intestinal barrier function in cultured Caco-2 epithelial cell monolayers. *Mol. Biol. Rep.* **2022**, *49*, 1817–1825. [CrossRef]
50. Wu, M.; Tian, T.; Mao, Q.; Zou, T.; Chen, J.J. Associations between disordered gut microbiota and changes of neurotransmitters and short-chain fatty acids in depressed mice. *Transl. Psychiatry* **2020**, *10*, 112–132. [CrossRef]
51. Ahern, G.P. 5-HT and the immune system. *Curr. Opin. Pharmacol.* **2011**, *11*, 29–33. [CrossRef] [PubMed]
52. Wan, M.; Ding, L.; Wang, D.; Han, J.; Gao, P. Serotonin: A Potent Immune Cell Modulator in Autoimmune Diseases. *Front. Immunol.* **2020**, *11*, 186. [CrossRef] [PubMed]
53. Koopman, N.; Katsavelis, D. The Multifaceted Role of Serotonin in Intestinal Homeostasis. *Int. J. Mol. Sci.* **2021**, *22*, 9487. [CrossRef] [PubMed]
54. de Bie, T.; Balvers, M.; Jongsma, M.; Witkamp, R. Dietary Neurotransmitters: The Relative Oral Bioavailability of GABA and Glutamic Acid From Tomato in Healthy Human Volunteers. *Curr. Dev. Nutr.* **2021**, *5*, 311. [CrossRef]
55. Motaghi, S.; Sirchi, M.M.; Hosseininasab, N.s.; Abbasnejad, M.; Esmaili-Mahani, S.; Sepehri, G. Age-Related Changes in Glutamic Acid Decarboxylase 1 Gene Expression in the Medial Prefrontal Cortex and Ventral Hippocampus of Fear-Potentiated Rats Subjected to Isolation Stress. *Behav. Brain Res.* **2023**, *453*, 114630. [CrossRef]
56. Coëffier, M.; Marion, R.; Leplingard, A.; Lerebours, E.; Ducrotté, P.; Déchelotte, P. Glutamine decreases interleukin-8 and interleukin-6 but not nitric oxide and prostaglandins e(2) production by human gut in-vitro. *Cytokine* **2002**, *18*, 92–97. [CrossRef]

Disclaimer/Publisher's Note: The statements, opinions and data contained in all publications are solely those of the individual author(s) and contributor(s) and not of MDPI and/or the editor(s). MDPI and/or the editor(s) disclaim responsibility for any injury to people or property resulting from any ideas, methods, instructions or products referred to in the content.

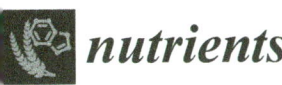

Article

Protective Effect of the Polyphenol Ligustroside on Colitis Induced with Dextran Sulfate Sodium in Mice

Ruonan Gao [1,2], Yilin Ren [1,2,3,*], Peng Xue [4], Yingyue Sheng [1], Qin Yang [2], Yuanyuan Dai [1], Xiaoyue Zhang [1,2], Ziming Lin [1,2], Tianhao Liu [1], Yan Geng [5] and Yuzheng Xue [1,*]

1. Department of Gastroenterology, Affiliated Hospital of Jiangnan University, Wuxi 214122, China
2. Wuxi School of Medicine, Jiangnan University, Wuxi 214122, China
3. Key Laboratory of Industrial Biotechnology of Ministry of Education, School of Biotechnology, Jiangnan University, Wuxi 214122, China
4. School of Medicine, Nantong University, Nantong 226001, China
5. School of Life Science and Health Engineering, Jiangnan University, Wuxi 214122, China; gengyan@jiangnan.edu.cn
* Correspondence: renyilin@jiangnan.edu.cn (Y.R.); 9862018034@jiangnan.edu.cn (Y.X.)

Abstract: Dietary polyphenols are reported to alleviate colitis by interacting with gut microbiota which plays an important role in maintaining the integrity of the intestinal barrier. As a type of dietary polyphenol, whether ligustroside (Lig) could alleviate colitis has not been explored yet. Here, we aimed to determine if supplementation of ligustroside could improve colitis. We explored the influence of ligustroside intake with different dosages on colitis induced with dextran sulfate sodium (DSS). Compared to the DSS group, supplementation of ligustroside could reduce body weight (BW) loss, decrease disease activity indices (DAI), and relieve colon damage in colitis mice. Furthermore, ligustroside intake with 2 mg/kg could decrease proinflammatory cytokine concentrations in serum and increase immunoglobulin content and antioxidant enzymes in colon tissue. In addition, supplementation of ligustroside (2 mg/kg) could reduce mucus secretion and prevent cell apoptosis. Also, changes were revealed in the bacterial community composition, microbiota functional profiles, and intestinal metabolite composition following ligustroside supplementation with 2 mg/kg using 16S rRNA sequencing and non-targeted lipidomics analysis. In conclusion, the results showed that ligustroside was very effective in preventing colitis through reduction in inflammation and the enhancement of the intestinal barrier. Furthermore, supplementation with ligustroside altered the gut microbiota and lipid composition of colitis mice.

Keywords: inflammatory bowel disease (IBD); ligustroside; colitis

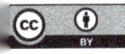

1. Introduction

Inflammatory bowel disease (IBD) is a chronic non-specific intestinal inflammatory disease. It mainly involves colonic mucosa and submucosa and presents as recurrent chronic intestinal inflammation. There are two subtypes of IBD, including ulcerative colitis (UC) and Crohn's disease (CD) [1,2]. The latest data show that IBD is still on the rise worldwide, with about 0.2% of the European population suffering from IBD, which has become a serious global health burden [3]. The pathogenesis of IBD is unknown at present, involving a variety of causes such as being heredity, the environmental diet, intestinal barrier, immunity, and microorganisms [4–6]. IBD is prone to recurrence and various systemic complications after treatment, which seriously affect patient's quality of life and survival rate. How to effectively solve the treatment difficulties of IBD has become a major research focus at present.

Several factors contribute to IBD pathogenesis, including genetic susceptibility and environmental factors, which can weaken the intestinal barrier and lead to inappropriate intestinal immune activation by affecting the microflora. An imbalance of intestinal microflora has been observed in patients with IBD [7]. The most common changes were that Firmicutes decreased and Enterobacteriaceae increased in IBD [8,9]. Compared with healthy individuals, *Faecalibacterium prausnitzii*, *Roseburia intestinalis*, Lachnospiraceae, and Ruminococcaceae decreased, while *B.fragilis*, *Escherichia coli*, and Enterobacteriaceae increased in CD. *Bifidobacterium*, *Roseburia hominis*, and *Faecalibacterium prausnitzii* decreased while Lachnospiraceae increased in UC [10,11]. In addition, an imbalance between intestinal mucosa and intestinal contents is also a cause of pathological changes in IBD. Intestinal mucosa consists of epithelial cells, goblet and Paneth cells, stroma, and immune cells. Goblet cells can produce a mucous matrix that covers epithelial cells and thus plays a role in mucosal defense and repair [12]. Innate immune cells, such as neutrophils and macrophages, can strengthen the physical and functional barriers of the intestinal barrier as the first line of defense of the well-developed mucosal innate immune system. Neutrophils can directly cause tissue damage by releasing neutrophil elastase, matrix metalloproteinases (MMPs), pro-inflammatory cytokines including tumor necrosis factor (TNF)-α and interleukin (IL)-1β, and superoxide dismutase (SOD) in IBD. Furthermore, these factors lead to damage to the epithelial barrier as well as recruiting neutrophils and other immune cells to the inflamed area [13,14]. In addition, macrophages were expressed at high levels of pro-inflammatory molecules including TNF-α, IL-1β, IL-6, and inducible nitric oxide synthase (iNOS) during IBD [15].

Polyphenols are organic compounds containing oxygen heterocycles. Researchers have found that polyphenols and their derivatives can play antioxidant and anti-inflammatory roles by regulating intestinal barrier function, changing the composition of intestinal flora, or activating congenital and adaptive immune responses [16–18]. On the one hand, colonic microbes extensively metabolize polyphenols [19]. Polyphenols can shape the composition of the intestinal bacteria, such as through increasing probiotics *Bifidobacterium* and inhibiting the growth of several pathogenic bacteria [20]. On the other hand, it has been demonstrated that polyphenols have protective effects on intestinal barrier functions by modulating mucus production and antimicrobial peptide secretion [21,22]. As a functional food, ligustroside is one of the common polyphenolic compounds which can be extracted from extra virgin olive oil (EVOO) [17,23]. Diets including EVOO in mice colitis have been extensively studied [24,25]. The prospect of ligustroside being a complementary therapy for IBD has attracted more attention in recent years. Therefore, considering that the effects of ligustroside on colitis are unclear, we investigated the potential effects of ligustroside on DSS-induced colitis in mice.

2. Materials and Methods

2.1. Animal Experimental Design

Male C57BL/6 mice (aged 7–8 weeks, weighing about 20 ± 2 g) were purchased from Gempharmatech Co., Ltd. (Nanjing, China) The drug ligustroside (CAS35897-92-8, purity ≥ 98%, store at 2–8 °C) and 5-aminosalicylic acid (5-ASA, CAS89-57-6, purity ≥ 99%, store at RT) were purchased from Shanghai Yuanye Bio-Technology Co., Ltd. (Shanghai, China), and dextran sulfate sodium (DSS, CAS9011-18-1, store at 2–8 °C, M.W 40,000) was purchased from Shanghai Macklin Biochemical Co., Ltd. (Shanghai, China). As shown in Figure 1A, a total of 30 C57BL/6 male mice were randomly divided into six groups ($n = 5$ per group).

After 7 days of adaption, mice in the Control and DSS groups received phosphate-buffered saline (PBS) solution while mice in the DSS + 5-ASA group received oral administration of 5-ASA dissolved in distilled water (150 mg/kg BW) and mice in the DSS + Lig groups received different dosages of ligustroside dissolved in distilled water daily for 14 days. On Day 8, 2.5% DSS (w/v) was added to the water for mice except for the Control group for an additional 7 days. All mice were raised in the Experimental Animal Centre of the Medical College of Jiangnan University. Mice were fed a rodent chow diet, and the daily food intake of the mice was about 5–10 g/mouse. The mice ate and drank freely every day. The feeding conditions were as follows: 12 h light/dark cycle, temperature 22 ± 2 °C, humidity 55 ± 5%, and noise level ≤ 60 dB. All mice were anesthetized through inhalation of 3% isoflurane and then euthanatized using cervical dislocation on the 15th day of the experiment. A review and approval of the animal study was conducted by Jiangnan University's Institutional Animal Care and Use Committee [Approval No. 20220330c1440615 (114)].

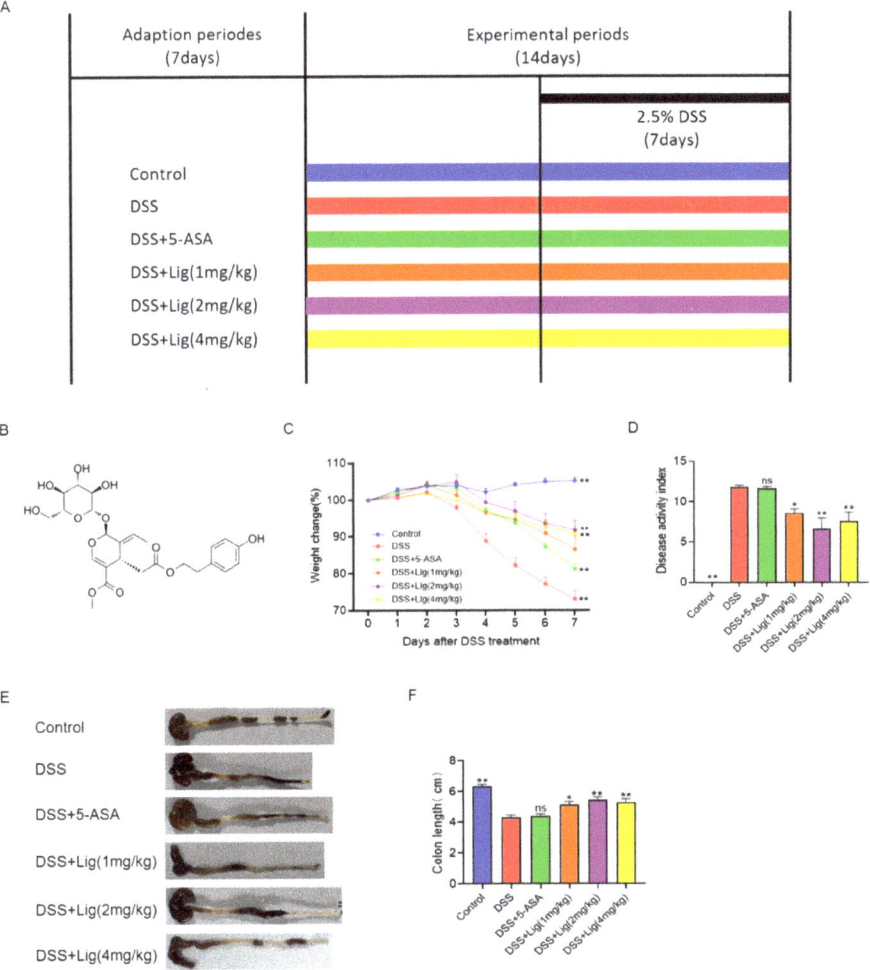

Figure 1. Supplementation of ligustroside alleviated colitis symptoms in DSS-treated mice. (**A**) Treatment timeline for the experiment, (**B**) chemical structure of ligustroside, (**C**) body weight change (%), (**D**) disease activity index scores, (**E,F**) colon lengths of the mice. * $p < 0.05$ and ** $p < 0.01$ vs. DSS group, ns means $p > 0.05$ vs. DSS group, $n = 5$.

2.2. Disease Activity Index (DAI)

The disease changes in mice were observed by evaluating their DAI, including weight loss, occult blood or blood stool and shape of feces, as described in previous research article [26].

2.3. Analysis of Colon Histology in Mice

After the experiment, mice's colons were dissected. The lengths of the colons were measured. Ice-cold phosphate-buffered saline was used to wash the lumen of the colons. A neutral tissue fixation solution was then applied to the tissues. After dehydration with ethanol, paraffin was used to embed the sample. After preparing 4 mm thick paraffin sections, hematoxylin and eosin staining, and Alcian blue/periodic acid-Schiff (AB/PAS) staining were conducted. Under the microscope, colon morphology was observed. As previously described, the degree of tissue injury was based on the degree of inflammatory cell infiltration (0–3) and tissue injury (0–3) [27]. A TUNEL assay was used to determine the apoptosis level in colonic cells. The nuclei of the cells were stained with DAPI and observed using a fluorescence microscope.

2.4. Enzyme-Linked Immunosorbent Assay (ELISA)

We separated mouse serum from blood with centrifugation at $1500\times g$ for 15 min and stored at -20 °C. The contents of proinflammatory cytokines IL-6, IL-1β, TNF-α, and immunoglobulin IgA, IgG, and IgM in serum were detected using an ELISA kit (Thermo Scientific, Shanghai, China). The colonic tissue of mice was homogenized in ice-cold phosphate-buffered saline and centrifuged at $13,000\times g$ for 20 min at 4 °C. The supernatant of colonic tissue was collected, and the content of the secretory immunoglobulin (SIgA) and superoxide dismutase (SOD) in the colonic tissue supernatant was detected using an ELISA kit.

2.5. Gut Microbiota Analysis

DNA from the stool microbial community was extracted using MagPure Stool DNA KF kit B (Magen, Foshan, China), and then it was quantified with a Qubit Fluorometer using the Qubit dsDNA BR Assay kit (Invitrogen, Waltham, MA, USA). The PCR products were sequenced on the Illumina MiSeq platform (BGI, Shenzhen, China). Tags with 100% similarity were clustered to the same ASV. The Ribosomal Database Project Bayesian classifier algorithm was used to analyze the ASV representative sequences. Alpha and beta diversity analyses were assessed using MOTHUR and QIIME (v2022.2). Linear Discriminant Analysis Effect Size (LEfSe) was used to analyze the biomarkers of different groups. Microbial functions were also predicted using Phylogenetic Investigation of Communities through Reconstruction of Unobserved States (PICRUSt).

2.6. Non-Targeted Lipidomic Analysis

To extract metabolites from the contents of the mouse colons, 300 μL methanol, 1000 μL methyl tert-butyl ether, and 250 μL ultra-pure water extraction solvent was added to the sample and thoroughly vortexed. Then, the samples were incubated for 10 min, followed by centrifugation at $1000\times g$ for 5 min at 10 °C. We collected the supernatant, and a vacuum centrifuge was used to collect and dry the elution. For a liquid chromatography mass spectrometer (LC-MS) analysis, the samples were redissolved in 50 μL chloroform/methanol ($v{:}v$ = 2:1) solvent and transferred to vials.

An ultra-high-performance liquid chromatography (UHPLC) system (ThermoFisherQ Exactive™ Plus, Waltham, MA, USA) was used to analyze the samples. The sample was separated using a UPLC BEH C18 column (100 mm × 2.1 mm, 1.7 μm). Separation was initiated at a flow rate of 250 μL/min. During the whole analysis process, the sample was kept at 4 °C. Detection of metabolites was performed using ThermoFisherQ Exactive™ Plus with an ESI ion source. Raw data were processed using LipidSearch v.4.1 (Thermo Fisher Scientific, Waltham, MA, USA). The data were imported into MetaboAnalysit 5.0 for sparse PLS-DA (sPLSDA), volcano map, and hierarchical clustering heatmap analysis.

2.7. Statistical Analyses

The data are shown as means $\pm$ standard error of the mean (SEM). The statistical difference between two groups was assessed using unpaired two-tailed Student's t-tests, and the differences of more than two groups were assessed using ordinary one-way analysis of variance, using GraphPad Prism 8.4 (Graphpad Software, Inc., La Jolla, CA, USA). A difference of $p < 0.05$ was considered statistically significant. * $p < 0.05$ and ** $p < 0.01$ vs. DSS group, ns means $p > 0.05$ vs. DSS group, $n = 5$.

3. Results

3.1. Ligustroside Can Relieve DSS-Induced Colitis in Mice

The chemical structure of ligustroside is shown in Figure 1B. The timeline of the experiment is shown in Figure 1A. After drinking 2.5% DSS solution for one week, mice developed severe acute colitis, including loss of weight (Figure 1C), an increase in the DAI (Figure 1D), diarrhea, and bleeding in feces. DSS stimulation significantly shortened the length of the colon in mice (Figure 1E,F). After the administration of DSS solution for one week, the weight of the mice significantly dropped, which was alleviated through the oral administration of ligustroside (Figure 1C). In colitis mice induced with DSS, ligustroside also significantly decreased the DAI scores (Figure 1D). Ligustroside increased the length of the colon (Figure 1E,F). To summarize, DSS-induced colitis could be significantly improved with oral ligustroside supplementation.

3.2. Ligustroside Can Ameliorate Colonic Injury Induced with DSS

A histopathological analysis showed that mucosal injury, inflammatory cell infiltration, and crypt loss were significantly alleviated in the mice treated with ligustroside (Figure 2A), while the histopathological scores of colons from the DSS group were significantly higher than the Control group. A significant decrease in the histopathological scores of the colon tissue was observed in mice after supplementation with ligustroside (Figure 2B).

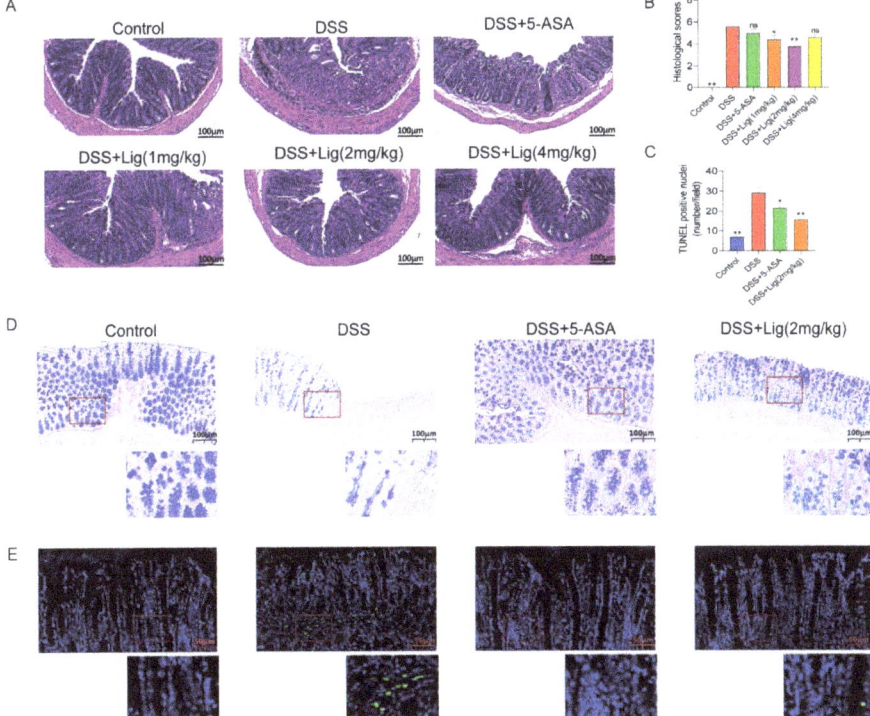

Figure 2. Supplementation of ligustroside alleviated histological changes in colitis mice. (A) Mouse colon morphology stained with hematoxylin and eosin. (B) The histological scores of mouse colon tissue. (C) The number of TUNEL-positive nuclei per field in mouse colon. (D) AB/PAS staining. (E) The TUNEL staining of colon cells. * $p < 0.05$ and ** $p < 0.01$ vs. DSS group, ns means $p > 0.05$ vs. DSS group, $n = 5$.

Based on the results of the above data, we found that the DSS + Lig (2 mg/kg) group had the best effect on alleviating colitis induced with DSS. Therefore, we conducted further analysis on the mice in the DSS + Lig (2 mg/kg) group. AB-PAS staining analysis showed that the protective substances secreted by the mucus layer in the colon of mice decreased in the DSS group (Figure 2D), and the intestinal barrier was damaged. Furthermore, a large number of apoptotic cells were seen in the DSS group using TUNEL staining (Figure 2C,F), which could be reversed through the supplementation of ligustroside.

3.3. Effects of Ligustroside on the Secretion of Cytokines, Immunoglobulins, and the Oxidation Index

The concentrations of proinflammatory cytokines IL-6, IL-1β, and TNF-α significantly increased in the serum of mice with colitis induced with DSS (Figure 3A–C), while the concentration of immunoglobulin IgA in serum was decreased in the DSS group (Figure 3D). Furthermore, the concentration of SIgA (Figure 3E) and the activity of the antioxidant SOD (Figure 3F) in the mouse colon were decreased in the DSS-induced colitis mice. However, after supplementing with ligustroside, the changes in these indicators can be reversed and were similar to the Control group.

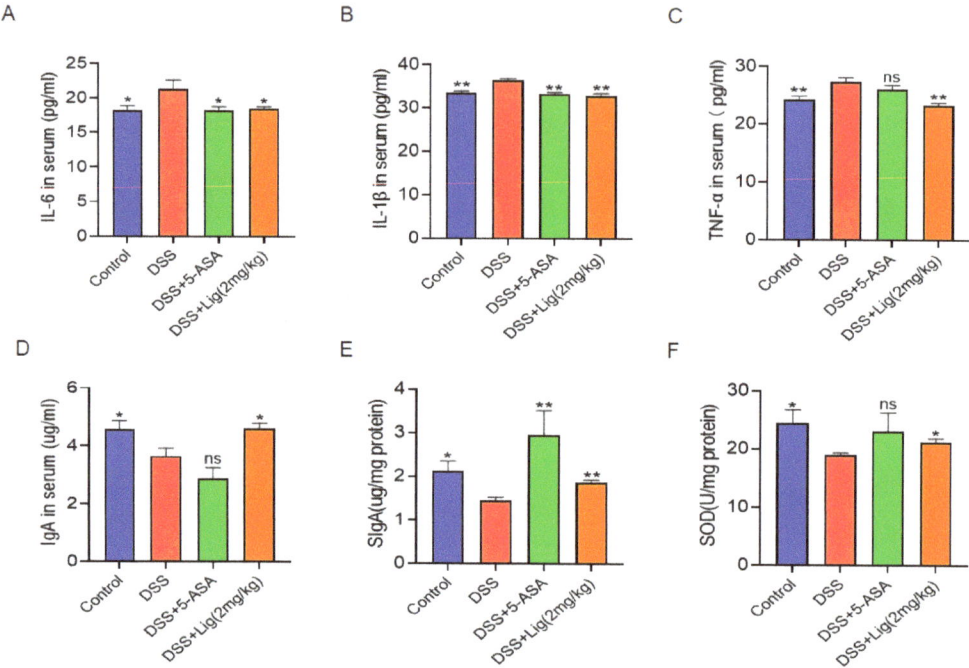

Figure 3. (**A**–**D**) Concentrations of IL-6, IL-1β, TNF-α, and IgA in the serum of colitis mice. (**E**,**F**) Concentrations of SIgA and SOD in colon tissue of colitis mice. * $p < 0.05$ and ** $p < 0.01$ vs. DSS group, ns means $p > 0.05$ vs. DSS group, $n = 5$.

3.4. Gut Microbiota Profiling

In total, 16s rRNA was sequenced from the feces of mice. Alpha diversity was shown using the Shannon and Simpson indices. We found that the Shannon index decreased significantly (Figure 4A), while the Simpson index increased (Figure 4B) after treatment with DSS. Principal co-ordinate analysis showed that the intestinal microflora of mice changed significantly after treatment with DSS. The intestinal microbial composition of the mice treated with ligustroside was more similar to that of the 5-ASA group (Figure 4C). At the same time, an unweighted_UniFrac cluster tree analysis showed that the microbial composition of the Control group, DSS + 5-ASA group, and DSS + Lig (2 mg/kg) group were more similar (Figure 4D). Using functional difference analysis, it was found that there were significant differences in glycerophospholipid metabolism and linoleic acid metabolism pathways between the Control and DSS groups (Figure 4E). In view of this change, we decided to explore the effect of ligustroside intervention on lipid metabolism in colitis mice.

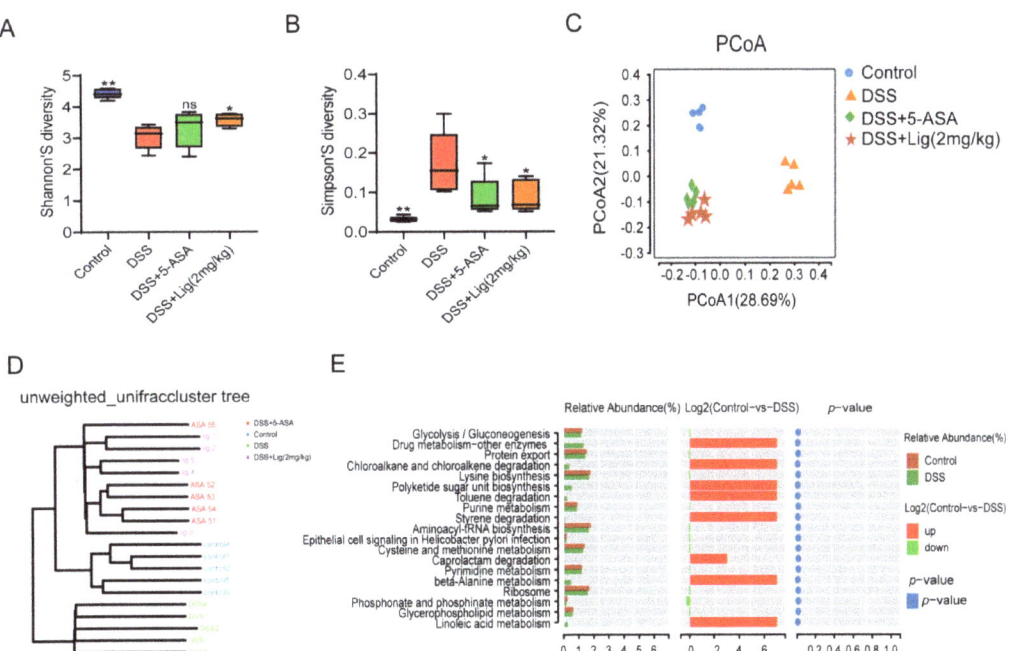

Figure 4. The microbiota of mice suffering from colitis were altered by supplementation with ligustroside. (**A,B**) Shannon and Simpson indices showed alpha diversity, (**C**) principal co-ordinate analysis of gut microbiota, (**D**) unweighted_UniFrac cluster tree, (**E**) functional difference analysis between Control and DSS groups. * $p < 0.05$ and ** $p < 0.01$ vs. DSS group, ns means $p > 0.05$ vs. DSS group, $n = 5$.

Then, LEfSe analysis was used to analyze the differences between groups. It was found that Actinobacteriota, Actinobacteria, Bifidobacteriales, Bifidobacteriaceae, and *Bifidobacterium* were the key differential species in the Control group, but Proteobacteria, Gammaproteobacteria, Enterobacterales, Enterobacteriaceae, Bacteriodaceae, and *Bacteroides* are the key differential species in the DSS group (Figure 5A, Supplementary Figure S2A). The LEfSe analysis of the DSS + Lig (2 mg/kg) group and DSS group showed that the key differential species in the DSS + Lig (2 mg/kg) group were similar to those in the Control group, in which the main differential bacteria were *Bifidobacterium*, while *Bacteroides* was still the key differential species in the DSS group (Figure 5B, Supplementary Figure S2B). In addition, these key different species also had significant differences among the four groups, and they were statistically significant (Figure 5C,D, Supplementary Figure S3A–I). Then, by analyzing the correlation between different key bacteria and inflammation-related indexes (Figure 5E), it was found that *Bifidobacterium* had a positive correlation with index SIgA and SOD after the intervention of ligustroside, and had a significant positive correlation with SIgA. In addition, it was negatively correlated with IL-6, IL-1β, and TNF-α and significantly negatively correlated with IL-6. On the contrary, *Bacteroides* showed the opposite trend. Based on the above results, we speculated that ligustroside could reshape the gut microbiota and restore a damaged intestinal barrier. Furthermore, ligustroside can increase the proportion of beneficial bacteria *Bifidobacterium* in the intestine that have anti-inflammatory effects. In addition, the improvement of the intestinal microenvironment can also reduce abnormal activation of innate immunity, prevent abnormal activation and aggregation of neutrophils, and thus reduce the production of pro-inflammatory cytokines such as IL-6 to alleviate damage to the intestinal barrier.

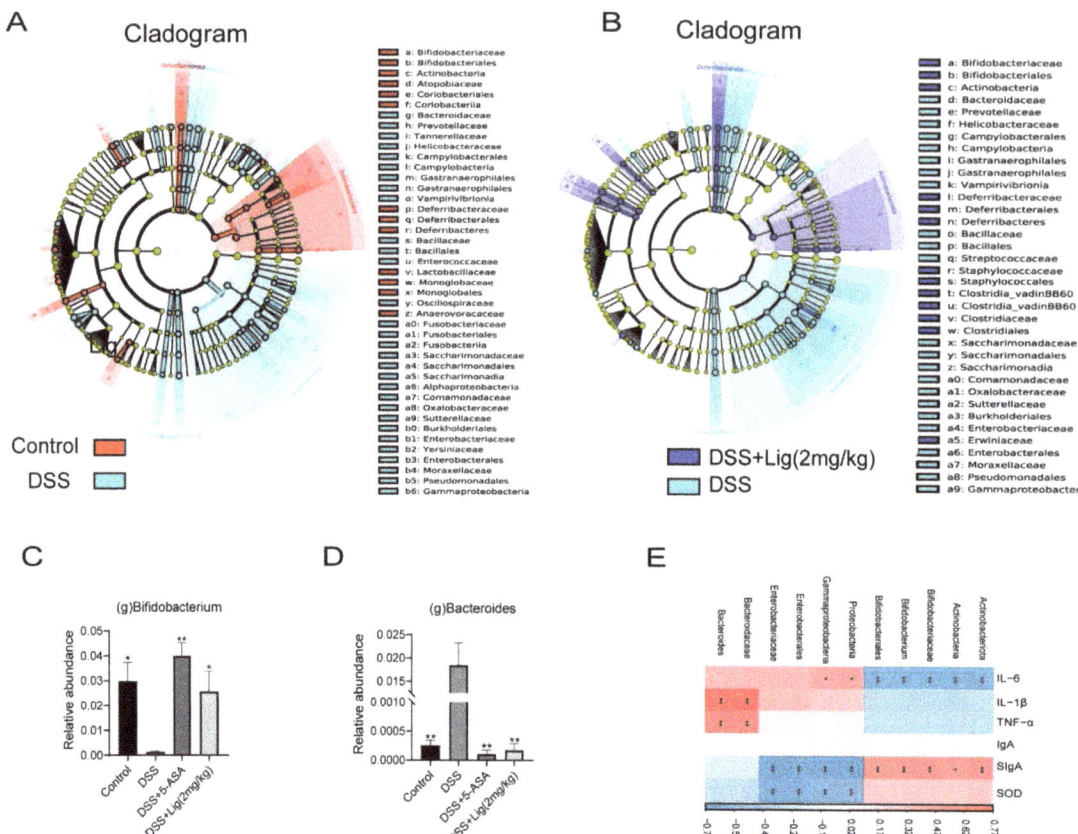

Figure 5. (**A**) Taxonomic cladogram of LEfSe analysis between Control and DSS groups. Biomarker taxa are shown in different colors, where Linear discriminant analysis (LDA) score > 2 and $p < 0.05$, (**B**) taxonomic cladogram of LEfSe analysis between the DSS + Lig (2 mg/kg) and DSS groups. Biomarker taxa are shown in different colors, where LDA score > 2 and $p < 0.05$. Relative abundance of Bifidobacterium (**C**) and Bacteroides (**D**) are shown. (**E**) Correlation between different key bacteria and inflammation-related indices. * $p < 0.05$ and ** $p < 0.01$ vs. DSS group, ns means $p > 0.05$ vs. DSS group, $n = 5$.

3.5. Non-Targeted Lipidomic Analysis

Using UHPLC-QE-MS to analyze the colonic contents of mice, a total of 914 peaks were obtained in positive and negative ion mode. sPLSDA found a significant difference between the composition of metabolites in the DSS + Lig (2 mg/kg) group and the DSS group (Figure 6A). Furthermore, the lipidomic metabolites in the DSS + Lig (2 mg/kg) group were nearer to the Control group than the DSS group. Then, we detected the differential metabolites between the Control and DSS groups using a volcano map. We found that there were 130 key different metabolites between the Control and DSS groups. Among these metabolites, 57 metabolites were significantly decreased and 73 metabolites were significantly up-regulated (Figure 6B). In addition, among the top 10 metabolites with the most obvious changes in Hierarchical Clustering Heatmaps (Figure 6C), Lyso-phosphatidylglycerol (LPG) (18:0), Lyso-phosphatidylcholine (LPC) (18:0p), and LPC (20:0p) decreased significantly in the DSS group. The other seven substances, Digalactosyldiacylglycerol (DGDG)

(36:0), Phosphatidylinositol (PI) (18:2/18:2), Phosphatidylcholine (PC) (16:0/15:2), Phosphatidylethanolamine (PE) (34:3), Cholesteryl Ester (ChE) (18:2), Phosphatidylglycerol (PG) (16:0/12:0), and PG (12:0/14:0) significantly increased in the DSS group.

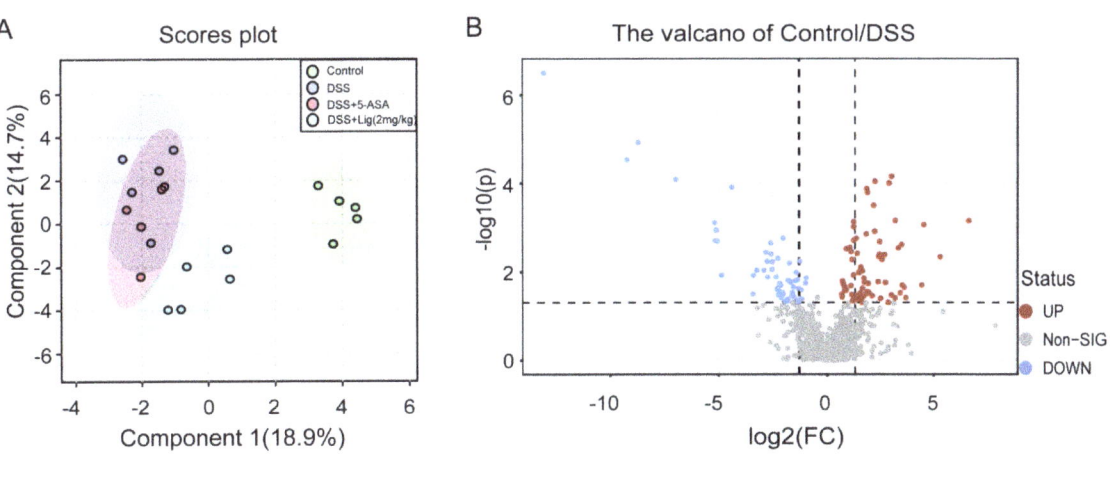

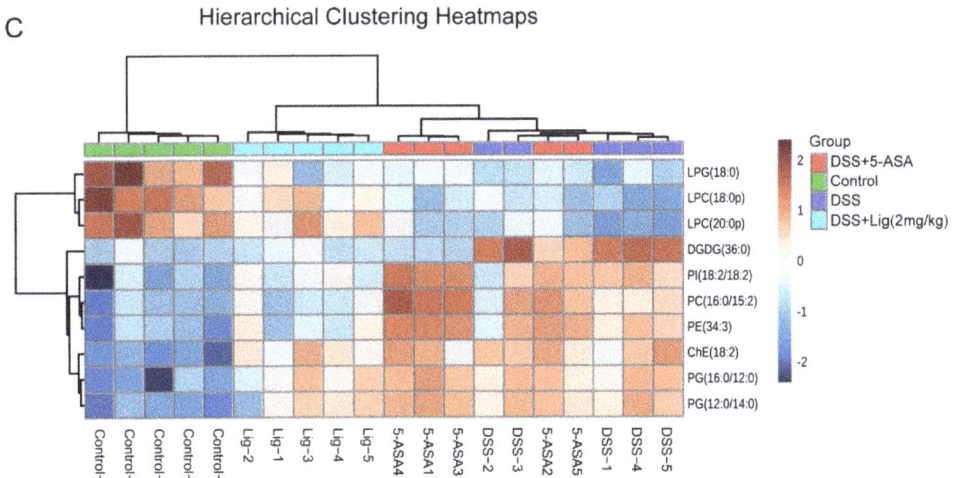

Figure 6. (**A**) Score plots for the sPLSDA model of metabolites in the intestinal content of mice, (**B**) volcano plot of significantly different metabolites between the Control and DSS groups (fold change > 1.5 and $p < 0.05$), (**C**) hierarchical clustering heatmaps of differential metabolites in intestinal luminal contents of mice between different groups. The red color indicates a metabolite concentration higher than the mean concentration of all samples, and the blue color indicates a metabolite concentration lower than the mean concentration of all samples, $n = 5$.

4. Discussion

In this study, the polyphenolic compound ligustroside was used as an intervention for the first time, to the best of our knowledge, to explore its supplementary therapeutic effects on DSS-induced colitis in mice.

IBD, as chronic intestinal inflammation, has become an important worldwide public health problem [28]. At present, IBD sufferers are still prone to relapse after treatment, and the course of the disease is protracted, seriously affecting the quality of life of patients. Therefore, we have attempted to find new compounds, derived from food or other substances, that can be used as supplementary treatment to improve the treatment of IBD. Several studies have shown that among people who suffer from certain chronic diseases associated with oxidative stress, inflammation, and the immune system, the Mediterranean diet, which contains ligustroside, may have protective effects [23].

DSS has been widely used to induce colitis and IBD in mice [29]. The mice utilized in this study developed acute colitis after drinking a solution of 2.5% DSS, resulting in diarrhea, hematochezia, weight loss, and colon shortening. 5-ASA is a classic drug used for the treatment of IBD, and it has been used in many studies to treat acute colitis induced with DSS [30,31]. In this study, it was found that supplementation of 5-ASA and ligustroside could significantly improve intestinal inflammation in mice with colitis, increase BW and colon length along with a reduction in DAI scores.

Many studies have shown that cytokines IL-6, IL-1β, and TNF-α play an important role in colitis [28]. Their increased expression can lead to intestinal dysfunction [32]. Oxidative stress is also involved in the pathogenesis and aggravation of IBD [33]. In this study, mice with colitis had more serious colonic mucosal damage than mice in the Control group, as well as an increased number of inflammatory cells. Significantly higher concentrations of proinflammatory cytokines were found in the serum of colitis mice than in the serum from Control group mice, and these inflammatory symptoms could be alleviated after intervention with ligustroside. The change of SOD content is an important index of oxidative stress in vivo, and DSS treatment can reduce the activity of SOD [34]. The intestine is rich in a large amount of SIgA, which is very important for mucosal immunity. It protects the mesentery and has therapeutic effects against IBD [20]. The content of SIgA in the intestinal tissue and immunoglobulin IgA in the serum of colitis mice decreased, but recovered after the intervention with ligustroside.

In DSS-induced colitis mice, DSS can directly target intestinal mucosa, destroy intestinal epithelial cells of the basal recess, damage the integrity of the mucosal barrier, and significantly change the composition of intestinal microorganisms [35]. Therefore, we studied the effect of ligustroside on the histopathological changes in the colon and on intestinal microfloral imbalance after DSS intervention. Our results showed that the intestinal integrity and intestinal microfloral composition in the DSS-treated mice were improved with supplementation of ligustroside. Compared with the Control group, supplementation of ligustroside changed the composition of lipid metabolites in the intestinal contents of the mice. In this study, we also found that the total number of microbial species in colitis mice decreased compared with the Control group. In the LEfSe analysis between Control and DSS groups, we found that *Bifidobacterium*, one of the bacteria beneficial to colitis [36], became the key differential microorganism in the Control group, and the proportion of *Bifidobacterium* was different between the Control and DSS groups. In contrast, in the DSS group, *Bacteroides* became the key differential genus, and the genus level was higher than that of the Control group, a finding which is similar to the previous research [37]. According to our findings, supplementation of ligustroside can improve species composition and species diversity in the gut of DSS-induced colitis mice.

As previous studies have shown, the lipid metabolism profiles of patients with IBD change [38]. Chronic inflammation on the surface of the intestinal epithelium has been found to be regulated by lipids in IBD [39]. Compared with healthy mice, the lipid metabolism spectrum of colitis mice induced with DSS also changed significantly. In addition, as important structural components of cell membranes, lipids have significant effects on different metabolic pathways and cell functions, which are important components of the intestinal barrier. In our results, a significant difference was found in the composition of colonic contents between the Lig and DSS groups. The composition of colonic contents in the Lig group was more similar to that of the Control group than the DSS group. Based on these findings, it is clear that DSS treatment can cause disruption of the lipid metabolism by altering the colonic lipid profile, and ligustroside protected it by reversing this process. Furthermore, endogenous bioactive lipids are widely recognized as pro-inflammatory mediators and triggers of inflammatory bowel disease [40,41]. These results revealed a close relationship between lipid metabolism and inflammation, suggesting that exploring lipid metabolism further may provide a way to regulate IBD's inflammatory response.

5. Conclusions

Under the existing treatment methods for IBD, ligustroside may be useful as a supplementary treatment to improve the treatment effect and long-term quality of life for IBD patients. In conclusion, supplementation of ligustroside could improve the occurrence of colitis in mice by reducing inflammation, enhancing the intestinal barrier, improving intestinal microbial composition, and altering lipid metabolism composition. However, it is not without its limitations: results from animals need to be extrapolated to humans, potential gaps need to be filled, other IBD models need to be validated, and so forth. These issues deserve further study and in-depth analyses from researchers.

Supplementary Materials: The following supporting information can be downloaded at: https://www.mdpi.com/article/10.3390/nu16040522/s1, Figure S1. The concentrations of IgG (A) and IgM (B) in serum. Data were presented as means ± SEM. * $p < 0.05$ and ** $p < 0.01$ vs. DSS group, ns means $p > 0.05$ vs. DSS group, $n = 5$. Figure S2. Top ten Linear discriminant analysis (LDA) score for different taxa abundances (A) between control and DSS groups and (B) between DSS + Lig (2 mg/kg) and DSS groups, $n = 5$. Figure S3. Relative abundance of predominant bacteria is shown for the phylum (A,B), class (C,D), order (E,F) and family (G–I) levels. Data are presented as means ± SEM. * $p < 0.05$ and ** $p < 0.01$ vs. DSS group, ns means $p > 0.05$ vs. DSS group, $n = 5$. Figure S4. (A) The quantification of AB/PAS Positive cells/crypt in colon tissue. (B) Mucus thickness of colon tissue. Data are presented as means ± SEM. * $p < 0.05$ and ** $p < 0.01$ vs. DSS group, ns means $p > 0.05$ vs. DSS group, $n = 5$. Table S1. The composition of diet for mice.

Author Contributions: Conceptualization, Y.R., Y.S. and Y.X.; methodology, R.G., P.X., Y.S., Q.Y., Y.D., X.Z. and Z.L.; validation, R.G., P.X. and T.L.; data curation, R.G., P.X. and Y.R.; writing of original draft preparation, R.G., P.X. and Y.R.; writing, review, and editing, R.G., Y.G. and Y.R.; supervision, Y.R. and Y.X. All authors have read and agreed to the published version of the manuscript.

Funding: Funding for this work was provided by the National Natural Science Foundation of China (Grant No. 32101964, 32372302, 31970746), China Postdoctoral Science Foundation (Grant No. 339576), Top Talent Support Program for young and middle-aged people of Wuxi Health Committee (Grant No. BJ2023046, HB2023043), Wuxi Municipal Health Commission (M202027), and the Wuxi Science and Technology Bureau (N20202022).

Institutional Review Board Statement: The animal study was reviewed and approved by the Institutional Animal Care and Use Committee of Jiangnan University, Wuxi, China [Approval No. JN. No20220330c1440615 (114)] on 30 March 2022.

Informed Consent Statement: Not applicable.

Data Availability Statement: Data are contained within the article and Supplementary Materials.

Conflicts of Interest: The authors declare no conflict of interest.

References

1. Graham, D.B.; Xavier, R.J. Pathway paradigms revealed from the genetics of inflammatory bowel disease. *Nature* **2020**, *578*, 527–539. [CrossRef]
2. Franzosa, E.A.; Sirota-Madi, A.; Avila-Pacheco, J.; Fornelos, N.; Haiser, H.J.; Reinker, S.; Vatanen, T.; Hall, A.B.; Mallick, H.; McIver, L.J.; et al. Gut microbiome structure and metabolic activity in inflammatory bowel disease. *Nat. Microbiol.* **2019**, *4*, 293–305. [CrossRef]
3. Zhao, M.; Gönczi, L.; Lakatos, P.L.; Burisch, J. The Burden of Inflammatory Bowel Disease in Europe in 2020. *J. Crohn's Colitis* **2021**, *15*, 1573–1587. [CrossRef]
4. Lloyd-Price, J.; Arze, C.; Ananthakrishnan, A.N.; Schirmer, M.; Avila-Pacheco, J.; Poon, T.W.; Andrews, E.; Ajami, N.J.; Bonham, K.S.; Brislawn, C.J.; et al. Multi-omics of the gut microbial ecosystem in inflammatory bowel diseases. *Nature* **2019**, *569*, 655–662. [CrossRef]
5. Ramos, G.P.; Papadakis, K.A. Mechanisms of Disease: Inflammatory Bowel Diseases. *Mayo Clin. Proc.* **2019**, *94*, 155–165. [CrossRef]

6. Levine, A.; Sigall Boneh, R.; Wine, E. Evolving role of diet in the pathogenesis and treatment of inflammatory bowel diseases. *Gut* **2018**, *67*, 1726–1738. [CrossRef]
7. Sartor, R.B.; Wu, G.D. Roles for Intestinal Bacteria, Viruses, and Fungi in Pathogenesis of Inflammatory Bowel Diseases and Therapeutic Approaches. *Gastroenterology* **2017**, *152*, 327–339.e324. [CrossRef]
8. Nishida, A.; Inoue, R.; Inatomi, O.; Bamba, S.; Naito, Y.; Andoh, A. Gut microbiota in the pathogenesis of inflammatory bowel disease. *Clin. J. Gastroenterol.* **2018**, *11*, 1–10. [CrossRef]
9. Huang, L.; Zheng, J.; Sun, G.; Yang, H.; Sun, X.; Yao, X.; Lin, A.; Liu, H. 5-Aminosalicylic acid ameliorates dextran sulfate sodium-induced colitis in mice by modulating gut microbiota and bile acid metabolism. *Cell Mol. Life Sci.* **2022**, *79*, 460. [CrossRef]
10. Schirmer, M.; Garner, A.; Vlamakis, H.; Xavier, R.J. Microbial genes and pathways in inflammatory bowel disease. *Nat. Rev. Microbiol.* **2019**, *17*, 497–511. [CrossRef]
11. Machiels, K.; Joossens, M.; Sabino, J.; De Preter, V.; Arijs, I.; Eeckhaut, V.; Ballet, V.; Claes, K.; Van Immerseel, F.; Verbeke, K.; et al. A decrease of the butyrate-producing species Roseburia hominis and Faecalibacterium prausnitzii defines dysbiosis in patients with ulcerative colitis. *Gut* **2014**, *63*, 1275–1283. [CrossRef]
12. Johansson, M.E.; Ambort, D.; Pelaseyed, T.; Schütte, A.; Gustafsson, J.K.; Ermund, A.; Subramani, D.B.; Holmén-Larsson, J.M.; Thomsson, K.A.; Bergström, J.H.; et al. Composition and functional role of the mucus layers in the intestine. *Cell Mol. Life Sci.* **2011**, *68*, 3635–3641. [CrossRef]
13. Drury, B.; Hardisty, G.; Gray, R.D.; Ho, G.T. Neutrophil Extracellular Traps in Inflammatory Bowel Disease: Pathogenic Mechanisms and Clinical Translation. *Cell Mol. Gastroenterol. Hepatol.* **2021**, *12*, 321–333. [CrossRef]
14. Zhou, G.X.; Liu, Z.J. Potential roles of neutrophils in regulating intestinal mucosal inflammation of inflammatory bowel disease. *J. Dig. Dis.* **2017**, *18*, 495–503. [CrossRef]
15. Saez, A.; Herrero-Fernandez, B.; Gomez-Bris, R.; Sánchez-Martinez, H.; Gonzalez-Granado, J.M. Pathophysiology of Inflammatory Bowel Disease: Innate Immune System. *Int. J. Mol. Sci.* **2023**, *24*, 1526. [CrossRef]
16. Lee, T.H.; Chen, J.L.; Liu, P.S.; Tsai, M.M.; Wang, S.J.; Hsieh, H.L. Rottlerin, a natural polyphenol compound, inhibits upregulation of matrix metalloproteinase-9 and brain astrocytic migration by reducing PKC-δ-dependent ROS signal. *J. Neuroinflamm.* **2020**, *17*, 177. [CrossRef]
17. Emma, M.R.; Augello, G.; Di Stefano, V.; Azzolina, A.; Giannitrapani, L.; Montalto, G.; Cervello, M.; Cusimano, A. Potential Uses of Olive Oil Secoiridoids for the Prevention and Treatment of Cancer: A Narrative Review of Preclinical Studies. *Int. J. Mol. Sci.* **2021**, *22*, 1234. [CrossRef]
18. Castejón, M.L.; Montoya, T.; Alarcón-de-la-Lastra, C.; Sánchez-Hidalgo, M. Potential Protective Role Exerted by Secoiridoids from Olea europaea L. in Cancer, Cardiovascular, Neurodegenerative, Aging-Related, and Immunoinflammatory Diseases. *Antioxidants* **2020**, *9*, 149. [CrossRef]
19. Cardona, F.; Andrés-Lacueva, C.; Tulipani, S.; Tinahones, F.J.; Queipo-Ortuño, M.I. Benefits of polyphenols on gut microbiota and implications in human health. *J. Nutr. Biochem.* **2013**, *24*, 1415–1422. [CrossRef]
20. Wan, M.L.Y.; Co, V.A.; El-Nezami, H. Dietary polyphenol impact on gut health and microbiota. *Crit. Rev. Food Sci. Nutr.* **2021**, *61*, 690–711. [CrossRef]
21. Georgiades, P.; Pudney, P.D.; Rogers, S.; Thornton, D.J.; Waigh, T.A. Tea derived galloylated polyphenols cross-link purified gastrointestinal mucins. *PLoS ONE* **2014**, *9*, e105302. [CrossRef]
22. Ling, K.H.; Wan, M.L.; El-Nezami, H.; Wang, M. Protective Capacity of Resveratrol, a Natural Polyphenolic Compound, against Deoxynivalenol-Induced Intestinal Barrier Dysfunction and Bacterial Translocation. *Chem. Res. Toxicol.* **2016**, *29*, 823–833. [CrossRef]
23. Cárdeno, A.; Sánchez-Hidalgo, M.; Alarcón-de-la-Lastra, C. An update of olive oil phenols in inflammation and cancer: Molecular mechanisms and clinical implications. *Curr. Med. Chem.* **2013**, *20*, 4758–4776. [CrossRef] [PubMed]
24. Sánchez-Fidalgo, S.; Villegas, I.; Aparicio-Soto, M.; Cárdeno, A.; Rosillo, M.; González-Benjumea, A.; Marset, A.; López, Ó.; Maya, I.; Fernández-Bolaños, J.G.; et al. Effects of dietary virgin olive oil polyphenols: Hydroxytyrosyl acetate and 3, 4-dihydroxyphenylglycol on DSS-induced acute colitis in mice. *J. Nutr. Biochem.* **2015**, *26*, 513–520. [CrossRef] [PubMed]
25. Sánchez-Fidalgo, S.; Cárdeno, A.; Sánchez-Hidalgo, M.; Aparicio-Soto, M.; de la Lastra, C.A. Dietary extra virgin olive oil polyphenols supplementation modulates DSS-induced chronic colitis in mice. *J. Nutr. Biochem.* **2013**, *24*, 1401–1413. [CrossRef] [PubMed]
26. Ren, Q.; Yang, B.; Zhang, H.; Ross, R.P.; Stanton, C.; Chen, H.; Chen, W. c9, t11, c15-CLNA and t9, t11, c15-CLNA from Lactobacillus plantarum ZS2058 Ameliorate Dextran Sodium Sulfate-Induced Colitis in Mice. *J. Agric. Food Chem.* **2020**, *68*, 3758–3769. [CrossRef] [PubMed]
27. Wang, K.; Jin, X.; Li, Q.; Sawaya, A.; Le Leu, R.K.; Conlon, M.A.; Wu, L.; Hu, F. Propolis from Different Geographic Origins Decreases Intestinal Inflammation and *Bacteroides* spp. Populations in a Model of DSS-Induced Colitis. *Mol. Nutr. Food Res.* **2018**, *62*, e1800080. [CrossRef] [PubMed]
28. Zhu, W.; Ren, L.; Zhang, L.; Qiao, Q.; Farooq, M.Z.; Xu, Q. The Potential of Food Protein-Derived Bioactive Peptides against Chronic Intestinal Inflammation. *Mediators Inflamm.* **2020**, *2020*, 6817156. [CrossRef] [PubMed]
29. Wirtz, S.; Popp, V.; Kindermann, M.; Gerlach, K.; Weigmann, B.; Fichtner-Feigl, S.; Neurath, M.F. Chemically induced mouse models of acute and chronic intestinal inflammation. *Nat. Protoc.* **2017**, *12*, 1295–1309. [CrossRef] [PubMed]

30. Cevallos, S.A.; Lee, J.Y.; Velazquez, E.M.; Foegeding, N.J.; Shelton, C.D.; Tiffany, C.R.; Parry, B.H.; Stull-Lane, A.R.; Olsan, E.E.; Savage, H.P.; et al. 5-Aminosalicylic Acid Ameliorates Colitis and Checks Dysbiotic Escherichia coli Expansion by Activating PPAR-γ Signaling in the Intestinal Epithelium. *mBio* **2021**, *12*, e03227-20. [CrossRef]
31. Tang, S.; Liu, W.; Zhao, Q.; Li, K.; Zhu, J.; Yao, W.; Gao, X. Combination of polysaccharides from Astragalus membranaceus and Codonopsis pilosula ameliorated mice colitis and underlying mechanisms. *J. Ethnopharmacol.* **2021**, *264*, 113280. [CrossRef]
32. Zhang, H.; Hua, R.; Zhang, B.; Zhang, X.; Yang, H.; Zhou, X. Serine Alleviates Dextran Sulfate Sodium-Induced Colitis and Regulates the Gut Microbiota in Mice. *Front. Microbiol.* **2018**, *9*, 3062. [CrossRef]
33. Samsamikor, M.; Daryani, N.E.; Asl, P.R.; Hekmatdoost, A. Resveratrol Supplementation and Oxidative/Anti-Oxidative Status in Patients with Ulcerative Colitis: A Randomized, Double-Blind, Placebo-controlled Pilot Study. *Arch. Med. Res.* **2016**, *47*, 304–309. [CrossRef]
34. Liu, G.; Yan, W.; Ding, S.; Jiang, H.; Ma, Y.; Wang, H.; Fang, J. Effects of IRW and IQW on Oxidative Stress and Gut Microbiota in Dextran Sodium Sulfate-Induced Colitis. *Cell Physiol. Biochem.* **2018**, *51*, 441–451. [CrossRef] [PubMed]
35. Munyaka, P.M.; Rabbi, M.F.; Khafipour, E.; Ghia, J.E. Acute dextran sulfate sodium (DSS)-induced colitis promotes gut microbial dysbiosis in mice. *J. Basic. Microbiol.* **2016**, *56*, 986–998. [CrossRef] [PubMed]
36. Zhao, B.; Wu, J.; Li, J.; Bai, Y.; Luo, Y.; Ji, B.; Xia, B.; Liu, Z.; Tan, X.; Lv, J.; et al. Lycopene Alleviates DSS-Induced Colitis and Behavioral Disorders via Mediating Microbes-Gut-Brain Axis Balance. *J. Agric. Food Chem.* **2020**, *68*, 3963–3975. [CrossRef] [PubMed]
37. Hu, L.; Jin, L.; Xia, D.; Zhang, Q.; Ma, L.; Zheng, H.; Xu, T.; Chang, S.; Li, X.; Xun, Z.; et al. Nitrate ameliorates dextran sodium sulfate-induced colitis by regulating the homeostasis of the intestinal microbiota. *Free Radic. Biol. Med.* **2020**, *152*, 609–621. [CrossRef] [PubMed]
38. Li, Q.; Chen, G.; Zhu, D.; Zhang, W.; Qi, S.; Xue, X.; Wang, K.; Wu, L. Effects of dietary phosphatidylcholine and sphingomyelin on DSS-induced colitis by regulating metabolism and gut microbiota in mice. *J. Nutr. Biochem.* **2022**, *105*, 109004. [CrossRef] [PubMed]
39. Hyder, A. PGlyRP3 concerts with PPARγ to attenuate DSS-induced colitis in mice. *Int. Immunopharmacol.* **2019**, *67*, 46–53. [CrossRef] [PubMed]
40. Yang, P.; Chan, D.; Felix, E.; Madden, T.; Klein, R.D.; Shureiqi, I.; Chen, X.; Dannenberg, A.J.; Newman, R.A. Determination of endogenous tissue inflammation profiles by LC/MS/MS: COX- and LOX-derived bioactive lipids. *Prostaglandins Leukot. Essent. Fatty Acids* **2006**, *75*, 385–395. [CrossRef] [PubMed]
41. Chiurchiù, V.; Leuti, A.; Maccarrone, M. Bioactive Lipids and Chronic Inflammation: Managing the Fire Within. *Front. Immunol.* **2018**, *9*, 38. [CrossRef] [PubMed]

Disclaimer/Publisher's Note: The statements, opinions and data contained in all publications are solely those of the individual author(s) and contributor(s) and not of MDPI and/or the editor(s). MDPI and/or the editor(s) disclaim responsibility for any injury to people or property resulting from any ideas, methods, instructions or products referred to in the content.

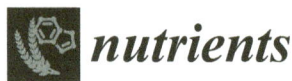

Article

Hydrophobic Components in Light-Yellow Pulp Sweet Potato (*Ipomoea batatas* (L.) Lam.) Tubers Suppress LPS-Induced Inflammatory Responses in RAW264.7 Cells via Activation of the Nrf2 Pathway

Yuma Matsumoto, Mari Suto, Io Umebara, Hirofumi Masutomi * and Katsuyuki Ishihara

Research and Development Division, Calbee, Inc., 23-6 Kiyohara-Kogyodanchi, Utsunomiya 321-3231, Japan; y_matsumoto1@calbee.co.jp (Y.M.)
* Correspondence: h_masutomi@calbee.co.jp; Tel.: +81-70-3872-7681

Abstract: Sweet potato is a crop that is widely consumed all over the world and is thought to contribute to health maintenance due to its abundant nutrients and phytochemicals. Previous studies on the functionality of sweet potatoes have focused on varieties that have colored pulp, such as purple and orange, which contain high levels of specific phytochemicals. Therefore, in the present study, we evaluated the anti-inflammatory effects of light-yellow-fleshed sweet potatoes, which have received little attention. After freeze-drying sweet potatoes harvested in 2020, extracts were prepared from the leaves, stems, roots, and tubers in 100% ethanol. Mouse macrophage-like cell line RAW264.7 cells were cultured with 10 μg/mL of the extracts and induced lipopolysaccharide (LPS)-stimulated inflammation. Of the extracts, the tuber extracts showed the highest suppression of LPS-induced interleukin-6 (IL-6) gene expression and production in RAW264.7, which was attributed to the activation of the nuclear factor erythroid 2-related factor 2 (Nrf2) oxidative stress response pathway. In addition, preparative high-performance liquid chromatography (HPLC) experiments suggested that hydrophobic components specific to the tuber were the main body of activity. In previous studies, it has been shown that the tubers and leaves of sweet potatoes with colored pulp exhibit anti-inflammatory effects due to their rich phytochemicals, and our results show that the tubers with light-yellow pulp also exhibit the effects. Furthermore, we were able to show a part of the mechanism, which may contribute to the fundamental understanding of the treatment and prevention of inflammation by food-derived components.

Keywords: anti-inflammation; sweet potato (*Ipomoea batatas* (L.); Nrf2; RAW264.7

Citation: Matsumoto, Y.; Suto, M.; Umebara, I.; Masutomi, H.; Ishihara, K. Hydrophobic Components in Light-Yellow Pulp Sweet Potato (*Ipomoea batatas* (L.) Lam.) Tubers Suppress LPS-Induced Inflammatory Responses in RAW264.7 Cells via Activation of the Nrf2 Pathway. *Nutrients* **2024**, *16*, 563. https://doi.org/10.3390/nu16040563

Academic Editor: Rita Businaro

Received: 1 February 2024
Revised: 14 February 2024
Accepted: 16 February 2024
Published: 18 February 2024

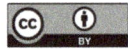

Copyright: © 2024 by the authors. Licensee MDPI, Basel, Switzerland. This article is an open access article distributed under the terms and conditions of the Creative Commons Attribution (CC BY) license (https://creativecommons.org/licenses/by/4.0/).

1. Introduction

Inflammation is a defense response in the body, and macrophages play a role in this response by phagocytosing targets and secreting molecules such as nitric oxide, cytokines, and chemokines, thereby activating the immune response. Although inflammation is, in essence, a response to protect the organism, various studies in recent years have shown that chronic inflammation causes various problems in the tissues of the body and is closely related to the onset and worsening of age-related diseases, such as diabetes and cancer [1–3]. Although the most effective treatment for such chronic inflammation is probably the suppression of inflammation with drugs, from the perspective of social problems, such as increased medical costs, we should also pay attention to improvements in symptoms due to food-derived ingredients. It is believed that food-derived ingredients with anti-inflammatory effects can prevent or treat diseases, and there have been many reports on their effects, including one that examined the relationship between dietary flavonoid intake and the risk of developing chronic diseases [4,5]. In that report, it was mentioned that quercetin and other flavonoids may reduce the risk of heart disease and type II diabetes mellitus.

The anti-inflammatory effects of food-derived ingredients are often related to their antioxidant properties [5,6]. When inflammatory signals are activated in macrophages, reactive oxygen species (ROS) are generated, which are involved in signal transduction as secondary messengers, and play important roles in metabolism and proliferation; however, they can also cause oxidative stress and damage DNA and cells [7]. Some food-derived components are reported to have antioxidant effects by scavenging ROS and activating oxidative stress response pathways [8–10].

NF-E2-related factor 2 (Nrf2) is a key transcription factor that plays a central role in the oxidative stress response pathway. Its function is inhibited under normal conditions, as it binds to Kelch-like ECH-associated protein 1 (Keap1). It is released and translocated into the nucleus upon activation, and it recognizes antioxidant response element (ARE) sequences that activate the transcription of antioxidant factors such as Heme Oxygenase 1 (HO-1) and NAD(P)H quinone oxidoreductase 1 (NQO-1) [11]. In addition to suppressing inflammatory responses by reducing ROS through HO-1 and other functions, it has also been reported to inhibit NF-κB, which transduces inflammatory signals [12–14].

Sweet potato is a perennial herbaceous plant found in the *Ipomoea* genus of the Hirudoaceae family; it is drought tolerant and produces high yields, even on barren land. Globally, it is mostly produced in China and African regions, but its tuberous roots are eaten in many parts of the world and are expected to have a positive effect on health due to their high dietary fiber, vitamin, and mineral content [15]. There is diversity in pulp color among cultivars, which are mainly light yellow, orange, and purple. The colored cultivars are rich in phytochemicals, with the orange ones containing more carotenoids and the purple ones containing more anthocyanin [16,17]. These colored sweet potatoes have various functional properties, and there have been many reports dedicated to their relationship with the immune system, which has attracted much attention in recent years [18–20]. Sugata et al. reported that anthocyanin in purple sweet potatoes reduced the production of lipopolysaccharide (LPS)-induced inflammatory cytokines (tumor necrosis factor α(TNFα), interleukin-6 (IL-6), and nitric oxide (NO)) in RAW264.7 cells and inhibited the growth of several cancer cell lines. Similarly, Bae et al. reported that β-carotene in orange sweet potatoes also inhibited LPS-induced production of IL-6, NO, and prostaglandin E2 (PGE2) in RAW 264.7. However, these colored sweet potatoes are still not commonly eaten, at least in Japan, and reports on the functional properties of light-yellow-fleshed cultivars, which are mainly consumed, are still poor. In order to benefit from functional food components, it is important that they be found in commonly consumed foods. Therefore, the present study focused on the light-yellow cultivar Beniharuka, whose tubers are widely consumed in Japan, and verified whether it also has the anti-inflammatory effects that have been confirmed with colored sweet potatoes. In the results, we found that extracts from tuberous roots of light-yellow pulp sweet potato suppressed the expression of pro-inflammatory genes via the Nrf2 oxidative stress response pathway.

2. Materials and Methods

2.1. Preparation of Sweet Potato Samples and Extracts

The sweet potatoes used in this study were sampled from Ibaraki, Japan, in July 2020. Samples were collected from 10 plants, washed immediately in water, and the leaves, stems, roots, and tuberous roots were separated and freeze-dried. The samples were then pulverized and extracted using 100% ethanol (Kanto Chemical, Tokyo, Japan); the solvent was evaporated in an evaporator and suspended in dimethyl sulfoxide (DMSO; Fujifilm Wako Pure Chemicals, Osaka, Japan) to create a 10 mg/mL extract.

2.2. Reagents and Antibodies

LPS (*Escherichia. coli* O127) was purchased from Fujifilm Wako Pure Chemicals (Osaka, Japan). Anti-Lamin B1 (ab16048), anti-Nrf2 (ab2352), and anti-HO-1 (ab68477) were from Abcam (Cambridge, UK), and anti-NF-κB (#8242), anti-β-Actin (#4967) and anti-rabbit

IgG-HRP (#7074) were purchased from Cell Signaling Technology (Danvers, MA). Nrf2 inhibitor ML385 was purchased from Selleck (Houston, TX, USA).

2.3. Cell Culture and Stimulation Conditions

RAW264.7 murine macrophage cells were obtained from KAC (Kyoto, Japan). Cells were cultured in Dulbecco's Modified Eagle Medium (DMEM; Sigma-Aldrich, St. Louis, MO, USA) plus 10% deactivated fetal bovine serum (FBS; Biowest, Nuaillé, France) and 1% penicillin–streptomycin (Gibco, Grand Island, NY, USA) at 37 °C in 5% CO_2. Extracts were added to the medium at a final concentration of 10 µg/mL (1000×) and incubated for 1 h, after which LPS (final concentration 50 ng/mL) was added. Unless otherwise mentioned, these conditions were standardized for all cell cultures and stimulation.

2.4. Cell Viability Assay

RAW264.7 cells were cultured in 96-well plates (AGC Technoglass, Shizuoka, Japan) at a density of 1.0×10^4 cells/well for 24 h and each extract was added at final concentrations of 1, 10, and 100 µg/mL. After 1 h of incubation, LPS stimulation was performed, and the cells were incubated for 24 h. Then, the WST-1 reagent (Cayman Chemical, Ann Arbor, MI, USA) was added, and the cells were incubated for another 2 h. Finally, the absorbance of the culture supernatant at 450 nm was measured by a microplate reader (model 680, Bio-rad, Hercules, CA, USA) to determine the cell survival rate.

2.5. Enzyme-Linked Immunosorben Assay (ELISA)

RAW264.7 cells were cultured in 96-well plates at a density of 1.0×10^4 cells/well. After 24 h of incubation, each extract and LPS were added. After incubation for another 24 h, the supernatant was collected and used for the assay. An ELISA MAX™ Deluxe Set Mouse IL-6 (BioLegend, San Diego, CA, USA) was used for the experiments, following the described protocol.

2.6. Intracellular ROS Observation

RAW264.7 cells were cultured in 96-well plates at a density of 1.0×10^4 cells/well for 24 h, and then each extract and LPS were added. After incubation for another 20 h, intracellular ROS was stained using an ROS Assay Kit-Highly Sensitive DCFH-DA (Dojindo Laboratories, Kumamoto, Japan) and observed using a fluorescence microscope (BZ-X810, Keyence, Osaka, Japan).

2.7. RT-qPCR

RAW264.7 cells were cultured in 96-well plates at a density of 1.0×10^4 cells/well, and each extract and LPS were added after 24 h of culture. After another 24 h of culture, cells were collected, and cDNA was prepared using the SuperPrep® Cell Lysis & RT Kit for qPCR (TOYOBO, Osaka, Japan). RT-qPCR was performed using THUNDERBIRD® Next SYBR® qPCR Mix (TOYOBO) and QuantStudio 5 real-time PCR system (Thermo Fisher Scientific, Waltham, MA, USA), and the relative expression levels between samples were evaluated using the ΔΔCt method. Primer information is shown in Table 1.

Table 1. Primer information.

Gene		Primer Sequence
IL-6	Forward:	AGAGGATACCACTCCCAACAGA
	Reverse:	CTGCAAGTGCATCATCGTTGTTC
Tnf	Forward:	ATTCGAGTGACAAGCCTGTAG
	Reverse:	TGAAGAGAACCTGGGAGTAGAC

Table 1. *Cont.*

Gene		Primer Sequence
iNOS (Nos2)	Forward:	AGGCTGGAAGCTGTAACAAAGG
	Reverse:	GCTGAAACATTTCCTGTGCTGTG
Actb	Forward:	ACTATTGGCAACGAGCGGTTC
	Reverse:	TCAGCAATGCCTGGGTACATG

2.8. Western Blotting

RAW264.7 cells were cultured in 60 mm tissue culture dishes (AGC Technoglass, Shizuoka, Japan) at a density of 2.0×10^5 cells/dish, and extracts and LPS were added after 24 h. After LPS stimulation, the cells were sampled at predetermined time points.

For whole-cell sampling, cells were lysed in 250 µL lysis buffer (50 mM Tris-HCl (pH 7.5), 150 mM NaCl, 0.5% sodium dodecyl sulfate (SDS), protease inhibitor cocktail (cOmplete™ Mini, Roche, Basel, Switzerland), and phosphatase inhibitor cocktail (PhosSTOP™, Roche, Basel, Switzerland), and the suspension was incubated on ice for at least 1 h. The supernatant obtained from centrifugation ($20,000 \times g$, 15 min, 4 °C) was mixed with 4× Laemmli's sample buffer (Bio-rad, Hercules, CA, USA) to make samples.

For separation of the nuclear and cytoplasmic fractions, cells were lysed in 200 µL cytoplasmic lysis buffer (10 mM HEPES (pH 7.9), 10 mM KCl, 1.5 mM $MgCl_2$, 1 mM dithiothreitol (DTT), 0.5% NP-40, protease inhibitors, and phosphatase inhibitors). The suspension was incubated on ice for at least 15 min, and the supernatant was centrifuged ($800 \times g$, 10 min, 4 °C) to obtain the cytoplasmic fraction. The precipitated pellet was dissolved in 100 µL nucleolytic buffer (20 mM HEPES (pH 7.9), 400 mM NaCl, 1.5 mM $MgCl_2$, 0.2 mM EDTA, 1 mM DTT, 10% Glycerol, protease inhibitors, phosphatase inhibitors). The supernatant was then sonicated on ice and centrifuged ($14,000 \times g$, 30 min, 4 °C) to obtain the nuclear fraction. Each was mixed with 4× Laemmli's sample buffer to form the separated samples.

SDS-PAGE was performed on the prepared samples, which were transferred to Immobilon-P PVDF membranes (Merck, Darmstadt, Germany). The target proteins on the PVDF membrane were then labeled with antibodies, detected with SuperSignal™ West Femto Maximum Sensitivity Substrate (Thermo Fisher Scientific), and analyzed using a Lumino Image Analyzer (ImageQuant LAS 800, Cytiva, Marlborough, MA, USA). The intensity of each band was analyzed using ImageJ software (Ver. 1.53).

2.9. High-Performance Liquid Chromatography (HPLC)

Analysis of the properties of the components contained in the extract was performed with an Agilent 1260 Infinity (Agilent Technologies, Santa Clara, CA, USA) ODS column (Cadenza CD-C18 column, 250 × 4.6 mm, particle size 3 µm, Imtakt Corporation, Kyoto, Japan) at a constant temperature of 40 °C. In the mobile phase, a 5-fold-diluted extract in ethanol of 30 µL was applied to the column, and elution was performed at a flow rate of 1 mL/min with a mixture of solvents A (0.4% formic acid (Fujifilm Wako Pure Chemicals, Osaka, Japan)) and B (100% acetonitrile (Kanto Chemical, Tokyo, Japan)). Elution was performed under the following conditions: gradient from initial conditions to 40 min (0 min (A:B = 93:7), 33 min (A:B = 60:40), 40 min (A:B = 0:100)), from 40 to 70 min (A:B = 0:100). Spectra were detected with a diode array detector (DAD) at 280 and 326 nm. In parallel with the analysis, fraction collection was also performed. The preparative schedule was as follows: Fr.1: 8–15 min, Fr.2: 19–25 min, Fr.3: 42–51 min, Fr.4: 51–60 min, Fr.5: 60–69 min.

2.10. DPPH Radical Scavenging Activity Assay

To a 96-well plate, 50 µL of Trolox standard solution, a sweet potato extract sample (5 mg/mL in 50% ethanol) and a blank (50% ethanol) were added. Then, 150 µL of 200 µM 1,1-diphenyl-2-picrylhydrazyl (DPPH) solution was added to each well and agitated for 15 min. The absorbance at 540 nm was then measured using a microplate reader, and the DPPH radical scavenging activity per 100 g of sample was calculated as μmol Trolox equivalent.

2.11. Total Polyphenol Content Assay

As standard solutions, gallic acid was adjusted to 500, 250, 100, 50, and 25 μg/mL. To a test tube, 100 μL of each concentration of gallic acid standard or each sweet potato extract (10 mg/mL in 100% ethanol) was added, followed by 2 mL of distilled water. After adding 500 μL of Folin and Ciocalteu's phenol reagent (MP Biomedicals, Santa Ana, CA, USA), 500 μL of a 10% sodium carbonate solution was quickly added, mixed, and placed in the dark for 1 h at room temperature. The absorbance at 760 nm was measured, and the total polyphenol content per 100 g of sample was calculated.

2.12. Total Flavonoid Content Assay

As standard solutions, catechin hydrate was prepared at concentrations of 500, 250, 100, 50, and 25 μg/mL. To the test tubes, 250 μL of each concentration of catechin standard solution or sweet potato extract (10 mg/mL in 100% ethanol) was added. They were mixed with 1250 μL of distilled water and 75 μL of 5% sodium nitrite solution. After 5 min of incubation, 150 μL of 10% aluminum chloride solution was added and mixed. After another 6 min of incubation, 500 μL of 1 M sodium hydroxide solution and 275 μL of distilled water were added and mixed. The absorbance at 510 nm was then measured, and the total flavonoid content per 100 g of sample was calculated.

2.13. Statistical Analysis

Statistical analysis was performed with GraphPad Prism 9 (MDF, Tokyo, Japan). A Student's t-test was performed to compare the two groups, and one-way analysis of variance (ANOVA) was performed to test three or more groups, followed by Dunnett's or Tukey's post-hoc test. The significance level was set at 5%.

3. Results

3.1. Sweet Potato Tuber Extracts Suppressed the Production of Inflammatory Cytokines and Gene Expression

The effects of extracts of sweet potato leaf, stem, root, and tuber on the viability of RAW264.7 cells under LPS-stimulated conditions were determined. Up to a concentration of 10 μg/mL, no extract showed any change in viability, but at 100 μg/mL, the tuber extract showed a significant decrease in viability (Figure 1A). Therefore, we set 10 μg/mL as the prescribed concentration of the extracts in subsequent experiments. IL-6 is one of the main inflammatory markers whose expression is increased by LPS stimulation in macrophages, and we selected it as an indicator of inflammatory intensity in this study. Cells were stimulated in the presence of sweet potato extract, and the IL-6 concentration in the medium at 24 h after stimulation was significantly reduced by about 50% in the presence of the tuber extract (Figure 1B). The expression of the *IL-6* gene was also suppressed, as well as that of other proinflammatory genes such as *Tnf* and *iNOS* (Figure 1C). These results indicate that only the tuber extract suppressed LPS-induced inflammatory responses.

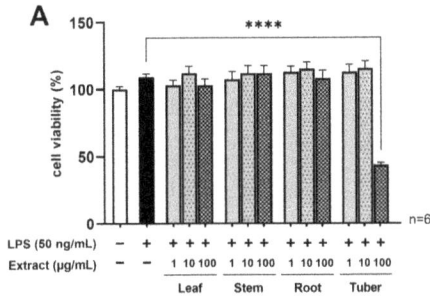
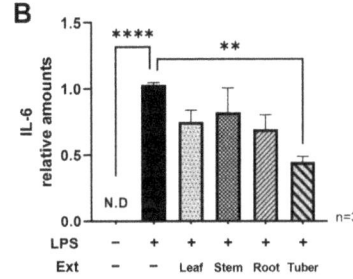
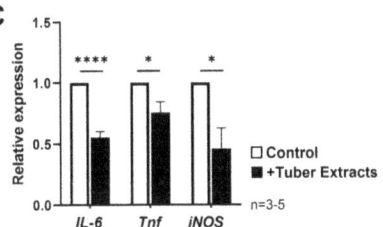

Figure 1. Cell viability and expression of LPS-induced pro-inflammatory cytokines under conditions with sweet potato extracts: (**A**) Cell viability at 24 h of incubation after the addition of the sweet potato extracts at concentrations of 1 µg/mL, 10 µg/mL, and 100 µg/mL; (**B**) Relative production level of IL-6 at 24 h after LPS stimulation with/without each sweet potato extracts; (**C**) Relative expression of pro-inflammatory genes (*IL-6, Tnf, iNOS(Nos2)*) at 24 h after LPS stimulation with/without sweet potato tuber extracts: (**A**,**B**) mean ± SEM, one-way ANOVA with Dunnett's post-hoc test (vs +LPS), **: $p < 0.01$, ****: $p < 0.0001$; (**C**) mean ± SEM, Student's *t*-test, *: $p < 0.05$, ****: $p < 0.0001$: LPS, lipopolysaccharide; Ext, extract.

3.2. Tuber Extracts Induce Activation of the Nrf2 Oxidative Stress Response Pathway and Inhibit the Function of NF-κB

We observed intracellular ROS using fluorescence microscopy and quantified the fluorescence intensity of each cell after 20 h of LPS stimulation in the presence of extracts of sweet potato tubers and found that the addition of the tuber extracts tended to decrease ROS (Figure 2A,B). Among the four extracts used in this study, the highest values for total polyphenols, total flavonoids, and DPPH radical scavenging activity were found in the leaf extracts, and the other three extracts had significantly lower values (Figure S1). Thus, in the present study, the high antioxidant capacity of the extracts did not simply act to suppress inflammation. These results suggest that the tuber extract induced the activation of an intracellular antioxidant function. Therefore, we focused on Nrf2, which is known to be an oxidative stress response factor. We used Western blotting to examine nuclear Nrf2 180 min after LPS stimulation and found that nuclear Nrf2 increased with tuber extract addition (Figure 2C,D). At the same time, nuclear NF-κB was reduced (Figure 2E). We also found an increase in downstream-regulated HO-1 in the cytoplasmic fraction (Figure 2F), suggesting that the tuber extract somehow activates the Nrf2 pathway and suppresses the expression of pro-inflammatory genes through NF-κB.

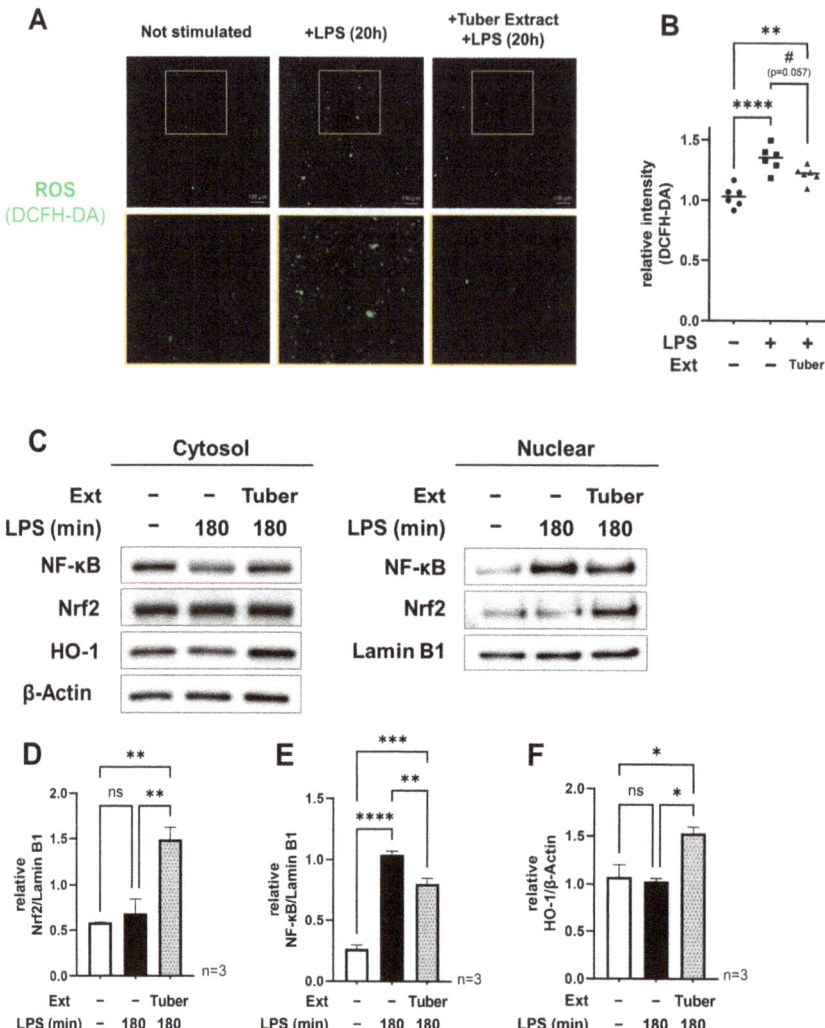

Figure 2. Analysis of intracellular ROS, NF-κB, and Nrf2 oxidative stress response pathway under tuber extract conditions: (**A**,**B**) Fluorescence microscopy images of intracellular ROS at 20 h after LPS stimulation with/without tuber extracts and comparison of its fluorescence intensity per cell; (**C**) Western blot of nuclear and cytoplasmic fractions at 180 min after LPS stimulation in the presence of tuber extracts; (**D**–**F**) Relative quantification of nuclear NF-κB, Nrf2, and cytoplasmic HO-1: mean ± SEM, one-way ANOVA with Tukey's post-hoc test, #: $p < 0.1$, *: $p < 0.05$, **: $p < 0.01$, ***: $p < 0.001$, ****: $p < 0.0001$, ns: not significant : LPS, lipopolysaccharide; Ext, extract; ROS, reactive oxygen species.

3.3. Nrf2 Inhibition Cancels the Anti-Inflammatory Effect of the Tuber Extracts

To verify the involvement of Nrf2 in the suppression of inflammation-related gene expression by tuber extracts, we conducted experiments using ML385, a small molecule compound known as an Nrf2 inhibitor. ML385 binds to the CNC-bZIP domain of Nrf2, Neh1, thereby blocking its ability to bind to the small molecule protein Maf and inhibiting the activity of Nrf2 as a transcription factor [21]. We conducted an experiment in which the inhibitor ML385 was added to the medium 1 h before the addition of tuber extract and evaluated LPS-induced IL-6 production, the expression of inflammation-related genes, and the nuclear translocation of Nrf2 and NF-κB. As a result, the concentration of IL-6 in the medium after 24 h of LPS stimulation with ML385 was almost the same as that without the extract (Figure 3A). Furthermore, we confirmed that ML385 canceled out the extract-induced decrease in *IL-6* gene expression (Figure 3B). However, no significant changes were observed in the expression of other inflammation-related genes (*Tnf* and *iNOS*), suggesting that the decreased expression of these genes was regulated by a different pathway. Under the conditions with added ML385, nuclear Nrf2, NF-κB, and cytoplasmic HO-1 levels were similar to those without the extract, suggesting that NF-κB's function was inhibited by the activation of the Nrf2 pathway (Figure 3C–F). These results for the addition of ML385 suggest that the components in the sweet potato tuber inhibited the function of NF-κB via the activation of the Nrf2 pathway, leading to the suppression of LPS-induced IL-6 expression.

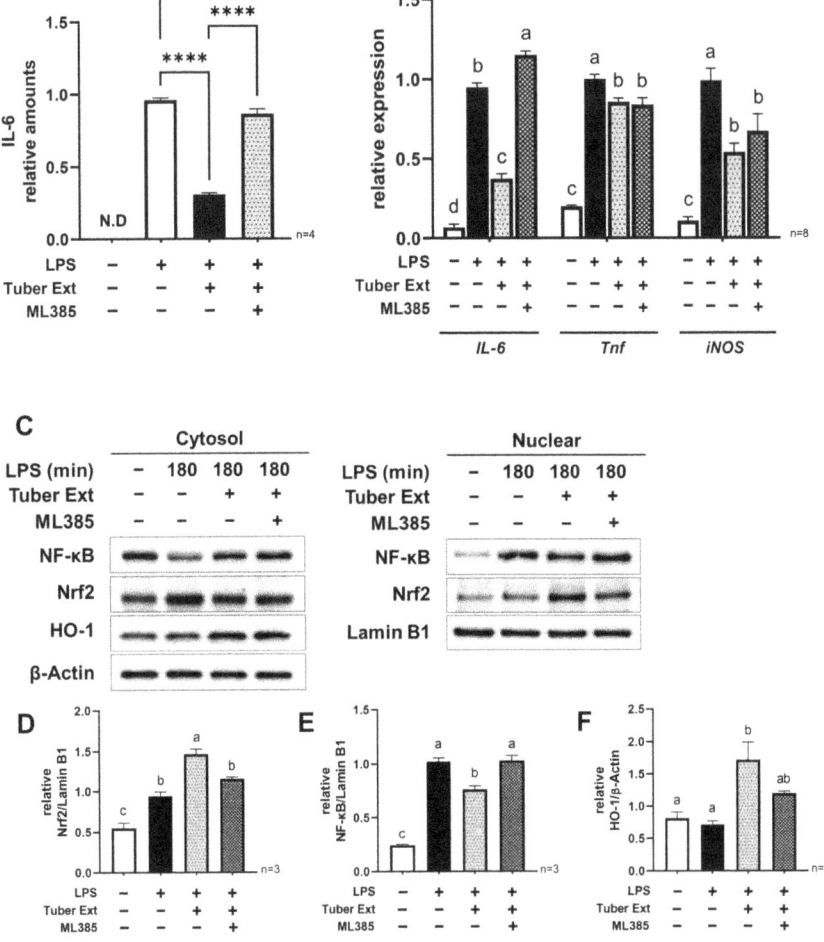

Figure 3. Analysis of the effects of Nrf2 inhibition on the suppression of LPS-induced inflammation by tuber extracts: (**A**) Relative production level of IL-6 at 24 h after LPS stimulation with/without tuber extracts and ML385; (**B**) Relative expression of pro-inflammatory genes (*IL-6, Tnf, iNOS(Nos2)*) at 24 h after LPS stimulation with/without tuber extracts and ML385; (**C**) Western blot of nuclear and cytoplasmic fractions at 180 min after LPS stimulation in the presence of tuber extracts and ML385;

(**D–F**) Relative quantification of nuclear NF-κB, Nrf2 and cytoplasmic HO-1 under each condition: (**A,B,D–F**) mean ± SEM, one-way ANOVA with Tukey's post-hoc test, *: $p < 0.05$, ****: $p < 0.0001$, Distinct symbols (a, b, c, d) are used to denote significant differences between groups: LPS, lipopolysaccharide; Ext, extract.

3.4. Hydrophobic Components in the Tuber Contribute to Its Anti-Inflammatory Properties

To characterize the active components in the extract, we fractionated the extract based on high-performance liquid chromatography (HPLC) analysis. HPLC analysis revealed multiple peaks, both under elution with 0.4% formic acid and with acetonitrile alone (Figure 4A). Based on the data we obtained, the extracts were collected in five fractions (Fr.1–Fr.5), as shown in Figure 4A. After drying and solidifying, each fraction was resuspended to a concentration equivalent to that of the original extract. In the IL-6 ELISA assay, a similar level of reduction was observed under conditions with added Fr.4 as in the original tuber extract (Figure 4B). In addition, among the five fractions, the addition of Fr.4 resulted in the greatest reduction in *IL-6* and *iNOS* expression (Figure 4C). The HPLC conditions for eluting Fr.4 were "0.4% formic acid:acetonitrile = 0:100", suggesting that the main component in Fraction 4 is a hydrophobic component. Moreover, when extracts of leaves, stems, and roots were analyzed by HPLC under the same conditions, most of the peaks in these fractions were undetectable (Figure S2). Therefore, the hydrophobic component that is only contained within the tuber may contribute to the anti-inflammatory effect confirmed in this study.

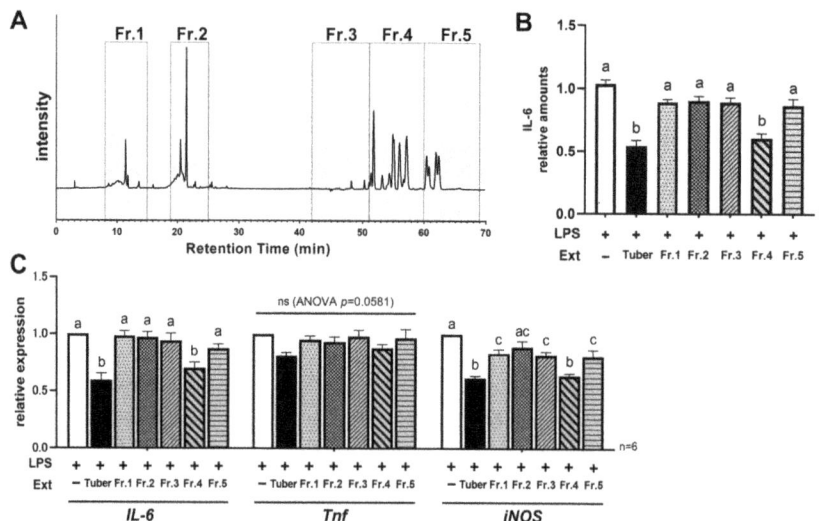

Figure 4. Characterization of the components responsible for anti-inflammatory activity in tuber extracts: (**A**) Peaks observed in HPLC analysis of tuber extracts and fraction settings; (**B**) Relative production level of IL-6 at 24 h after LPS stimulation with/without tuber extracts or each fraction; (**C**) Relative expression of pro-inflammatory genes (*IL-6*, *Tnf*, *iNOS*(*Nos2*)) at 24 h after LPS stimulation with/without tuber extracts or each fraction: (**B,C**) mean ± SEM, one-way ANOVA with Tukey's post-hoc test, Distinct symbols (a, b, c) are used to denote significant differences between groups: LPS, lipopolysaccharide; Ext, extract; Fr., fraction.

4. Discussion

In this study, we evaluated the anti-inflammatory activity of different parts of light-yellow pulp sweet potato, which have received little attention thus far. Among the leaves, stems, roots, and tubers, only extracts from tubers, the edible part of the plant, showed significant anti-inflammatory activity. Furthermore, the suppression of IL-6 production and expression was shown to be mediated by the activation of the Nrf2 pathway. It was also suggested that the hydrophobic component of the tuber extract contributed to its anti-inflammatory effects.

Previous studies have shown that many of the anti-inflammatory effects of foods or plants are associated with components with high antioxidant capacity [5,6]. It has been reported that anthocyanins in purple sweet potatoes and β-carotene in orange sweet potatoes inhibit LPS-induced inflammatory cytokine production in RAW264.7 cells [18,19]. Thus, phytochemicals with high antioxidant capacities are known to be involved in anti-inflammation in vitro. It should be noted, however, that high antioxidant capacity does not mean high anti-inflammatory activity. In the present study, the leaf extract had the highest values of total polyphenols, total flavonoids, and DPPH radical scavenging activity among the four extracts (Figure S1). Makori et al. also reported that among the parts of several cultivars of sweet potatoes, the leaves contain the highest amount of polyphenols and flavonoids, and exhibit high antioxidant activity [22]. In their report, they also showed that the same tendency was observed in purple and orange sweet potatoes. Nevertheless, in the present study, we found that the expression of inflammatory cytokines is more suppressed with tuber extracts. In addition, as shown in Figure 4, most of the peaks in the hydrophobic fraction, which is thought to play a central role in the anti-inflammatory activity, were detected in the tuber but not in the other three extracts (Figure S2). Therefore, these suggest that the key to anti-inflammation is not the antioxidant capacity of the extract, but the components it contains and that the component contributing to the anti-inflammatory activity is likely to be present only in the tubers in sweet potatoes. Although we were unable to identify the components responsible for this activity in this study, previous studies have reported that some carotenoids, flavonoids, and lipid-soluble polyphenols are contained in sweet potato tuber [23–25], which may be related to our findings. For instance, caffeic acid ethyl ester, one of the lipid-soluble polyphenols, has been reported to exhibit anticancer effects [25], and a number of other components are expected to have such activity via biochemical mechanisms. Identifying the components is an important issue to be addressed in future research, as it is a key factor in applying our findings to the prevention and improvement of chronic inflammation.

The present study also indicated that the activation of the Nrf2 pathway is, at least, involved in the suppression of *IL-6* gene expression. We hypothesize that the increased nuclear translocation of Nrf2 and the function of downstream factors contribute to this. First, the promoter region upstream of the *IL-6* gene contains a common binding site for Nrf2 and NF-κB, and Nrf2 binding in this site inhibits the function of Pol II [14], suggesting that the increased nuclear translocation of activated Nrf2 simply reduced IL-6 expression. We also observed increased expression of the downstream factor (Figure 2C,F). As HO-1 and NQO-1, which are downstream factors, have been reported to inhibit the NF-κB signaling pathway [12,26], we believe that this indirectly led to the suppression of inflammation-related gene expression. There are many reports of anti-inflammatory effects mediated by Nrf2 activation. Some of them have been linked to medicinal plants or herbs, such as Chinese sweet plum (*Sageretia thea* (Osbek.)), Ginseng (*Penax ginseng* (C. A. Mey.)), Elecampane (*Inula helenium* (L.)) [27–29], and other components in commonly consumed foods, such as pyrocatechol in roasted coffee [10], indicating that effects on daily food intake may also be expected.

In this study, we showed that components in light-yellow pulp sweet potato tuber extract suppressed LPS-induced inflammation in RAW264.7 cells via the Nrf2 pathway, but the specific components responsible for the activity, upstream of Nrf2 activation, and in vivo effects remain unclear. However, sweet potato is a daily consumed crop in many regions, and these results may help to encourage consumption as a dietary approach against inflammation. In the future, we plan to examine the effects of heat processing on the activity.

5. Conclusions

While it has been known that sweet potatoes with purple or orange pulp have anti-inflammatory effects due to the plant metabolites contained abundantly in them, we described the anti-inflammatory effects of light-yellow pulp sweet potatoes in this study. We found that only extracts from the tuber, among the four parts of the plant (leaf, stem, root, and tuber), suppressed LPS-induced inflammation in RAW264.7 cells, and this effect may be attributed to the inhibition of NF-κB associated with the activation of the Nrf2 pathway. It was also shown that the hydrophobic components of the tuber are responsible for the activity, but the specific components remained unknown within this study and remain an issue to be addressed in the future. However, we believe that these results expand the potential of sweet potato as a food-derived approach to inflammation.

Supplementary Materials: The following supporting information can be downloaded at: https://www.mdpi.com/article/10.3390/nu16040563/s1, Figure S1: Total polyphenols, total flavonoids, and DPPH radical scavenging activity of sweet potato extracts; Figure S2: Comparison of peaks observed in HPLC analysis of sweet potato extracts.

Author Contributions: Conceptualization, Y.M.; methodology, Y.M., M.S. and I.U.; formal analysis, Y.M.; writing—original draft preparation, Y.M.; writing—review and editing, H.M. and K.I.; visualization, Y.M.; supervision, H.M. and K.I. All authors have read and agreed to the published version of the manuscript.

Funding: This research received no external funding.

Institutional Review Board Statement: Not applicable.

Informed Consent Statement: Not applicable.

Data Availability Statement: The raw data supporting the conclusions of this article will be made available by the authors on request.

Acknowledgments: We would like to thank Calbee Kaitsuka Sweet Potato, Inc. for the provision of plant samples.

Conflicts of Interest: Y.M, M.S, I.U, H.M and K.I are employees of Calbee, Inc.

References

1. Franceschi, C.; Campisi, J. Chronic inflammation (inflammaging) and its potential contribution to age-associated diseases. *J. Gerontol. A Biol. Sci. Med. Sci.* **2014**, *69* (Suppl. S1), S4–S9. [CrossRef]
2. Boutens, L.; Hooiveld, G.J.; Dhingra, S.; Cramer, R.A.; Netea, M.G.; Stienstra, R. Unique metabolic activation of adipose tissue macrophages in obesity promotes inflammatory responses. *Diabetologia* **2018**, *61*, 942–953. [CrossRef]
3. Giallongo, C.; Tibullo, D.; Camiolo, G.; Parrinello, N.L.; Romano, A.; Puglisi, F.; Barbato, A.; Conticello, C.; Lupo, G.; Anfuso, C.D.; et al. TLR4 signaling drives mesenchymal stromal cells commitment to promote tumor microenvironment transformation in multiple myeloma. *Cell Death. Dis.* **2019**, *10*, 704. [CrossRef]
4. Knekt, P.; Kumpulainen, J.; Jarvinen, R.; Rissanen, H.; Heliovaara, M.; Reunanen, A.; Hakulinen, T.; Aromaa, A. Flavonoid intake and risk of chronic diseases. *Am. J. Clin. Nutr.* **2002**, *76*, 560–568. [CrossRef]
5. Rudrapal, M.; Khairnar, S.J.; Khan, J.; Dukhyil, A.B.; Ansari, M.A.; Alomary, M.N.; Alshabrmi, F.M.; Palai, S.; Deb, P.K.; Devi, R. Dietary Polyphenols and Their Role in Oxidative Stress-Induced Human Diseases: Insights Into Protective Effects, Antioxidant Potentials and Mechanism(s) of Action. *Front. Pharmacol.* **2022**, *13*, 806470. [CrossRef] [PubMed]
6. Maleki, S.J.; Crespo, J.F.; Cabanillas, B. Anti-inflammatory effects of flavonoids. *Food. Chem.* **2019**, *299*, 125124. [CrossRef] [PubMed]
7. Schieber, M.; Chandel, N.S. ROS function in redox signaling and oxidative stress. *Curr. Biol.* **2014**, *24*, R453–R462. [CrossRef] [PubMed]
8. Na, H.K.; Surh, Y.J. Modulation of Nrf2-mediated antioxidant and detoxifying enzyme induction by the green tea polyphenol EGCG. *Food Chem. Toxicol.* **2008**, *46*, 1271–1278. [CrossRef] [PubMed]
9. Cardozo, L.F.; Pedruzzi, L.M.; Stenvinkel, P.; Stockler-Pinto, M.B.; Daleprane, J.B.; Leite, M., Jr.; Mafra, D. Nutritional strategies to modulate inflammation and oxidative stress pathways via activation of the master antioxidant switch Nrf2. *Biochimie* **2013**, *95*, 1525–1533. [CrossRef] [PubMed]
10. Funakoshi-Tago, M.; Nonaka, Y.; Tago, K.; Takeda, M.; Ishihara, Y.; Sakai, A.; Matsutaka, M.; Kobata, K.; Tamura, H. Pyrocatechol, a component of coffee, suppresses LPS-induced inflammatory responses by inhibiting NF-kappaB and activating Nrf2. *Sci. Rep.* **2020**, *10*, 2584. [CrossRef]

11. Bellezza, I.; Giambanco, I.; Minelli, A.; Donato, R. Nrf2-Keap1 signaling in oxidative and reductive stress. *Biochim. Biophys. Acta Mol. Cell. Res.* **2018**, *1865*, 721–733. [CrossRef]
12. Willis, D.; Moore, A.R.; Frederick, R.; Willoughby, D.A. Heme oxygenase: A novel target for the modulation of the inflammatory response. *Nat. Med.* **1996**, *2*, 87–90. [CrossRef]
13. Liu, G.H.; Qu, J.; Shen, X. NF-kappaB/p65 antagonizes Nrf2-ARE pathway by depriving CBP from Nrf2 and facilitating recruitment of HDAC3 to MafK. *Biochim. Biophys. Acta* **2008**, *1783*, 713–727. [CrossRef] [PubMed]
14. Kobayashi, E.H.; Suzuki, T.; Funayama, R.; Nagashima, T.; Hayashi, M.; Sekine, H.; Tanaka, N.; Moriguchi, T.; Motohashi, H.; Nakayama, K.; et al. Nrf2 suppresses macrophage inflammatory response by blocking proinflammatory cytokine transcription. *Nat. Commun.* **2016**, *7*, 11624. [CrossRef] [PubMed]
15. Oin, Y.; Naumovski, N.; Ranasheera, C.S.; D'Cunha, N.M. Nutrition-related health outcomes of sweet potato (*Ipomoea batatas*) consumption: A systematic review. *Food Biosci.* **2022**, *50*, 102208. [CrossRef]
16. Islam, S.N.; Nusrat, T.; Begum, P.; Ahsan, M. Carotenoids and beta-carotene in orange fleshed sweet potato: A possible solution to vitamin A deficiency. *Food Chem.* **2016**, *199*, 628–631. [CrossRef]
17. Chen, C.C.; Lin, C.; Chen, M.H.; Chiang, P.Y. Stability and Quality of Anthocyanin in Purple Sweet Potato Extracts. *Foods* **2019**, *8*, 393. [CrossRef] [PubMed]
18. Sugata, M.; Lin, C.Y.; Shih, Y.C. Anti-Inflammatory and Anticancer Activities of Taiwanese Purple-Fleshed Sweet Potatoes (*Ipomoea batatas* L. Lam) Extracts. *Biomed Res. Int.* **2015**, *2015*, 768093. [CrossRef] [PubMed]
19. Bae, J.Y.; Park, W.S.; Kim, H.J.; Kim, H.S.; Kang, K.K.; Kwak, S.S.; Ahn, M.J. Protective Effect of Carotenoid Extract from Orange-Fleshed Sweet Potato on Gastric Ulcer in Mice by Inhibition of NO, IL-6 and PGE(2) Production. *Pharmaceuticals* **2021**, *14*, 1320. [CrossRef] [PubMed]
20. Jiang, T.; Zhou, J.; Liu, W.; Tao, W.; He, J.; Jin, W.; Guo, H.; Yang, N.; Li, Y. The anti-inflammatory potential of protein-bound anthocyanin compounds from purple sweet potato in LPS-induced RAW264.7 macrophages. *Food Res. Int.* **2020**, *137*, 109647. [CrossRef]
21. Singh, A.; Venkannagari, S.; Oh, K.H.; Zhang, Y.Q.; Rohde, J.M.; Liu, L.; Nimmagadda, S.; Sudini, K.; Brimacombe, K.R.; Gajghate, S.; et al. Small Molecule Inhibitor of NRF2 Selectively Intervenes Therapeutic Resistance in KEAP1-Deficient NSCLC Tumors. *ACS Chem. Biol.* **2016**, *11*, 3214–3225. [CrossRef]
22. Makori, S.; Mu, T.-H.; Sun, H.-N. Total Polyphenol Content, Antioxidant Activity, and Individual Phenolic Composition of Different Edible Parts of 4 Sweet Potato Cultivars. *Nat. Prod. Commun.* **2020**, *15*. [CrossRef]
23. Ishiguro, K.; Yoshinaga, M.; Kai, Y.; Maoka, T.; Yoshimoto, M. Composition, content and antioxidative activity of the carotenoids in yellow-fleshed sweetpotato (*Ipomoea batatas* L.). *Breed. Sci.* **2010**, *60*, 324–329. [CrossRef]
24. Wang, A.; Li, R.; Ren, L.; Gao, X.; Zhang, Y.; Ma, Z.; Ma, D.; Luo, Y. A comparative metabolomics study of flavonoids in sweet potato with different flesh colors (*Ipomoea batatas* (L.) Lam). *Food Chem.* **2018**, *260*, 124–134. [CrossRef] [PubMed]
25. Kato, K.; Nagane, M.; Aihara, N.; Kamiie, J.; Miyanabe, M.; Hiraki, S.; Luo, X.; Nakanishi, I.; Shoji, Y.; Matsumoto, K.I.; et al. Lipid-soluble polyphenols from sweet potato exert antitumor activity and enhance chemosensitivity in breast cancer. *J. Clin. Biochem. Nutr.* **2021**, *68*, 193–200. [CrossRef] [PubMed]
26. Kimura, A.; Kitajima, M.; Nishida, K.; Serada, S.; Fujimoto, M.; Naka, T.; Fujii-Kuriyama, Y.; Sakamato, T.; Ito, T.; Handa, H.; et al. NQO1 inhibits the TLR-dependent production of selective cytokines by promoting IkappaB-zeta degradation. *J. Exp. Med.* **2018**, *215*, 2197–2209. [CrossRef] [PubMed]
27. Yang, S.; Li, F.; Lu, S.; Ren, L.; Bian, S.; Liu, M.; Zhao, D.; Wang, S.; Wang, J. Ginseng root extract attenuates inflammation by inhibiting the MAPK/NF-kappaB signaling pathway and activating autophagy and p62-Nrf2-Keap1 signaling in vitro and in vivo. *J. Ethnopharmacol.* **2022**, *283*, 114739. [CrossRef]
28. Kim, H.N.; Park, G.H.; Park, S.B.; Kim, J.D.; Eo, H.J.; Son, H.J.; Song, J.H.; Jeong, J.B. Sageretia thea Inhibits Inflammation through Suppression of NF-kappa B and MAPK and Activation of Nrf2/HO-1 Signaling Pathways in RAW264.7 Cells. *Am. J. Chin. Med.* **2019**, *47*, 385–403. [CrossRef]
29. Park, E.J.; Kim, Y.M.; Park, S.W.; Kim, H.J.; Lee, J.H.; Lee, D.U.; Chang, K.C. Induction of HO-1 through p38 MAPK/Nrf2 signaling pathway by ethanol extract of *Inula helenium* L. reduces inflammation in LPS-activated RAW 264.7 cells and CLP-induced septic mice. *Food Chem. Toxicol.* **2013**, *55*, 386–395. [CrossRef] [PubMed]

Disclaimer/Publisher's Note: The statements, opinions and data contained in all publications are solely those of the individual author(s) and contributor(s) and not of MDPI and/or the editor(s). MDPI and/or the editor(s) disclaim responsibility for any injury to people or property resulting from any ideas, methods, instructions or products referred to in the content.

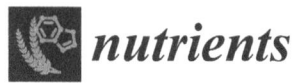

Article

Novel Fermentates Can Enhance Key Immune Responses Associated with Viral Immunity

Dearbhla Finnegan [1,2], Monica A. Mechoud [1,3], Jamie A. FitzGerald [1,4], Tom Beresford [1,3], Harsh Mathur [1,3], Paul D. Cotter [1,3,5,6] and Christine Loscher [1,2,*]

1. Food for Health Ireland, Science Centre South (S2.79), University College Dublin, Dublin 4, Ireland; dearbhla.finnegan7@mail.dcu.ie (D.F.); monica.mechoud@teagasc.ie (M.A.M.); jamie.fitzgerald@ucd.ie (J.A.F.); tom.beresford@teagasc.ie (T.B.); harsh.mathur@teagasc.ie (H.M.); paul.cotter@teagasc.ie (P.D.C.)
2. School of Biotechnology, Faculty of Science, Glasnevin Campus, Dublin City University, D09 DX63 Dublin, Ireland
3. Teagasc Food Research Centre, Moorepark, Fermoy, P61 C996 Co. Cork, Ireland
4. College of Health and Agricultural Sciences, School of Medicine, University College Dublin, D04 V1W8 Dublin, Ireland
5. APC Microbiome Ireland, Biosciences Institute, Biosciences Research Institute, University College Cork, T12 R229 Cork, Ireland
6. VistaMilk, Teagasc, Moorepark, Shanacloon, Fermoy, P61 C996 Co. Cork, Ireland
* Correspondence: christine.loscher@dcu.ie; Tel.: +353-(01)7008515

Abstract: Fermented foods have long been known to have immunomodulatory capabilities, and fermentates derived from the lactic acid bacteria of dairy products can modulate the immune system. We have used skimmed milk powder to generate novel fermentates using *Lb. helveticus* strains SC234 and SC232 and we demonstrate here that these fermentates can enhance key immune mechanisms that are critical to the immune response to viruses. We show that our novel fermentates, SC234 and SC232, can positively impact on cytokine and chemokine secretion, nitric oxide (NO) production, cell surface marker expression, and phagocytosis in macrophage models. We demonstrate that the fermentates SC234 and SC232 increase the secretion of cytokines IL-1β, IL-6, TNF-α, IL-27, and IL-10; promote an M1 pro-inflammatory phenotype for viral immunity via NO induction; decrease chemokine expression of Monocyte Chemoattractant Protein (MCP); increase cell surface marker expression; and enhance phagocytosis in comparison to their starting material. These data suggest that these novel fermentates have potential as novel functional food ingredients for the treatment, management, and control of viral infection.

Keywords: fermentates; functional food; immune boosting; immunomodulation; macrophage; viral immunity

Citation: Finnegan, D.; Mechoud, M.A.; FitzGerald, J.A.; Beresford, T.; Mathur, H.; Cotter, P.D.; Loscher, C. Novel Fermentates Can Enhance Key Immune Responses Associated with Viral Immunity. *Nutrients* 2024, 16, 1212. https://doi.org/10.3390/nu16081212

Academic Editor: Ping Zhang

Received: 22 March 2024
Revised: 16 April 2024
Accepted: 17 April 2024
Published: 19 April 2024

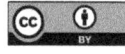

Copyright: © 2024 by the authors. Licensee MDPI, Basel, Switzerland. This article is an open access article distributed under the terms and conditions of the Creative Commons Attribution (CC BY) license (https://creativecommons.org/licenses/by/4.0/).

1. Introduction

The term "fermentates" generally refers to "a powdered preparation, derived from a fermented [food] product and which can contain the fermenting microorganisms, components of these microorganisms, culture supernatants, fermented substrates, and a range of metabolites and bioactive components" [1]. In recent years, such fermented food products have been of ever-increasing interest, as they can exhibit health benefits including protection against infectious agents, immunomodulatory effects, anti-allergenic effects, anti-obesity effects, anti-oxidant effects and anti-anxiety effects [1]. Lactic acid bacteria (LAB), including *Lactobacilli* and *Bifidobacteria*, are responsible for the fermentation process within fermented foods, are generally regarded as safe (GRAS), and thus can be used in the production of functional foods [2]. Different strains of LAB can produce different fermentation products that can interact with microorganisms during intestinal transit and have the ability to therefore interact with the cells of the intestinal wall [3]. In the generation of these fermentates, the LAB undergo a heat killing phase, creating a fermentate or postbiotic ingredient that has bioactivity associated with the secondary metabolites present, as opposed to a viable LAB strain. Postbiotics are ideal components for the development of a large range of novel health-promoting consumable products, as functional foods and potential nutraceuticals [4].

With recent viral outbreaks like that of the SARS-CoV-2 virus, Monkeypox virus, and most recently the Langya virus, as well as the yearly outbreaks of seasonal influenza, there is a need to explore new ways of enhancing viral immunity [5]. This study is one of the first to explore the effects of novel milk fermentates, derived from *Lb. helveticus*, to impact on immune mechanisms that are critical to viral immunity. The objective of this study was to examine the effects of two milk fermentates made using *Lb. helveticus* SC234 or SC232 (sourced from Lallemand, Quebec, CA) on murine macrophage cells challenged with the viral immune stimulus Loxoribine (LOX), or an inflammatory immune stimulus lipopolysaccharide (LPS; *Escherichia coli* 055:B5). The effects of these novel fermentates on cell viability, cytokine secretion interleukin-1β (IL-1β), IL-6, IL-10, tumour necrosis factor (TNF)-α, IL-12p40, IL-27, nitric oxide production (NO) and arginase activity in M1- and M2-polarised macrophages, chemokine secretion (MIP)-1, MIP-2, Monocyte Chemoattractant Protein (MCP), cell surface marker expression (major histocompatibility complex (MHC) II, CD86, Toll-like receptor ligand (TLR) 4, cluster-differentiated (CD) 80, CD14, TLR2, CD40, and MHCI), and phagocytosis were investigated in LOX- and LPS-activated murine-derived macrophage. We demonstrate that fermentates SC234 and SC232 increase the secretion of cytokines IL-1β, IL-6, TNF-α, IL-27, and IL-10; promote an M1 pro-inflammatory phenotype for viral immunity via NO induction; decrease chemokine expression of MCP; increase cell surface marker expression; and enhance phagocytosis in comparison to their starting material.

2. Materials and Methods

2.1. Generation of Dairy-Based Fermentates

Skim Milk Powder (SMP) was used as a substrate for the generation of the fermentates used in this study. SMP was reconstituted at 10% w/v in distilled water to generate Reconstituted Skim Milk (RSM), autoclaved, cooled, and stored at 4 °C for a maximum of 7 days. An inoculum of frozen mother culture stocks of the individual strains *Lb. helveticus* SC232 and *Lb. helveticus* Lafti L10 SC234 (which were previously prepared in 10% w/v RSM) was added to 10% RSM and incubated for 24 h at 37 °C under aerobic conditions without agitation, to generate these individual fermentates derived from the above-mentioned individual strains. From these cultures, a further inoculum was added to 10% w/v RSM and incubated for 24 h at 37 °C under aerobic conditions again without agitation. These fermentates were subjected to a heat treatment step to generate the fermentates which contained one of the heat-killed LAB strains mentioned above. After cooling to room temperature, the pH of the fermentates was neutralized. These fermentates were aliquoted and immediately frozen at −80 °C until further analysis. Non-fermented RSM samples subjected to the same heat-treatment mentioned above were used as negative controls for all experiments described herein.

2.2. Cell Culture

J774.A.1 Murine Macrophage, purchased from the European Collection of Animal Cell Cultures (Salisbury, UK), were maintained in Dulbecco Modified Eagle Medium (DMEM) supplemented with 10% heat-inactivated foetal bovine serum (FBS), and 1% Penicillin–Streptomycin Antibiotic obtained from Biosciences (Dublin, Ireland), and incubated at 37 °C, with 5% CO_2 and 95% humidified air. Cells were passaged every three to four days at a confluence of 80–90%. Cells were sub-cultured at a ratio of 1:10. Bone Marrow-Derived Macrophage cells (BMDMs), harvested from the bone marrow of 6–8-week-old female BALB/c mice obtained from Charles River (Margate, UK), were cultured in complete Roswell Park Memorial Institute (RPMI) 1640 medium, containing 25 ng/mL rM-CSF (Merck, Haverhill, UK).

2.3. Cell Viability

Cell viability was determined using the CellTiter 96® AQueous One Solution Cell Proliferation Assay and conducted as per the manufacturer's instructions (MyBio, Kilkenny, Ireland). Macrophages were seeded at a concentration of 1×10^6 cells/mL in a flat-bottom 96-well plate, and incubated for 24 h at 37 °C in a 95% humidified air and 5% CO_2 atmosphere. Cells were treated with 25 mg/mL of the fermentate sample for 1 h and incubated under the same conditions, before stimulation with LOX 0.5 mM and LPS 100 ng/mL for 24 h. DMSO was included as a positive control to induce cell death. After 24 h, 20 µL of the thawed CellTiter96® Aqueous One Solution was added to each well of the 96-well plate, and incubated at 37 °C for 3 h in a humidified 5% CO_2 atmosphere. Absorbance was read at 490 nm using Versamax™ 96-well plate reader (VWR, Dublin, Ireland). Cell viability was expressed as the percentage viability of the treatment group relative to the control group.

2.4. Enzyme-Linked ImmunoSorbent Assay (ELISA)

Determination of the effects of the fermentate samples on cytokine and chemokine production in the activated macrophages required harvesting of the cell supernatants, and subsequent analysis using commercial DuoSet ELISA kits (R&D Systems Europe, Abdingdon, Oxon, UK), according to the manufacturer's instructions. This allowed for the quantification of the cytokines IL-1β, IL-6, IL-10, TNF-α, IL-12p40, and IL-27, as well as the chemokines MCP, MIP-1, and MIP-2.

2.5. Nitric Oxide (NO) and Arginase Assay

NO production was determined by measuring the NO_2^- in the cell supernatants of the cultured macrophage via a Griess assay, carried out as per manufacturer's instructions (MyBio, Kilkenny, Ireland). Cell lysates were prepared and analysed for arginase activity via the proportional detection of urea, a direct result of arginase catalysing the conversion of arginine to urea and ornithine, using a commercial kit and following the manufacturer's instructions (Merck, Haverhill, UK). BMDM cells were seeded at a concentration of 5×10^5 cells per well in 24-well plates and incubated for 30 min at 37 °C. BMDMs were stimulated with 25 mg/mL fermentates for 3 h and incubated under the same conditions. BMDM cells were polarised towards M1 macrophages by adding LPS (100 ng/mL) in the presence of 20 ng/mL rIFN-γ or towards M2 cells by adding 20 ng/mL rIL-4, 20 ng/mL IL-13, and 20 ng/mL rTGF-B and incubated for 24 h at 37 °C. After 24 h, supernatant was harvested and Griess assay was carried out to quantify the NO_2^- present, while an arginase assay was carried out to determine the arginase activity within the cell.

2.6. Cell Surface Marker Expression Analysis

The determination of cell surface markers present on the J774.A.1 macrophage was carried out via cell surface marker staining using the fluorescently labelled antibodies FITC, APC, and PE. J774.A.1 macrophages were seeded at a concentration of 1×10^6 cells/mL in a 6-well plate, stimulated with appropriate treatments and incubated at 37 °C, with 5% CO_2 and 95% humidified air. Cells were blocked with FBS for 15 min, before being harvested via centrifugation at 2000 rpm for 5 min at 4 °C. Cells were resuspended in FACS buffer. Cell suspension was plated in a 96-well round-bottom plate and centrifuged. Supernatant was aspirated, and cells resuspended in 1:1000 dilutions of antibodies (FITC, APC, PE) and incubated for 30 min at 4 °C. Cells were centrifuged and washed 3 times in FACS buffer. Cells were resuspended in FACS buffer and transferred to FACS loading tubes. Cells were analysed using a BD FACSAria 1 system flow cytometer. Raw FCS files were analysed, and data were graphed using V10.0 FlowJo software. Cell surface marker expression was determined for cell surface markers MHCI, MHCII, TLR2, TLR4, CD40, CD14, CD80, and CD86.

2.7. Phagocytosis Assay

J774A.1 macrophages were seeded at 1×10^6 cells/mL in 6-well plates and incubated overnight at 37 °C in a humidified, 5% CO_2 atmosphere. Cells were stimulated with sample for 1 h, incubated under the same conditions. Subsequently, cells were stimulated with 100 ng/mL LPS and LOX for 4 h. Cells were incubated with 1 μm fluorescent latex beads (Merck, Haverhill, UK) at a concentration of 20 beads per cell for 1 h at 37 °C in a humidified 5% CO_2 atmosphere. Cells were scraped from the cell culture plate and pelleted via centrifugation at 4 °C at 2000 rpm for 5 min. Cells were resuspended and washed twice in 1 mL FACs buffer via centrifugation. Cells were resuspended in FACs buffer and added to FACs tubes. The uptake of beads was measured by flow cytometry on a FACSAria™ flow cytometer. Data were analysed using FlowJo software (Treestar, Woodburn, OR, USA). MFI and percentage of phagocytosing cells were the two outputs measured.

Data were represented as the MPI. This is a representation to incorporate the MFI from the phagocytosed beads as well as the percentage of phagocytosing cells in the viable population of cells and compare them to the control, which represents baseline phagocytosis. The MPI is calculated as follows:

$$MPI = \frac{\% \text{ phagocytes} \times MFI}{\text{control phagocytes} \times \text{control MFI}}$$

2.8. Statistical Analysis

Statistical analysis was carried out using a one-way ANOVA to compare variance among the means of different sample groups. A Newman–Keuls post-test was used to determine significance among the samples. The level of statistical significance was indicated by * ($p < 0.05$), ** ($p < 0.01$), and *** ($p < 0.001$).

2.9. Ethical Statement

The care, treatment, and experiments involved in this study were approved by the Research Ethics Committee (REC) of Dublin City University (Approval ID: DCUREC/2011/008).

3. Results

3.1. Immune-Boosting Effects of Fermentates on Cytokine Secretion

Initially, in the preliminary experiments carried out by the laboratory, an MTS assay confirmed that the fermentates SC232 and SC234 in the presence/absence of LOX or LPS had no effect on the viability of either J774.A.1 cells and BMDMs.

Additionally, an ELISA was performed on the cell line J774.A.1 macrophage to assess the bioactivity of fermentates SC232 and SC234 in the presence/absence of LOX or LPS. The novel fermentates altered the secretion of cytokines in response to LOX and LPS when compared to the respective controls in J774.A.1s. With this knowledge, we were then able to carry out the study in question.

In order to confirm the effects of our fermentates in macrophages, we assessed their effects in primary cells. SC234 and SC232 significantly affected the secretion of cytokines in response to LOX and LPS when compared to the respective controls in BMDMs (Figure 1). IL-1β ($p < 0.001$), IL-6 ($p < 0.001$), IL-12p40 ($p < 0.033$), IL-10 ($p < 0.033$), and TNF-α ($p < 0.001$) were increased in the presence of LOX with only low levels of IL-27 detected. IL-6 ($p < 0.001$), TNF-α ($p < 0.001$), and IL-27 ($p < 0.001$) were increased in the presence of LPS with only low levels of IL-1β, IL-10, and IL-12p40.

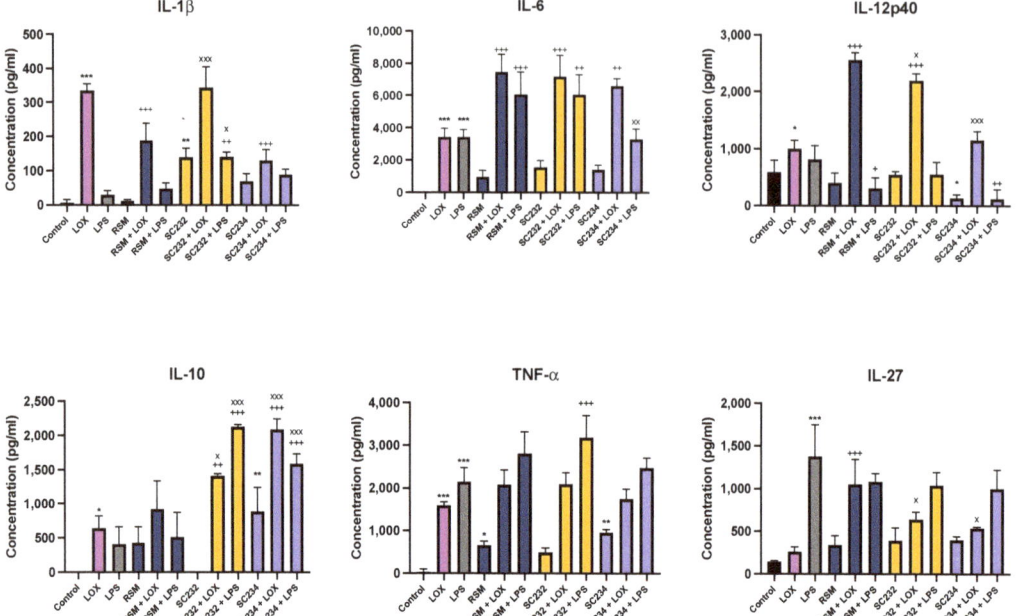

Figure 1. Exposure of LOX- and LPS-activated BMDM to 25 mg/mL fermentates results in the secretion of cytokines. BMDM cells were seeded at 1×10^6 cells/mL and incubated overnight at 37 °C in 5% CO_2. The following day, cells were stimulated with 25 mg/mL fermentate, incubated for 1 h at 37 °C in 5% CO_2 and subsequently exposed to LOX 0.5 mM; LPS 100 ng/mL before incubating overnight under the same conditions. Non-fermented RSM was the fermentate control. Supernatants were removed after 24 h and ELISA was performed for cytokines IL-1β, IL-6, IL-10, TNF-α, IL-12p40, and IL-27. Data are presented as mean ± SEM of three replicates. Significance determined using one-way ANOVA with a Newman–Keuls post-test. Output p value style APA: 0.12 nonsignificant (unlabelled), 0.033 somewhat significant (*), 0.002 significant (**), and <0.001 highly significant (***); where the following symbols represent; (1) comparing control cells to LOX and LPS and unstimulated samples "*", (2) comparing TLR to sample + TLR "+", and (3) comparing RSM +/− TLR to sample +/− TLR "x".

In the presence of LOX, SC234 significantly enhanced IL-6, and IL-10 secretion ($p < 0.002$; $p < 0.001$), but decreased IL-1β secretion ($p < 0.001$), with no significant effects on the other cytokines measured when compared to control cells. In contrast, SC232 significantly increased IL-6 ($p < 0.001$), IL-12p40 ($p < 0.001$), and IL-10 ($p < 0.001$), with no significant effect on the other cytokines. The exposure of cells to SC234 in the presence of LPS resulted in an increase in IL-10 ($p < 0.001$), but a decrease in IL-12p40 ($p < 0.002$), with no significant effect on the other cytokines. SC232 in the presence of LPS resulted in an increase in IL-1β ($p < 0.002$), IL-6 ($p < 0.002$), IL-10 ($p < 0.001$), and TNF-α ($p < 0.001$) but no change in IL-12p40 or IL-27. Interestingly, the exposure of cells to SC234 alone, in the absence of either LOX or LPS stimulation, resulted in enhanced secretion of IL-10 ($p < 0.001$), but decreased IL-12p40 ($p < 0.033$) and TNF-α secretion ($p < 0.002$), and the exposure of cells to SC232 alone resulted in decreased secretion of IL-1β ($p < 0.002$).

The non-fermented RSM, used as a negative control, did affect cytokine secretion in the presence of LOX with an increase in IL-6 ($p < 0.001$), IL-12p40 ($p < 0.001$), and IL-27 ($p < 0.001$), but a decrease in IL-1β ($p < 0.001$). Furthermore, RSM enhanced IL-6 ($p < 0.001$), but decreased IL-12p40 ($p < 0.033$) in the presence of LPS. RSM, in the absence of TLR stimulation, increased TNF-α ($p < 0.033$).

Given that RSM itself had some effects, we also compared the fermentates to the RSM. In the absence of TLR stimulation, SC232 increased IL-10 ($p < 0.002$). In the presence of LOX, SC234 increased IL-10 ($p < 0.001$) but decreased IL-12p40 ($p < 0.001$) and IL-27 ($p < 0.001$) relative to the RSM. In the presence of LOX, SC232 increased IL-1β ($p < 0.001$) and IL-10 ($p < 0.033$), but decreased IL-12p40 ($p < 0.033$) and IL-27 ($p < 0.001$). In the presence of LPS, SC234 increased IL-10 ($p < 0.001$), but decreased IL-6 ($p < 0.002$), and SC232 increased IL-1β ($p < 0.033$) and IL-10 ($p < 0.001$), relative to the RSM.

Given that the fermentates had clear effects on macrophages, we sought to determine if they could exert specific effects on M1- and M2-polarised macrophages. In Figure 2, A shows the cytokine secretion profiles of M0-, M1-, and M2-polarised macrophages. M1 macrophages secrete high levels of IL-6 and TNF-α ($p < 0.001$; $p < 0.001$), while M2 macrophages secrete only small concentrations of IL-6 and TNF-α but secrete higher concentrations of IL-10 compared with the M0-unpolarised macrophages and the M1-polarised macrophages which secrete undetectable levels. The M0 macrophages secrete undetectable levels of IL-6, TNF-α, or IL-10.

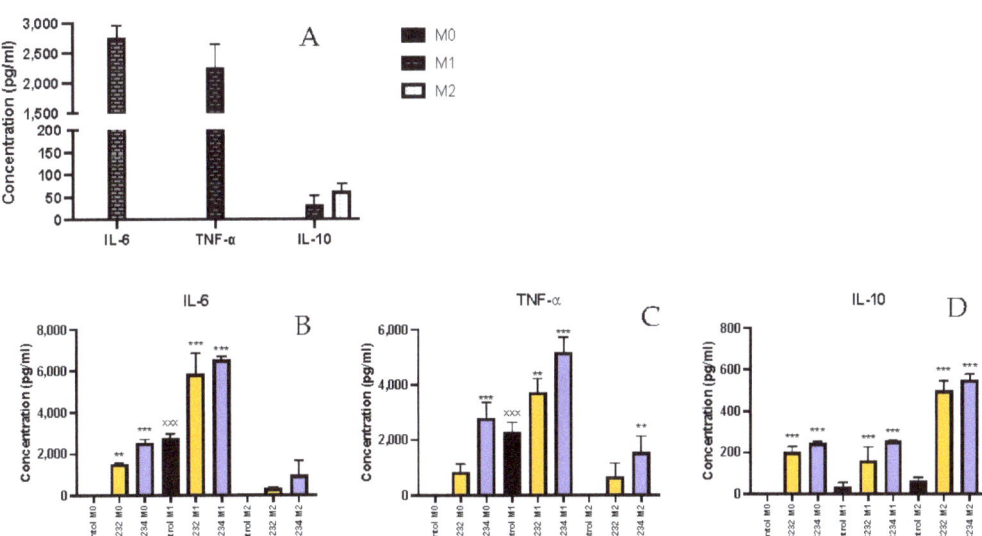

Figure 2. Exposure of M1/M2-polarised BMDMs to 25 mg/mL fermentates results in the secretion of cytokines IL-6, TNF-α, and IL-10. BMDM cells were seeded at 5×10^5 cells/mL and incubated for 1 h at 37 °C in 5% CO_2. Cells were stimulated with 25 mg/mL fermentates, incubated for 3 h at 37 °C in 5% CO_2. The cells were either polarised to the M1 phenotype by stimulating with LPS (100 ng/mL) in the presence of 20 ng/mL rIFN-γ or towards M2 cells by adding 20 ng/mL rIL-4, 20 ng/mL IL-13, and 20 ng/mL rTGF-B and incubating for 24 h at 37 °C. Supernatants were removed after 24 h and ELISA was performed for IL-6, IL-10, and TNF-α. Data are presented as mean ± SEM of three replicates. (**A**) represent the M0, M1, and M2 profiles for each cytokine. (**B**–**D**) represent cytokine output in response to sample presence. Significance determined using one-way ANOVA with a Newman–Keuls post-test. Output p value style APA: 0.12 nonsignificant (unlabelled), 0.033 somewhat significant (*), 0.002 significant (**), and <0.001 highly significant (***); where the following symbols represent; (1) comparing fermentates to polarised control cells "*", and (2) comparing M0 to M1 and M2 controls "x".

SC234 increased IL-6 ($p < 0.001$), IL-10 ($p < 0.001$), and TNF-α ($p < 0.001$) in M0 BMDMs (Figure 2A–D). M0 BMDMs in the presence of SC232 showed increased IL-6 ($p < 0.002$) and

IL-10 ($p < 0.001$) relative to the M0 control. In M1-polarised BMDMs, SC234 increased IL-6 ($p < 0.001$), IL-10 ($p < 0.001$), and TNF-α ($p < 0.001$), and SC232 increased IL-6 ($p < 0.001$), IL-10 ($p < 0.001$), and TNF-α ($p < 0.002$), relative to the M1 control. In M2-polarised BMDMs, SC234 increased IL-10 ($p < 0.001$) and TNF-α ($p < 0.002$), and SC232 increased IL-10 ($p < 0.001$), relative to the M2 control.

3.2. Immune-Boosting Effects of Fermentates on Nitric Oxide Production and Arginase Activity

Nitric oxide production and arginase activity are classical markers of M1 and M2 macrophages.

Figure 3A exhibits that M1 macrophages secreted high levels of NO ($p < 0.001$), while M0 and M2 macrophages secreted only small concentrations of NO.

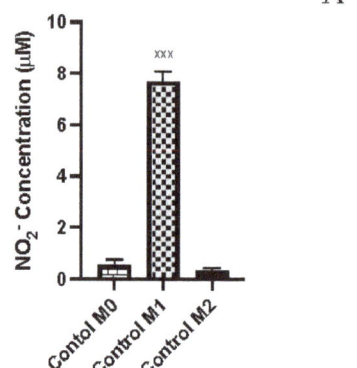
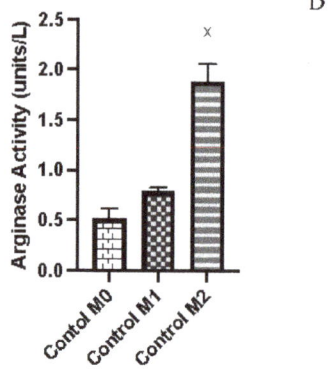
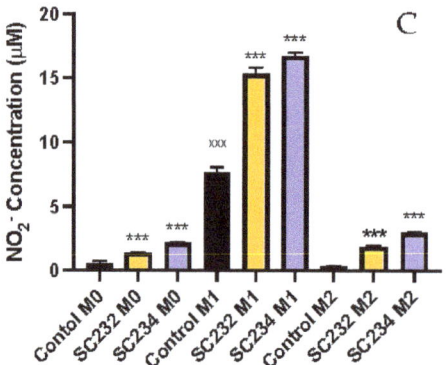
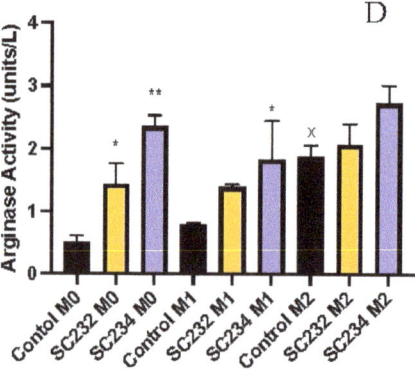

Figure 3. Exposure of M0, M1, and M2 BMDMs to 25 mg/mL fermentates affects production of NO production and arginase activity. BMDM cells were seeded at 5×10^5 cells/mL and incubated for 1 h at 37 °C in 5% CO_2. Cells were stimulated with 25 mg/mL fermentates and incubated for 3 h at 37 °C in 5% CO_2. The cells were either polarised to the M1 phenotype by stimulating with LPS (100 ng/mL) in the presence of 20 ng/mL rIFN-γ or towards M2 cells by adding 20 ng/mL rIL-4,

20 ng/mL IL-13, and 20 ng/mL rTGF-B and incubating for 24 h at 37 °C. Supernatants were removed after 24 h and Griess assay was performed as per manufacturer's instructions for determination of NO production (**A,C**). Cell lysates were prepared, and arginase assay carried out to determine arginase activity (**B,D**). Data are presented as mean ± SEM of three replicates. (**A,B**) represent the NO and arginase activity profiles for M0-, M1-, and M2-polarised cells, respectively. Significance determined using one-way ANOVA with a Newman–Keuls post-test. Output p value style APA: 0.12 nonsignificant (unlabelled), 0.033 somewhat significant (*), 0.002 significant (**), and <0.001 highly significant (***); where the following symbols represent; (1) comparing fermentates to polarised control cells "*" and (2) comparing M0 to M1 and M2 controls "x".

Figure 3B shows that M2 macrophages have high levels of arginase activity ($p < 0.033$), while M0 and M1 macrophages have much lower levels of arginase activity.

Figure 3C demonstrates that SC234 and SC232 significantly increased NO production in M0 ($p < 0.001$; $p < 0.001$), M1 ($p < 0.001$; $p < 0.001$), and M2 macrophages ($p < 0.001$; $p < 0.001$). However, it was the M1 BMDMs in the presence of SC234 and SC232 that produced the highest concentration of NO.

Figure 3D exhibits that SC234 and SC232 increased arginase activity in M0 ($p < 0.002$; $p < 0.033$). In M1 BMDMs, only SC234 increased arginase activity ($p < 0.033$), and in M2 BMDMs there was no significant effect.

3.3. Immune-Boosting Effects of Fermentates on Chemokine Secretion

Figure 4 exhibits that our novel fermentates significantly affected the secretion of chemokines in response to LOX and LPS in BMDMs. MCP ($p < 0.001$), MIP-1 ($p < 0.001$), and MIP-2 ($p < 0.001$) were increased in the presence of LOX relative to LOX control. MCP ($p < 0.001$) and MIP-2 ($p < 0.001$) were increased in the presence of LPS, with only a small increase seen in MIP-1 relative to LPS control.

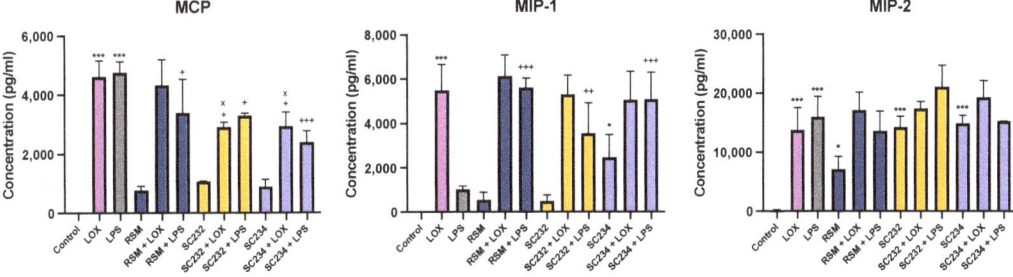

Figure 4. Exposure of LOX- and LPS-activated BMDMs to 25 mg/mL fermentates results in the secretion of chemokines. BMDM cells were seeded at 1×10^6 cells/mL and left overnight at 37 °C in 5% CO_2. The following day, cells were stimulated with 25 mg/mL raw sample fermentate, incubated for 1 h at 37 °C in 5% CO_2, and subsequently exposed to LOX 0.5 mM; LPS 100 ng/mL before incubating overnight under the same conditions. RSM was the fermentate control. Supernatants were removed after 24 h and ELISA was performed for MCP, MIP-1, and MIP-2. Data are presented as mean ± SEM of three replicates. Significance determined using one-way ANOVA with a Newman–Keuls post-test. Output p value style APA: 0.12 nonsignificant (unlabelled), 0.033 somewhat significant (*), 0.002 significant (**), and <0.001 highly significant (***); where the following symbols represent; (1) comparing control cells to LOX and LPS, and unstimulated samples"*", (2) comparing TLR to sample + TLR "+", and (3) comparing RSM +/− TLR to sample +/− TLR "x".

In the presence of LOX, SC234 and SC232 significantly decreased MCP ($p < 0.033$). Exposure of cells to SC234 in the presence of LPS resulted in an increase in MIP-1 ($p < 0.001$), but a decrease in MCP ($p < 0.001$), relative to LOX control. Similarly, SC232 in the presence of LPS resulted in an increase in MIP-1 ($p < 0.002$), but a decrease in MCP ($p < 0.033$), relative to LPS control. Interestingly, exposure of cells to SC234 alone, in the absence of either LOX or LPS stimulation, resulted in enhanced secretion of MIP-1 ($p < 0.033$) and

MIP-2 ($p < 0.001$) relative to control cells. Exposure of cells to SC232 alone, in the absence of either LOX or LPS stimulation, resulted in increased secretion of MIP-2 ($p < 0.001$), relative to control cells.

The RSM control itself did affect chemokine secretion in the presence of LPS with an increase in MIP-1 ($p < 0.001$), but decreased MCP ($p < 0.033$), relative to LPS control. Furthermore, RSM in the absence of TLR stimulation enhanced MIP-2 ($p < 0.033$) relative to the control cells.

Given that RSM itself had some effects, we also compared the fermentates to RSM. In the presence of LOX, SC234 and SC232 decreased MCP ($p < 0.033$).

3.4. Immune-Boosting Effects of Fermentates on Cell Surface Marker Expression

Figure 5 exhibits that fermentates significantly affected the expression of cell surface markers in response to LOX and LPS. LOX significantly increased the expression of CD86, CD14, CD40, TLR4, and CD80 ($p < 0.001$), and LPS significantly increased the expression of CD86, CD14, CD40, TLR4, CD80, and MHCI ($p < 0.001$).

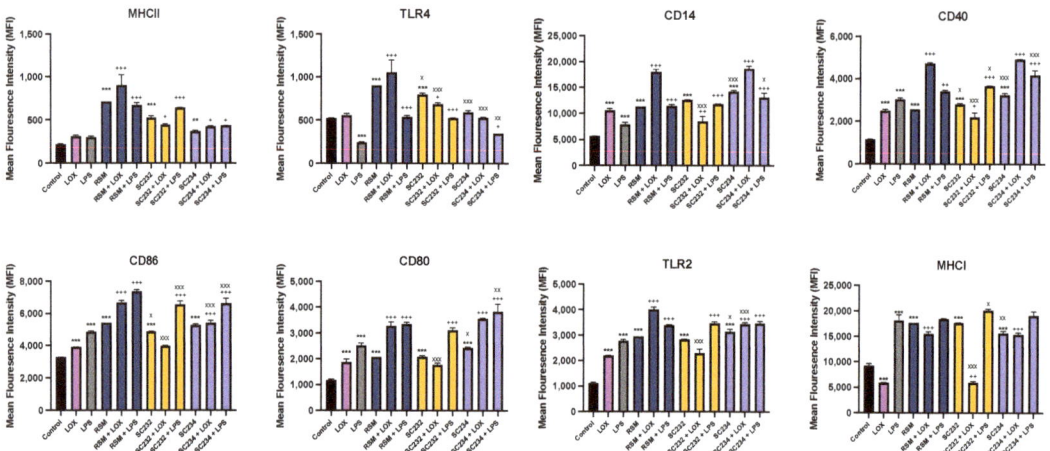

Figure 5. Exposure of LOX- and LPS-activated J774.A.1 to 25 mg/mL fermentates affect cell surface marker expression. J774.A.1 cells were seeded at 1×10^6 cells/mL and incubated overnight at 37 °C in 5% CO_2. After 24 h, cells were stimulated with 25 mg/mL fermentates and incubated for 1 h at 37 °C in 5% CO_2 before stimulating with LOX 0.5 mM or LPS 100 ng/mL. Cell suspensions were retained, and cell-staining protocol was carried out to assess the presence of cell surface markers MHCII, TLR4, CD86, CD80, CD14, CD40, TLR2, and MHCI in the presence of fermentate sample. Cells were analysed using a BD FACSAria 1 system flow cytometer, raw FCS files analysed, and data graphed using V10.0 FlowJo software. Data are presented as mean ± SEM of two replicates. Significance was determined using one-way ANOVA with a Newman–Keuls post-test. Output p value style APA: 0.12 nonsignificant (unlabelled), 0.033 somewhat significant (*), 0.002 significant (**), and <0.001 highly significant (***); where the following symbols represent; (1) comparing control cells to TLR controls and unstimulated samples "*", (2) comparing TLR controls to sample + TLR "+", and (3) comparing RSM +/− TLR to sample +/− TLR "x".

In the presence of LOX, SC234 further enhanced the expression of MHCII ($p < 0.033$), CD86 ($p < 0.001$), TLR2 ($p < 0.001$), MHCI ($p < 0.001$), CD14 ($p < 0.001$), CD40 ($p < 0.001$), and CD80 ($p < 0.001$). In the presence of LPS, SC234 further enhanced the expression of MHCII ($p < 0.033$), TLR4 ($p < 0.033$), CD86 ($p < 0.001$), TLR2 ($p < 0.001$), CD14 ($p < 0.001$), CD40 ($p < 0.001$), and CD80 ($p < 0.001$). In the absence of TLR, SC234 increased MHCII ($p < 0.002$), CD86 ($p < 0.001$), CD14 ($p < 0.001$), CD40 ($p < 0.001$), CD80 ($p < 0.001$), TLR2 ($p < 0.001$), and MHCI ($p < 0.001$).

In the presence of LOX, SC232 increased MHCII ($p < 0.033$) and TLR4 ($p < 0.033$) expression, but decreased CD14 ($p < 0.002$), CD40 ($p < 0.033$), and MHCI ($p < 0.002$) expression.

In the presence of LPS, R00352 further enhanced the expression of MHCII ($p < 0.001$), TLR4 ($p < 0.001$), CD14 ($p < 0.001$), CD86 ($p < 0.001$), CD80 ($p < 0.001$), TLR2 ($p < 0.001$), CD40 ($p < 0.001$), and MHCI ($p < 0.033$). In the absence of TLR, SC232 increased the expression of MHCII, CD14, CD80, TLR2, and MHCI ($p < 0.001$), and further enhanced TLR4, CD40, and CD86 ($p < 0.001$).

In the presence of LOX, RSM further enhanced the expression of MHCII ($p < 0.001$), TLR4 ($p < 0.001$), CD14 ($p < 0.001$), CD40 ($p < 0.001$), CD86 ($p < 0.001$), CD80 ($p < 0.001$), TLR2 ($p < 0.001$), and MHCI ($p < 0.001$). In the presence of LPS, RSM further enhanced the expression of MHCII ($p < 0.001$), TLR4 ($p < 0.001$), CD14 ($p < 0.001$), CD40 ($p < 0.002$), CD86 ($p < 0.001$), CD80 ($p < 0.001$), and TLR2 ($p < 0.001$). In the absence of TLR, RSM increased the expression of MHCII, TLR4, CD14, CD40, CD86, CD80, TLR2, and MHCI ($p < 0.001$).

Given that RSM itself had some effects, we also compared the fermentates to the RSM control. In the absence of TLR, SC234 decreased TLR4 and MHCI ($p < 0.001$; $p < 0.002$), but further increased CD14 ($p < 0.001$), CD40 ($p < 0.001$), CD80 ($p < 0.001$), and TLR2 ($p < 0.033$). In the absence of TLR, SC232 decreased TLR4 ($p < 0.033$) and CD86 ($p < 0.033$), but further increased CD40 ($p < 0.033$). In the presence of LOX, SC234 decreased TLR4, CD86, and TLR2 ($p < 0.001$). In the presence of LOX, SC232 decreased TLR4, CD14, CD40, CD86, CD80, TLR2, and MHCI ($p < 0.001$). In the presence of LPS, SC234 decreased TLR4 ($p < 0.002$) and CD86 ($p < 0.001$), but further increased CD40 ($p < 0.001$), CD80 ($p < 0.002$), and CD14 ($p < 0.033$). In the presence of LPS, SC232 decreased CD86 ($p < 0.001$), CD40 ($p < 0.033$), and MHCI ($p < 0.033$).

3.5. Stimulation of LOX and LPS Activated J774 with 25 mg/mL Fermentates Affect Phagocytosis

The procedure for phenotypic analysis of cell phagocytosis when stimulated with TLR ligands was carried out as previously described using 1 μm fluorescent FITC latex beads. MFI, percentage of phagocytosing cells, and MPI were measured.

3.5.1. MFI

Figure 6A–C demonstrate that stimulation of J774 cells with LOX and LPS significantly increased the MFI ($p < 0.033$; $p < 0.002$) and that the addition of SC234 or SC232 to LOX- and LPS-stimulated cells suppressed this increased MFI. SC234 and SC232 alone had no effect. Figure 6C demonstrates that the presence of RSM had a similar effect on LOX* and LPS-stimulated cells to SC234 and SC232 and RSM alone had no effect.

3.5.2. Percentage of Phagocytes

Figure 6D–F demonstrate that LOX and LPS increased the percentage of phagocytosing cells ($p < 0.002$; $p < 0.001$) which were suppressed by the presence of SC234 but not SC232. Interestingly, SC234 alone also increased the percentage of phagocytosing cells, and RSM alone or in the presence of LOX or LPS had no significant effect.

3.5.3. MPI

Figure 6G–I demonstrates that stimulation of J774 cells with LOX and LPS significantly increased the MPI ($p < 0.033$; $p < 0.001$) which was suppressed by the addition of SC234. However, SC234 alone enhanced the MPI. The addition of SC232 to LOX-stimulated cells also suppressed the increased MPI, in contrast to the maintained MPI in LPS-activated cells. SC232 alone had no effect and RSM had a similar effect on LOX- and LPS-stimulated cells to SC234.

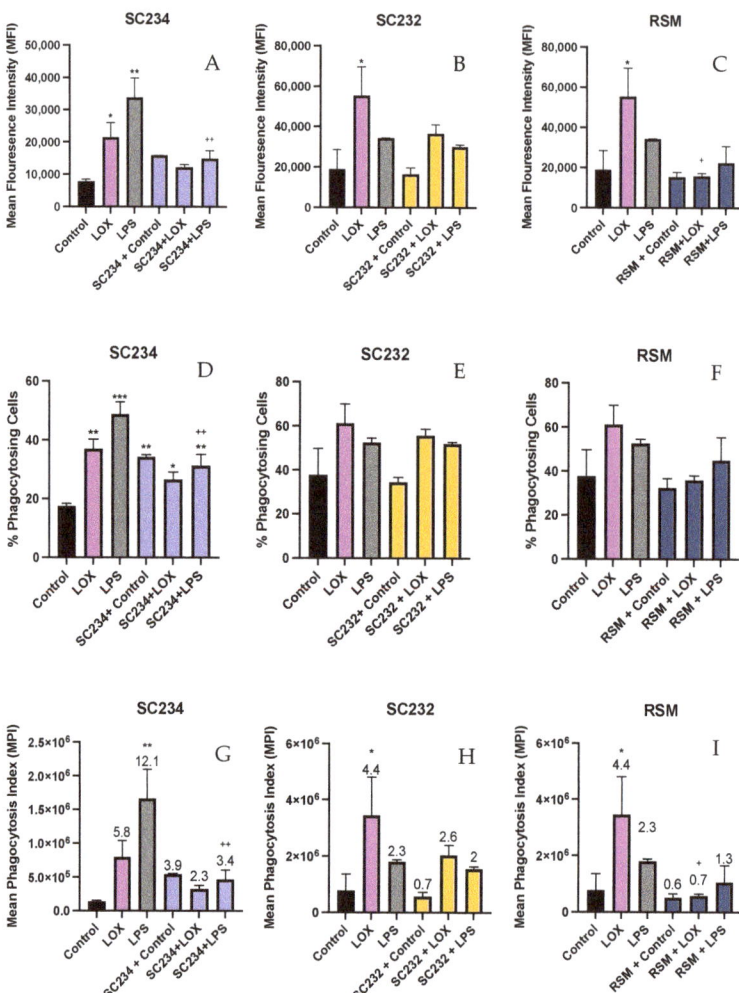

Figure 6. Exposure of LOX- and LPS-activated J774.A.1 to 25 mg/mL fermentates affects MFI, % phagocytosing cells, and MPI. J774.A.1. cells were seeded at 1×10^6 cells/mL and incubated overnight at 37 °C in 5% CO_2. The following day, cells were stimulated with 25 mg/mL fermentates for 1 h before activating with LPS 100 ng/mL and LOX 0.5 mM, and incubated for 4 h at 37 °C in 5% CO_2. Cell suspensions were retained, and cells were stimulated with 1 µm fluorescent latex beads at a concentration of 20 beads per cell for 1 h at 37 °C in 5% CO_2. Cells were analysed using a BD FACSAria 1 system flow cytometer, raw FCS files were analysed, and data graphed using V10.0 FlowJo software. Data are presented as mean ± SEM of two replicates. (**A**–**C**) represent MFI, (**D**–**F**) represent percentage of phagocytes, and (**G**–**I**) represent MPI. Significance determined using one-way ANOVA with a Newman–Keuls post-test. Output *p* value style APA0.12 nonsignificant (unlabelled), 0.033 somewhat significant (*), 0.002 significant (**), and <0.001 highly significant (***); where the following symbols represent; (1) comparing control cells to each test cell "*", (2) comparing each corresponding sample + TLR to TLR alone "+". MPI data analysed as a product of the percentage phagocytosing cells and MFI. Number indicated above bar is the MPI compared to the control cells, represented as 1.

4. Discussion

This study demonstrates the potential of the novel fermentates, SC232 and SC234, in modulating key macrophage functions, which are central to the protection and clearance of viral infections. Macrophages act as scavengers, enabled by the presence of pattern recognition receptors, to alert the immune system through chemokine and cytokine secretion and antigen presentation, and to engulf and destroy invading pathogens via phagocytosis [6]. Macrophages play a critical role in both innate and viral immunity and so are an important cell to target to enhance their capabilities.

Initially, preliminary studies carried out by the laboratory on a large panel of fermentates used a dose range of 5 mg/mL, 10 mg/mL, 25 mg/mL, and 50 mg/mL fermentates to reveal 25 mg/mL as the optimal dose for fermentate bioactivity, and thus this dose of 25 mg/mL was used for such further in-depth analysis. Following confirmation that the fermentates and the starting substrate, RSM, did not affect cell viability, we demonstrated that cytokine secretion in J774.A.1 and BMDM macrophages are positively affected by the presence of SC232 and SC234 when compared to the effects of the RSM. Furthermore, these effects differ depending on the mode of activation of the cell. J774.A.1 and BMDM cells, when activated with LOX and LPS in the presence of SC232 and SC234, showed enhanced levels of secretion of IL-1β, IL-6, IL-27, and IL-10. BMDM cells, when activated with LOX and LPS in the presence of SC232 and SC234, showed enhanced levels of secretion of IL-12p40 and IL-27 following LOX exposure, but decreased IL-12p40 and IL-27 secretion following LPS exposure. This suggests that they may have specific effects on the immune system in the presence of a viral ligand.

In polarised BMDMs, SC232 and SC234 show a similar profile of activity. M0- and M1-polarised BMDMs in the presence of SC232 and SC234 secreted high levels of IL-6 and TNF-α, and M0-, M1-, and M2-polarised BMDMs in the presence of SC232 and SC234 secrete high levels of IL-10.

Given the importance of IL-6, TNF-α, IL-12p40, and IL-27 in aiding the immune system during viral infections such as influenza, vaccinia virus, HIV, and herpes simplex [7–13] and supporting viral immunity, a fermentate that can enhance these cytokines could be beneficial. In response to a viral activation, the novel fermentates SC234 and SC232 can enhance not only IL-6, IL-12p40, and IL-27 in BMDMs, but also support IL-6 and TNF-α secretion in polarised BMDMs; thus, they have potential to support viral immunity. These effects are not the same in the presence of LPS with decreased IL-12p40 and IL-27, and so the unique bioactivity we see in the fermentates' ability to enhance cytokine response to viral ligands further supports their possible specificity in enhancing viral immunity.

Similarly, this anti-viral profile is seen in other classic markers of M1 and M2 macrophage, NO production, and arginase activity. M0, M1, and M2 BMDMs in the presence of SC232 and SC234 produce high levels of NO. M0 and M1 BMDMs in the presence of SC232 and SC234 promoted low levels of arginase activity. This emphasises the largely pro-inflammatory M1 profile of SC232 and SC234. The effect on NO production is of particular interest given that NO production is necessary for viral clearance via inducible NO synthase (iNOS), and depending on the virus can have direct antiviral properties, limiting the severity of virus-induced disease [14,15]. NO production is linked to the M1 killing/fighting phenotype, whereby arginine is metabolised via iNOS to NO and citrulline to aid M1 macrophages in the production of Th1 responses for fighting infection, and aiding in the drive and recruitment of pro-inflammatory cytokines useful for the defence of the immune system against viruses [16,17].

It has previously been demonstrated that an isolated acidic polysaccharide from the fungus *Cordyceps militaris* enhanced mRNA expression of IL-1β, IL-6, IL-10, and TNF-α, increased NO production, and induced iNOS mRNA and protein expression in RAW 264.7 macrophage cells, as well as increasing TNF-α and IFN-γ in mice, to decrease virus titres in the bronchoalveolar lavage fluid and the lungs of mice infected with influenza A virus to increase survival rate [18]. Similarly, a study involving *Lactobacillus helveticus* has showed a trending decrease in influenza-like illness in an elderly population, suggesting it could elicit a similar effect [19]. Another study showed that germinated *Rhynchosia nulubilis* fermented with *Pediococcus pentosaceus* SC11 has immune-enhancing and anti-viral effects, inhibiting 3CL protease activity in SARS-CoV in immunocompromised mice, increased T lymphocyte production and splenocyte proliferation, increased phagocytic activity, NO production via induction of iNOS, mRNA expression of IFN-γ, IFN-α, and ISG15 in RAW 264.7 macrophages, and subsequent increase in the expression of TNF-α [20], suggesting the role of GRC-SC11 in immunosuppressed patients for support against SARS-CoV. Similarly, *Grifola frondosa* extract can induce the expression of TNF-α mRNA in Madin–Darby canine kidney cells leading to the production of TNF-α, with subsequent inhibition of viral growth of influenza A/Aichi/2/68 virus [21]. TNF-α possesses anti-viral activity through its synergy with IFNs to induce resistance to DNA and RNA of viruses in diverse cell types, selectively killing the virus, necessary for the initiation and continuation of inflammation and immunity, adhesion molecule expression, and recruitment of leukocytes [22,23]. Other studies by Takeda et al. showed that LAB, in particular the strain *Lactiplantibacillus plantarum* 06CC2 from cow cheese, increased the production of IL-12 and IL-12p40 in vitro and in vivo [24]. *Lactiplantibacillus plantarum* 06CC2 has been associated with the enhancement of the Th1 response, and resulted in the alleviation of influenza virus infection in mice [25]. *Rapanea melanophloeos* has been shown to increase IL-27 production, ultimately increasing IL-10 production, to decrease the viral titre of influenza A virus in MDCK cells, suggesting its role as an anti-influenza treatment [26]. IL-27 activates and promotes the production of IFNs which are associated with various antiviral activities, support plasmacytoid DCs to sense viral DNA and RNA, promote macrophage differentiation and polarisation, increase TLR expression, and promote IL-10 cytokine production [7]. Therefore, not only is IL-27 important in viral immunity but IL-27 leads to subsequent enhanced IL-10 production for viral clearance, and thus where IL-27 is increased, IL-10 will often reflect this. IL-10 is a CD4-produced Th2 cytokine with the ability to indirectly suppress Th1 responses, downregulate the antigen-presenting capacities of APC, inhibit the activation and effector function of T cells, monocytes, and macrophages, therefore limiting host immune response to invading pathogens and ultimately preventing damage to the host from overactivation of the pro-inflammatory molecules, and provides a supportive role in effective virus clearance [27–30]. Additionally, in work carried out in our laboratory, we have further demonstrated the positive impact that fermentates SC232 and SC234 had on viral immunity [31]. SC232 and SC234 positively impacted on the secretion of the cytokines IL-6, TNF-α, IL-12p40, IL-23, IL-27, and IL-10, and decreased IL-1β in primary bone marrow-derived dendritic cells (BMDCs) stimulated with a viral ligand, thus further establishing their role as viral immune-boosting fermentates with positive effects in a range of immune cells [31].

Having established SC234 and SC232 as potential anti-viral fermentates that enhance viral immunity through their increased secretion of cytokines important for viral immune responses, we then extended our analysis to chemokines which are critical in supporting the immune system in response to viral infection and host protection. We demonstrate that chemokine secretion in BMDM macrophages is positively affected by the presence of SC232 and SC234 when compared to the activity of the RSM. Chemokines are critical in order to mediate macrophage chemotaxis, cell trafficking, and in the regulation of M1 and M2, and regulate differentiation of monocytes into dendritic cells (DCs), to attract macrophage towards the site of injury or infection [32–34]. MCP-1 (CCL2) is a key chemokine for the regulation of migration and infiltration of monocytes, playing a critical role in inflammation [33,35]. MIP-1 α (CCL3), on the other hand, plays a key role in viral immunity, being a chemotactic chemokine secreted by macrophages to aid in the recruitment of cells, wound healing, inhibition of stem cells, and maintaining of effector immune responses, and is a key mediator of virus-induced inflammation [36,37]. Similarly, MIP-2 (CXCL2) plays a role in viral immunity, aiding in neutrophil recruitment and activation, and is a potent chemoattractant secreted by macrophage and epithelial cells that plays a critical role in LPS-induced inflammation, as well as aiding in suppressing of viral replication [38–40]. Therefore, while MCP is important for inflammation, it is MIP-1 and MIP-2 that play critical roles in the context of viral infection, with roles in virus-induced inflammation and suppressing viral replication [33,36–40]. It is important, however, that these chemokines are not overexpressed, as this leads to pathogenesis of many inflammatory diseases including cancers and rheumatoid arthritis, and viruses such as coronavirus [34,36].

BMDMs, when activated with LOX in the presence of SC232 and SC234, decrease MCP. LOX-activated BMDMs in the presence of RSM, SC232, and SC234 maintain MIP-1 and MIP-2 concentrations. MCP, MIP-1, and MIP-2 are all enhanced in the presence of the fermentates alone. This again highlights the potential for SC232 and SC234 to be anti-viral, as they maintain concentrations of the viral-associated chemokines MIP-1 and MIP-2 and decrease MCP, which is often associated with pathogenesis of viral infections [34,36].

It is well established that decreases in MCP can be linked with the ability to inhibit viruses such as HIV [41]. The use of the Chinese herbal medicine Shikonin, from the dried root of *Lithospermum erythrorhizon*, has been linked to the ability to inhibit HIV-1 through its interactions inhibiting MCP and MIP-1 [41]. Lianhuaqingwen capsules from the traditional Chinese medicine prescriptions Maxing Shigan Tang and Yinqiao San decreased the expression of MCP-1, resulting in anti-viral activity for the treatment of influenza viral infection [42]. The similar activities of SC234 and SC232 on chemokines may highlight their anti-viral potential.

Next, we went on to assess the effect of the fermentates SC234 and SC232 on cell surface marker expression in J774.A.1. These cell surface proteins play a critical role in host immunity by enabling the cell to respond and interact with the environment around them, thus playing a critical role in intracellular signalling [43]. Therefore, enhancing any of these cells' surface markers would suggest further anti-viral activity for SC234 and SC232.

J774.A.1 cells, when activated with LOX or LPS in the presence of SC234 and SC232, positively impact cell surface marker expression. LOX- and LPS-activated J774.A.1 in the presence of SC234 showed increases in CD80, CD86, CD40, MHCII, TLR2, and CD14. LOX-activated J774.A.1 in the presence of SC234 also showed increased MHCI, highlighting the specificity in bioactivity whereby SC234 has unique specificity in increasing the viral-associated cell surface marker MHCI, not seen in LPS-activated cells. LOX- and LPS-activated J774.A.1 in the presence of SC232 increase MHCII and TLR4. LOX-activated J774.A.1 cells in the presence of SC232 decrease CD14, CD40, and MHCI. Our results clearly demonstrate different effects on cells depending on either Lox or LPS activation.

MHCI plays a particularly important role in viral immunity for the detection of virally infected cytotoxic T lymphocytes [44]. CD80 and CD86 interact on APC and CD28 on T cells as costimulatory signals for the activation of T cells, are key players in anti-viral humoral and cellular immune responses, and play a critical role in the control of chronic and latent infections [45]. CD40 in particular is important for the restriction of infection of a broad range of RNA viruses and is critical for the control of RNA viruses over the first 24 h of infection [46].

Furthermore, TLR2 has been identified to play a role in viral immunity with protective roles against viruses such as varicella zoster virus, hepatitis C virus, vaccinia virus, cytomegalovirus, and respiratory syncytial virus [47].

Exopolysaccharides (EPS) from Cordyceps sinensis induces the expression of MHCII, CD40, CD80, and CD86 in DC sarcoma cells, enhances their ability of antigen uptake, and increases the secretion of IL-12 and TNF-α, thus suggesting that EPS have a critical role in initiating anti-tumour immunity and pro-inflammatory immune modulation [48]. Carrot pomace has also been found to increase the expression of co-stimulatory molecules CD40 and CD80, and the fraction of cells CD11c+MHCII+ cells in BMDCs increase pro-inflammatory cytokine production; in cyclophosphamide-immunosuppressed mice administered with influenza vaccine challenge, it significantly enhanced the efficacy of the influenza vaccine [49]. Resveratrol has been shown to enhance antigen presentation of peritoneal macrophages via the upregulation of CD86, MHCII, and TLR4 levels, suggesting its role as a pseudorabies virus vaccine-adjuvant therapy, aiding in the host protection against viral infection [50]. The similar effects of our fermentates on key cell surface markers involved in viral immunity further support their potential as anti-viral ingredients.

Having assessed and confirmed the immuno-supportive roles of SC234 and SC232 as immune-boosting compounds for defence against viral infection, we also assessed the effects of these novel fermentates on phagocytosis. Phagocytosis is another critical function of the macrophage in the defence against viral infection. In setting up the model for phagocytosis, the MFI of the latex beads and the percentage of phagocytosing cells within the population were measured. These two parameters were then combined in order to form the overall mean MPI, the combined effect of the MFI and percentage of phagocytosing cells, for a collective outlook of sample effect on phagocytosis.

In contrast to the viral immune-supportive roles identified for SC234 and SC232 so far, these fermentates negatively impact on the MPI. There is a small decrease in the MPI, meaning that the macrophage's ability to phagocytose is negatively impacted in the presence of SC234 and SC232. This negative impact on phagocytosis is something to consider if these novel fermentates are to be considered for commercial development. However, it must be noted that the MPI for SC234 and R003 is enhanced in comparison to the RSM. This means that in comparison to the fermentate starting substrate, these novel fermentates in fact increase the ability of the macrophage to phagocytose. Phagocytosis is closely associated with bacterial and fungal clearance [51]. This critical role of phagocytosis in bacterial and fungal clearance highlights the importance of phagocytosis in the context of bacterial and fungal infections as opposed to viral infections, thus suggesting that in the context of viral immunity the role of phagocytosis may not be deemed as important as in the context of bacterial or fungal infection. Therefore, the decrease seen in the MPI as a result of the presence of fermentates SC234 and SC232 may still support the role of such novel fermentates in the context of viral immunity, as they provide an increase in MPI above the RSM non-fermented control.

It is clear from the literature that increases in phagocytotic activity through the use of functional foods can be linked with enhanced immunity. When RAW 264.7 murine macrophages are treated with wild simulated ginseng, increased phagocytotic activity is observed [52]. Panax ginseng Meyer, when administered to BALB/c mice, enhanced innate and adaptive immunity via the improved cell-mediated and humoral immunity, macrophage phagocytosis capacity, and NK cell activity [53]. In that study, He et al. hypothesised that the increased immunomodulating activity was due to the increased macrophage phagocytosis capacity, along with increased NK cell activity, enhancement of T and Th cells, as well as IL-2, IL-6, and IL-12 secretion and IgA, IgG1, and IgG2b production [53]. Fermenting *C. militaris* with *Pediococcus pentosaceus* ON89A (GRC-ON89A) can enhance phagocytosis in RAW 264.7 cells and primary peritoneal macrophages from normal mice and cyclophosphamide-immunosuppressed mice via the activation of MAPK and Lyn pathways [54]. It is suggested that GRC-ON89A has the potential to act as an immunostimulant for use as an immune-boosting therapy in immunosuppressed patients [54]. Whilst our findings demonstrate that SC234 and SC232 could impact positively on viral immune response, this study assessed this in comparison to any activity the RSM would have alone. This was in order to assess any advantage the fermentation of the RSM had in terms of bioactivity. A further comparison to other types of non-fermented substances will provide more information on how potent these fermentates are in supporting viral immunity.

5. Conclusions

As demonstrated from the current literature available on similar functional foods, we suggest a role for fermentates SC232 and SC234 as potential novel food ingredients for defence against viral infection in humans due to their overall positive effect on systemic immune responses. This is due to their ability to support the secretion of pro-inflammatory cytokines IL-1β, IL-6, TNF-α, IL-12p40, and IL-27 while increasing the anti-inflammatory cytokine IL-10 to maintain immune homeostasis, as well as via their NO induction to support the proliferation of the M1 pro-inflammatory phenotype for viral immunity. Overall, the samples' ability to largely maintain chemokine expression, and in the case of MCP where this expression can be decreased, suggests a potential use of SC232 and SC234 as novel anti-viral and immune-supporting therapies. It is clear that increasing cell surface marker expression has a range of positive effects on a cell that can aid in adjuvant vaccine therapy, anti-tumour therapy, and immune-stimulating properties for overall immune boosting results for its host. Furthermore, functional food components which have the ability to enhance phagocytosis, like SC234 and SC232, above that of their starting substrate may have the potential to aid in boosting the immune system to provide enhanced innate and adaptive immunity, acting as potential immune-boosting therapies. However, it is important to consider the rate to which the overall phagocytosis is affected before consideration for commercial use to ensure the host is not negatively impacted. Therefore, we suggest the deeply impactful potential that our novel fermentates SC234 and SC232 have for defence against viral infection in humans.

Author Contributions: D.F. designed all the experiments, conducted the bioassays reported herein, analysed the data, and wrote the initial draft of the manuscript. M.A.M. generated the dairy fermentates used for the bioassays and edited and revised the manuscript. J.A.F. edited and revised the manuscript. T.B. edited and revised the manuscript. H.M. generated the dairy fermentates used for the bioassays and edited and revised the manuscript. P.D.C. edited and revised the manuscript. C.L. acquired funding for the work, supervised the project, and edited and revised the manuscript. All authors have read and agreed to the published version of the manuscript.

Funding: This work was funded and supported by Food for Health Ireland (FHI) and Enterprise Ireland (Grant #: TC20180025).

Institutional Review Board Statement: The care, treatment, and experiments involved in this study were approved by the Research Ethics Committee (REC) of Dublin City University (Approval ID: DCUREC/2023/187), granted the 13 September 2023.

Informed Consent Statement: Not applicable.

Data Availability Statement: The raw data supporting the conclusions of this article will be made available by the authors on request.

Acknowledgments: The authors would like to thank Lallemand Health Solutions for supplying the strains used in this study to generate the dairy fermentates.

Conflicts of Interest: Authors Monica A. Mechoud, Tom Beresford, Harsh Mathur, Paul D. Cotter were employed by the company Teagasc. The remaining authors declare that the research was conducted in the absence of any commercial or financial relationships that could be construed as a potential conflict of interest.

References

1. Mathur, H.; Beresford, T.P.; Cotter, P.D. Health Benefits of Lactic Acid Bacteria (LAB) Fermentates. *Nutrients* **2020**, *12*, 1679. [CrossRef] [PubMed]
2. Pessione, E. Lactic Acid Bacteria Contribution to Gut Microbiota Complexity: Lights and Shadows. *Front. Cell. Infect. Microbiol.* **2012**, *2*, 86. [CrossRef] [PubMed]
3. Granier, A.; Goulet, O.; Hoarau, C. Fermentation Products: Immunological Effects on Human and Animal Models. *Pediatr. Res.* **2013**, *74*, 238–244. [CrossRef] [PubMed]
4. García-Burgos, M.; Moreno-Fernández, J.; Alférez, M.J.; Díaz-Castro, J.; López-Aliaga, I. New Perspectives in Fermented Dairy Products and Their Health Relevance. *J. Funct. Foods* **2020**, *72*, 104059. [CrossRef]
5. Finnegan, D.; Tocmo, R.; Loscher, C. Targeted Application of Functional Foods as Immune Fitness Boosters in the Defense against Viral Infection. *Nutrients* **2023**, *15*, 3371. [CrossRef] [PubMed]
6. Atmeh, P.A.; Mezouar, S.; Mège, J.-L.; Atmeh, P.A.; Mezouar, S.; Mège, J.-L. *Macrophage Polarization in Viral Infectious Diseases: Confrontation with the Reality*; IntechOpen: London, UK, 2022; ISBN 978-1-80355-625-3.
7. Amsden, H.; Kourko, O.; Roth, M.; Gee, K. Antiviral Activities of Interleukin-27: A Partner for Interferons? *Front. Immunol.* **2022**, *13*, 902853. [CrossRef]
8. Hamza, T.; Barnett, J.B.; Li, B. Interleukin 12 a Key Immunoregulatory Cytokine in Infection Applications. *Int. J. Mol. Sci.* **2010**, *11*, 789–806. [CrossRef]

9. Kim, S.Y.; Solomon, D.H. Tumor Necrosis Factor Blockade and the Risk of Viral Infection. *Nat. Rev. Rheumatol.* **2010**, *6*, 165–174. [CrossRef] [PubMed]
10. Novelli, F.; Casanova, J.-L. The Role of IL-12, IL-23 and IFN-γ in Immunity to Viruses. *Cytokine Growth Factor Rev.* **2004**, *15*, 367–377. [CrossRef]
11. Seo, S.H.; Webster, R.G. Tumor Necrosis Factor Alpha Exerts Powerful Anti-Influenza Virus Effects in Lung Epithelial Cells. *J. Virol.* **2002**, *76*, 1071–1076. [CrossRef]
12. Velazquez-Salinas, L.; Verdugo-Rodriguez, A.; Rodriguez, L.L.; Borca, M.V. The Role of Interleukin 6 During Viral Infections. *Front. Microbiol.* **2019**, *10*, 445678. [CrossRef] [PubMed]
13. Wang, Y.; Chaudhri, G.; Jackson, R.J.; Karupiah, G. IL-12p40 and IL-18 Play Pivotal Roles in Orchestrating the Cell-Mediated Immune Response to a Poxvirus Infection1. *J. Immunol.* **2009**, *183*, 3324–3331. [CrossRef] [PubMed]
14. Sodano, F.; Gazzano, E.; Fruttero, R.; Lazzarato, L. NO in Viral Infections: Role and Development of Antiviral Therapies. *Molecules* **2022**, *27*, 2337. [CrossRef] [PubMed]
15. Burrack, K.S.; Morrison, T.E. The Role of Myeloid Cell Activation and Arginine Metabolism in the Pathogenesis of Virus-Induced Diseases. *Front. Immunol.* **2014**, *5*, 428. [CrossRef] [PubMed]
16. Mills, C. M1 and M2 Macrophages: Oracles of Health and Disease. *Crit. Rev.™ Immunol.* **2012**, *32*, 463–488. [CrossRef] [PubMed]
17. Rath, M.; Müller, I.; Kropf, P.; Closs, E.I.; Munder, M. Metabolism via Arginase or Nitric Oxide Synthase: Two Competing Arginine Pathways in Macrophages. *Front. Immunol.* **2014**, *5*, 532. [CrossRef] [PubMed]
18. Ohta, Y.; Lee, J.-B.; Hayashi, K.; Fujita, A.; Park, D.K.; Hayashi, T. In Vivo Anti-Influenza Virus Activity of an Immunomodulatory Acidic Polysaccharide Isolated from Cordyceps Militaris Grown on Germinated Soybeans. *J. Agric. Food Chem.* **2007**, *55*, 10194–10199. [CrossRef] [PubMed]
19. Koesnoe, S.; Masjkuri, N.; Adisasmita, A.; Djauzi, S.; Kartasasmita, C.; Sundoro, J.; Nadjib, M.; Korib, M.; Muthia, A.N.; Muzellina, V.N.; et al. A Randomized Controlled Trial to Evaluate the Effect of Influenza Vaccination and Probiotic Supplementation on Immune Response and Incidence of Influenza-like Illness in an Elderly Population in Indonesia. *PLoS ONE* **2021**, *16*, e0250234. [CrossRef] [PubMed]
20. Dhong, K.-R.; Kwon, H.-K.; Park, H.-J. Immunostimulatory Activity of Cordyceps Militaris Fermented with Pediococcus Pentosaceus SC11 Isolated from a Salted Small Octopus in Cyclophosphamide-Induced Immunocompromised Mice and Its Inhibitory Activity against SARS-CoV 3CL Protease. *Microorganisms* **2022**, *10*, 2321. [CrossRef]
21. Obi, N.; Hayashi, K.; Miyahara, T.; Shimada, Y.; Terasawa, K.; Watanabe, M.; Takeyama, M.; Obi, R.; Ochiai, H. Inhibitory Effect of TNF-α Produced by Macrophages Stimulated with Grifola Frondosa Extract (ME) on the Growth of Influenza A/Aichi/2/68 Virus in MDCK Cells. *Am. J. Chin. Med.* **2008**, *36*, 1171–1183. [CrossRef]
22. Wong, G.H.W.; Goeddel, D.V. Tumour Necrosis Factors α and β Inhibit Virus Replication and Synergize with Interferons. *Nature* **1986**, *323*, 819–822. [CrossRef]
23. Wada, H.; Saito, K.; Kanda, T.; Kobayashi, I.; Fujii, H.; Fujigaki, S.; Maekawa, N.; Takatsu, H.; Fujiwara, H.; Sekikawa, K.; et al. Tumor Necrosis Factor-α (TNF-α) Plays a Protective Role in Acute Viral Myocarditis in Mice. *Circulation* **2001**, *103*, 743–749. [CrossRef] [PubMed]
24. Takeda, S.; Kawahara, S.; Hidaka, M.; Yoshida, H.; Watanabe, W.; Takeshita, M.; Kikuchi, Y.; Bumbein, D.; Muguruma, M.; Kurokawa, M. Effects of Oral Administration of Probiotics from Mongolian Dairy Products on the Th1 Immune Response in Mice. *Biosci. Biotechnol. Biochem.* **2013**, *77*, 1372–1378. [CrossRef]
25. Takeda, S.; Takeshita, M.; Kikuchi, Y.; Dashnyam, B.; Kawahara, S.; Yoshida, H.; Watanabe, W.; Muguruma, M.; Kurokawa, M. Efficacy of Oral Administration of Heat-Killed Probiotics from Mongolian Dairy Products against Influenza Infection in Mice: Alleviation of Influenza Infection by Its Immunomodulatory Activity through Intestinal Immunity. *Int. Immunopharmacol.* **2011**, *11*, 1976–1983. [CrossRef]
26. Mehrbod, P.; Abdalla, M.A.; Fotouhi, F.; Heidarzadeh, M.; Aro, A.O.; Eloff, J.N.; McGaw, L.J.; Fasina, F.O. Immunomodulatory Properties of Quercetin-3-O-α-L-Rhamnopyranoside from Rapanea Melanophloeos against Influenza a Virus. *BMC Complement. Altern. Med.* **2018**, *18*, 184. [CrossRef]
27. Wilson, E.B.; Brooks, D.G. The Role of IL-10 in Regulating Immunity to Persistent Viral Infections. *Curr. Top. Microbiol. Immunol.* **2011**, *350*, 39–65. [CrossRef] [PubMed]
28. Rojas, J.M.; Avia, M.; Martín, V.; Sevilla, N. IL-10: A Multifunctional Cytokine in Viral Infections. *J. Immunol. Res.* **2017**, *2017*, 6104054. [CrossRef]
29. Moore, K.W.; de Waal Malefyt, R.; Coffman, R.L.; O'Garra, A. Interleukin-10 and the Interleukin-10 Receptor. *Annu. Rev. Immunol.* **2001**, *19*, 683–765. [CrossRef] [PubMed]
30. Iyer, S.S.; Cheng, G. Role of Interleukin 10 Transcriptional Regulation in Inflammation and Autoimmune Disease. *Crit. Rev. Immunol.* **2012**, *32*, 23–63. [CrossRef]
31. Finnegan, D.; Mechoud, M.A.; Connolly, C.; FitzGerald, J.A.; Beresford, T.; Mathur, H.; Brennan, L.; Cotter, P.D.; Loscher, C. Novel Dairy Fermentates Have Differential Effects on Key Immune Responses Associated with Viral Immunity and Inflammation. *Preprints* **2024**, 2024040455. [CrossRef]
32. Xuan, W.; Qu, Q.; Zheng, B.; Xiong, S.; Fan, G.-H. The Chemotaxis of M1 and M2 Macrophages Is Regulated by Different Chemokines. *J. Leukoc. Biol.* **2015**, *97*, 61–69. [CrossRef]

33. Deshmane, S.L.; Kremlev, S.; Amini, S.; Sawaya, B.E. Monocyte Chemoattractant Protein-1 (MCP-1): An Overview. *J. Interferon Cytokine Res.* **2009**, *29*, 313–326. [CrossRef]
34. Singh, S.; Anshita, D.; Ravichandiran, V. MCP-1: Function, Regulation, and Involvement in Disease. *Int. Immunopharmacol.* **2021**, *101*, 107598. [CrossRef]
35. MacPherson, C.W.; Shastri, P.; Mathieu, O.; Tompkins, T.A.; Burguière, P. Genome-Wide Immune Modulation of TLR3-Mediated Inflammation in Intestinal Epithelial Cells Differs between Single and Multi-Strain Probiotic Combination. *PLoS ONE* **2017**, *12*, e0169847. [CrossRef]
36. Bhavsar, I.; Miller, C.S.; Al-Sabbagh, M. Macrophage Inflammatory Protein-1 Alpha (MIP-1 Alpha)/CCL3: As a BiomarkerMIP-1α/CCL3. In *General Methods in Biomarker Research and Their Applications*; Preedy, V.R., Patel, V.B., Eds.; Springer: Dordrecht, The Netherlands, 2014; pp. 1–22. ISBN 978-94-007-7740-8.
37. Cook, D.N.; Beck, M.A.; Coffman, T.M.; Kirby, S.L.; Sheridan, J.F.; Pragnell, L.B.; Smithies, O. Requirement of Mip-1α for an Inflammatory Response to Viral Infection. *Science* **1995**, *269*, 1583–1585. [CrossRef]
38. Han, X.-B.; Liu, X.; Hsueh, W.; De Plaen, I.G. Macrophage Inflammatory Protein-2 Mediates the Bowel Injury Induced by Platelet-Activating Factor. *Am. J. Physiol.-Gastrointest. Liver Physiol.* **2004**, *287*, G1220–G1226. [CrossRef]
39. Chaochao, Q.; Lou, G.; Yang, Y.; Liu, Y.; Hu, Y.; Min, Z.; Chen, P.; He, J.; Chen, Z. Macrophage Inflammatory Protein-2 in High Mobility Group Box 1 Secretion of Macrophage Cells Exposed to Lipopolysaccharide. *Cell. Physiol. Biochem.* **2017**, *42*, 913–928. [CrossRef]
40. Tumpey, T.M.; Fenton, R.; Molesworth-Kenyon, S.; Oakes, J.E.; Lausch, R.N. Role for Macrophage Inflammatory Protein 2 (MIP-2), MIP-1α, and Interleukin-1α in the Delayed-Type Hypersensitivity Response to Viral Antigen. *J. Virol.* **2002**, *76*, 8050–8057. [CrossRef]
41. Chen, X.; Yang, L.; Zhang, N.; Turpin, J.A.; Buckheit, R.W.; Osterling, C.; Oppenheim, J.J.; Howard, O.M.Z. Shikonin, a Component of Chinese Herbal Medicine, Inhibits Chemokine Receptor Function and Suppresses Human Immunodeficiency Virus Type 1. *Antimicrob. Agents Chemother.* **2003**, *47*, 2810–2816. [CrossRef]
42. Ding, Y.; Zeng, L.; Li, R.; Chen, Q.; Zhou, B.; Chen, Q.; Cheng, P.L.; Yutao, W.; Zheng, J.; Yang, Z.; et al. The Chinese Prescription Lianhuaqingwen Capsule Exerts Anti-Influenza Activity through the Inhibition of Viral Propagation and Impacts Immune Function. *BMC Complement. Altern. Med.* **2017**, *17*, 130. [CrossRef]
43. Bradley, Z. Technologies for Measuring Cell Surface Markers. *Cofactor Genom.* **2020**. Available online: https://cofactorgenomics.com/wk-9-2020-cell-surface-markers/ (accessed on 16 April 2024).
44. Askew, D.; Chu, R.S.; Krieg, A.M.; Harding, C.V. CpG DNA Induces Maturation of Dendritic Cells with Distinct Effects on Nascent and Recycling MHC-II Antigen-Processing Mechanisms. *J. Immunol.* **2000**, *165*, 6889–6895. [CrossRef]
45. Fuse, S.; Obar, J.J.; Bellfy, S.; Leung, E.K.; Zhang, W.; Usherwood, E.J. CD80 and CD86 Control Antiviral CD8+ T-Cell Function and Immune Surveillance of Murine Gammaherpesvirus 68. *J. Virol.* **2006**, *80*, 9159–9170. [CrossRef]
46. Rogers, K.J.; Shtanko, O.; Stunz, L.L.; Mallinger, L.N.; Arkee, T.; Schmidt, M.E.; Bohan, D.; Brunton, B.; White, J.M.; Varga, S.M.; et al. Frontline Science: CD40 Signaling Restricts RNA Virus Replication in Mϕs, Leading to Rapid Innate Immune Control of Acute Virus Infection. *J. Leukoc. Biol.* **2021**, *109*, 309–325. [CrossRef]
47. de Oliviera Nascimento, L.; Massari, P.; Wetzler, L. The Role of TLR2 in Infection and Immunity. *Front. Immunol.* **2012**, *3*, 79. [CrossRef]
48. Song, D.; He, Z.; Wang, C.; Yuan, F.; Dong, P.; Zhang, W. Regulation of the Exopolysaccharide from an Anamorph of Cordyceps Sinensis on Dendritic Cell Sarcoma (DCS) Cell Line. *Eur. J. Nutr.* **2013**, *52*, 687–694. [CrossRef]
49. Sun, P.; Kim, Y.; Lee, H.; Kim, J.; Han, B.K.; Go, E.; Kwon, S.; Kang, J.-G.; You, S.; Kwon, J. Carrot Pomace Polysaccharide (CPP) Improves Influenza Vaccine Efficacy in Immunosuppressed Mice via Dendritic Cell Activation. *Nutrients* **2020**, *12*, 2740. [CrossRef]
50. Chen, M.; Chen, X.; Song, X.; Muhammad, A.; Jia, R.; Zou, Y.; Yin, L.; Li, L.; He, C.; Ye, G.; et al. The Immune-Adjuvant Activity and the Mechanism of Resveratrol on Pseudorabies Virus Vaccine in a Mouse Model. *Int. Immunopharmacol.* **2019**, *76*, 105876. [CrossRef]
51. Tay, M.Z.; Wiehe, K.; Pollara, J. Antibody-Dependent Cellular Phagocytosis in Antiviral Immune Responses. *Front. Immunol.* **2019**, *10*, 332. [CrossRef]
52. Um, Y.; Eo, H.J.; Kim, H.J.; Kim, K.; Jeon, K.S.; Jeong, J.B. Wild Simulated Ginseng Activates Mouse Macrophage, RAW264.7 Cells through TRL2/4-Dependent Activation of MAPK, NF-κB and PI3K/AKT Pathways. *J. Ethnopharmacol.* **2020**, *263*, 113218. [CrossRef]
53. He, L.-X.; Ren, J.-W.; Liu, R.; Chen, Q.-H.; Zhao, J.; Wu, X.; Zhang, Z.-F.; Wang, J.-B.; Pettinato, G.; Li, Y. Ginseng (Panax Ginseng Meyer) Oligopeptides Regulate Innate and Adaptive Immune Responses in Mice via Increased Macrophage Phagocytosis Capacity, NK Cell Activity and Th Cells Secretion. *Food Funct.* **2017**, *8*, 3523–3532. [CrossRef]
54. Kwon, H.-K.; Jo, W.-R.; Park, H.-J. Immune-Enhancing Activity of *C. militaris* Fermented with Pediococcus Pentosaceus (GRC-ON89A) in CY-Induced Immunosuppressed Model. *BMC Complement. Altern. Med.* **2018**, *18*, 75. [CrossRef] [PubMed]

Disclaimer/Publisher's Note: The statements, opinions and data contained in all publications are solely those of the individual author(s) and contributor(s) and not of MDPI and/or the editor(s). MDPI and/or the editor(s) disclaim responsibility for any injury to people or property resulting from any ideas, methods, instructions or products referred to in the content.

MDPI AG
Grosspeteranlage 5
4052 Basel
Switzerland
Tel.: +41 61 683 77 34

Nutrients Editorial Office
E-mail: nutrients@mdpi.com
www.mdpi.com/journal/nutrients

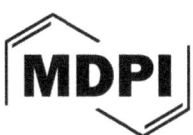

Disclaimer/Publisher's Note: The statements, opinions and data contained in all publications are solely those of the individual author(s) and contributor(s) and not of MDPI and/or the editor(s). MDPI and/or the editor(s) disclaim responsibility for any injury to people or property resulting from any ideas, methods, instructions or products referred to in the content.

www.ingramcontent.com/pod-product-compliance
Lightning Source LLC
LaVergne TN
LVHW070412100526
838202LV00014B/1441